Erdman B. Pal~~~
Laurence Branch
Diana K. Harris
Editors

Encyclopedia of Ageism

Pre-publication
REVIEWS,
COMMENTARIES,
EVALUATIONS . . .

"**W**hile our society is experiencing heightened sensitivity to sexism and racism, it is a wonder that the general public has limited awareness of ageism. Similar to sexism and racism, ageism is the discrimination, neglect, or simply assignment of negative stereotypes on older persons based on their age. Erdman Palmore has been a leading researcher and writer on ageism, and led a team of colleagues to compile a compendium of materials, in the form of an encyclopedia, to focus on available knowledge on this topic.

More than 45 gerontologists from the social and biomedical sciences contributed to this inaugural encyclopedia. Topics include definitions, measurements, sources, consequences, different environments and institutions that foster ageism, and ways to reduce ageism and change societal attitudes.

The co-editors, Erdman B. Palmore, Laurence Branch, and Diana K. Harris, are to be congratulated for undertaking this momentous effort. Changes in societal and individual attitudes are slow in coming; however, efforts such as this encyclopedia will definitely facilitate the study of ageism and educate all of us in ways of thinking about aging and the aged."

Leonard W. Poon, PhD, DrPhil (hc)
Professor of Psychology;
Chair, Faculty of Gerontology;
and Director, Gerontology Center,
University of Georgia

More pre-publication
REVIEWS, COMMENTARIES, EVALUATIONS . . .

"The *Encyclopedia of Ageism* provides timely documentation of why and how the concept of ageism continues to be widely used in gerontological research and training. Editor Erdman Palmore's pioneering research has stimulated other investigators to explore applications of his Facts on Aging Quiz, particularly in teaching situations designed to decrease age discrimination.

This volume not only documents the persistence of negative attitudes and behaviors toward older adults but also suggests practical ways to counter age discrimination. It not only brings together in a single source three decades of research about the origins and manifestations of ageism but also presents ways to combat it.

This is a valuable resource for investigators, teachers, and program managers interested in reducing age discrimination and promoting positive attitudes toward older adults."

George L. Maddox, PhD
Professor Emeritus of Medical Sociology,
Duke University Center for Aging

"That ageism warrants an encyclopedia is testimony to the reaches of this often-unwitting limitation of oneself and of others. This volume contains over 100 topic entries, a guide to related topics, measurement tools, as well as sources and consequences of ageism—enough to guide educators, practitioners, policymakers, and others through the tangle that the fact of ageism creates. This volume is not an idealistic tilting at windmills but, rather, a comprehensive assessment of a disposition that has insinuated itself into the nooks and crannies of everyday life.

This volume should serve as a ready resource and a launchpad for thoughtful discussion and debate. The contributors to this volume demonstrate the existence of both positive and negative ageism and examine ageism in health care, the social sciences, public policy, and elements of life at individual and societal levels."

Edward F. Ansello, PhD
Director, Virginia Center on Aging,
Virginia Commonwealth University

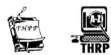

The Haworth Pastoral Press®
The Haworth Reference Press™
Imprints of The Haworth Press, Inc.
New York • London • Oxford

Encyclopedia of Ageism

THE HAWORTH PASTORAL PRESS®
Religion and Mental Health
Harold G. Koenig, MD
Senior Editor

"Martha, Martha": How Christians Worry by Elaine Leong Eng

Spiritual Care for Children Living in Specialized Settings: Breathing Underwater by Michael F. Friesen

Broken Bodies, Healing Hearts: Reflections of a Hospital Chaplain by Gretchen W. TenBrook

Shared Grace: Therapists and Clergy Working Together by Marion Bilich, Susan Bonfiglio, and Steven Carlson

The Pastor's Guide to Psychiatric Disorders and Mental Health Resources by W. Brad Johnson and William L. Johnson

Pastoral Counseling: A Gestalt Approach by Ward A. Knights

Christ-Centered Therapy: Empowering the Self by Russ Harris

Bioethics from a Faith Perspective: Ethics in Health Care for the Twenty-First Century by Jack Hanford

Family Abuse and the Bible: The Scriptural Perspective by Aimee K. Cassiday-Shaw

When the Caregiver Becomes the Patient: A Journey from a Mental Disorder to Recovery and Compassionate Insight by Daniel L. Langford and Emil J. Authelet

A Theology of God-Talk: The Language of the Heart by J. Timothy Allen

A Practical Guide to Hospital Ministry: Healing Ways by Junietta B. McCall

Pastoral Care for Post-Traumatic Stress Disorder: Healing the Shattered Soul by Daléne Fuller Rogers

Integrating Spirit and Psyche: Using Women's Narratives in Psychotherapy by Mary Pat Henehan

Chronic Pain: Biomedical and Spiritual Approaches by Harold G. Koenig

Spirituality in Pastoral Counseling and the Community Helping Professions by Charles Topper

Parish Nursing: A Handbook for the New Millennium edited by Sybil D. Smith

Mental Illness and Psychiatric Treatment: A Guide for Pastoral Counselors by Gregory B. Collins and Thomas Culbertson

A Christian Approach to Overcoming Disability: A Doctor's Story by Elaine Leong Eng

The Power of Spirituality in Therapy: Integrating Spiritual and Religious Beliefs in Mental Health Practice by Peter A. Kahle and John M. Robbins

Bereavement Counseling: Pastoral Care for Complicated Grieving by Junietta Baker McCall

Biblical Stories for Psychotherapy and Counseling: A Sourcebook by Matthew B. Schwartz and Kalman J. Kaplan

Faith, Medicine, and Science: A Festschrift in Honor of Dr. David B. Larson edited by Jeff Levin and Harold G. Koenig

Encyclopedia of Ageism edited by Erdman B. Palmore, Laurence Branch, and Diana K. Harris

Spirituality and Mental Health: Clinical Applications by Gary W. Hartz

Dying Declarations: Notes from a Hospice Volunteer by David B. Resnik

Maltreatment of Patients in Nursing Homes: There Is No Safe Place by Diana K. Harris and Michael L. Benson

Is There a God in Health Care? Toward a New Spirituality of Medicine by William F. Haynes and Geffrey B. Kelly

Dealing with the Psychological and Spiritual Aspects of Menopause: Finding Hope in the Midlife by Dana E. King, Melissa H. Hunter, and Jerri R. Harris

Guide to Ministering to Alzheimer's Patients and Their Families by Patricia A. Otwell

Encyclopedia of Ageism

Erdman B. Palmore
Laurence Branch
Diana K. Harris
Editors

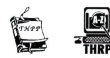

The Haworth Pastoral Press®
The Haworth Reference Press™
Imprints of The Haworth Press, Inc.
New York • London • Oxford

For more information on this book or to order, visit
http://www.haworthpress.com/store/product.asp?sku=5303

or call 1-800-HAWORTH (800-429-6784) in the United States and Canada
or (607) 722-5857 outside the United States and Canada

or contact orders@HaworthPress.com

Published by

The Haworth Pastoral Press® and The Haworth Reference Press™, imprints of The Haworth Press, Inc., 10 Alice Street, Binghamton, NY 13904-1580.

Cover design by Kerry E. Mack.

Library of Congress Cataloging-in-Publication Data

Encyclopedia of ageism / Erdman Palmore, Laurence Branch, Diana Harris, editors.
    p. cm.
    Includes bibliographical references and index.
    ISBN 0-7890-1889-6 (hard : alk. paper) — ISBN 0-7890-1890-X (pbk. : alk. paper)
    1. Ageism—Encyclopedia. I. Palmore, Erdman Ballagh, 1930- II. Branch, Laurence G. III. Harris, Diana K.

    HQ1061.E63 2004
    305.26'03—dc22

2004014795

CONTENTS

ABOUT THE EDITORS

Erdman B. Palmore, PhD, professor emeritus of medical sociology, edits the Center Report, the newsletter of the Duke University Center for the Study of Aging and Human Development at Duke University Medical Center in Durham, North Carolina. Dr. Palmore also writes a monthly column, "Vintage Years," for the newsmagazine *Fifty Plus*. His research includes retirement, longevity, life satisfaction, and international gerontology, as well as ageism. His current research and writing focuses on ageism: its nature, causes, consequences, and methods of reduction. Dr. Palmore has written or edited 16 books, including the *Normal Aging* series, the *International Handbook on the Aged,* the *Handbook on the Aged in the United States, The Honorable Elders Revisited, Retirement: Causes and Consequences, The Facts on Aging Quiz,* and *Ageism: Negative and Positive.* He has also published more than 100 articles or chapters in journals and other books. He has served as president of the Southern Gerontological Society and received the 1989 award for Distinguished Academic Gerontologist from the Southern Gerontological Society.

Laurence Branch, PhD, professor at the College of Public Health at the University of South Florida in Tampa, was Dean of the College of Public Health at the University of South Florida, a Research Professor at the Duke University Center for the Study of Aging and Human Development, and the Director of Duke's MD-MPH Program and its Long-Term Care Research Program. He has held faculty appointments from Harvard Medical School, Harvard's School of Public Health, and the Boston University School of Medicine. Dr. Branch has held adjunct appointments from Tufts University School of Medicine and the Harvard School of Dental Medicine. Dr. Branch contributes regularly to the health policy field with more than 150 articles in peer-reviewed journals and more than 50 book chapters and monographs. He currently is the co-editor of the *Journal of Aging & Health,* is a former editor in chief of *The Gerontologist,* and is on the editorial board or a reviewer for several other journals every year.

Diana K. Harris, MA, instructor of sociology, has taught at the University of Tennessee in the Department of Sociology for 38 years. Dr. Harris has written more than a half-dozen books, including *The Sociology of Aging, The Elderly in American Society, The Sociology of Aging: An Annotated Bibliography and Sourcebook,* and the *Dictionary of Gerontology.* In 1979 she founded the Cole Council on Aging at the University of Tennessee and served as its chair until 1991. She has received two awards from the National University Continuing Education Association for writing two independent study courses: "Working for the Elderly" and "Problems of Aging and Retirement." Dr. Harris was the series editor for Garland Publishing, Inc., for their series *Issues in Aging* from 1989 to 2000. In 1992 she received the National Alumni Public Service Award for her work with the elderly. Since 1992, her research and writing have focused on elder abuse, neglect, and exploitation. From 1997 to 1999 Dr. Harris co-directed the first national study on the theft of nursing home patients' possessions. Presently, she is co-authoring a book on elder maltreatment in nursing homes.

CONTRIBUTORS

Keith A. Anderson, MSW, PhD Program in Gerontology, The University of Kentucky, Lexington.

Jacqueline L. Angel, University of Texas, College Station, Texas

Ori Ashman, MA, Murdoch University, Australia.

Susan J. Aziz, MA, International Network for the Prevention of Elder Abuse, Newhall, California.

Mary M. Ball, PhD, Gerontology Center, Georgia State University, Atlanta.

Edna L. Ballard, MSW, Center for the Study of Aging and Human Development, Duke University, Durham, North Carolina.

Lucille B. Bearon, PhD, North Carolina Cooperative Extension Service, North Carolina State University, Raleigh.

Michael Beckerman, PhD, Department of Music, New York University, New York City.

Vern L. Bengtson, PhD, Andrus Gerontology Center, University of Southern California, Los Angeles.

Michael L. Benson, PhD, Division of Criminal Justice, University of Cincinnati, Cincinnati, Ohio.

Robert H. Binstock, PhD, School of Medicine, Case Western Reserve University, Cleveland, Ohio.

Charles F. Blanchard, JD, North Carolina Bar Association, Raleigh.

Dan G. Blazer, MD, PhD, Department of Psychiatry, Duke University, Durham, North Carolina.

David E. Boaz, DDS, Dentist, Chapel Hill, North Carolina.

Hayden B. Bosworth, PhD, Center for the Study of Aging and Human Development, Duke University, Durham, North Carolina.

Bruce M. Burchett, PhD, JD, Center for the Study of Aging and Human Development, Duke University, Durham, North Carolina.

Anna Burdin, MA, Department of Social and Behavioral Sciences, University of California, San Francisco.

Elias S. Cohen, MPA, JD, retired, Wynnewood, Pennsylvania.

Eric Collier, MS, RN, Department of Social and Behavioral Sciences, University of California, San Francisco.

Stephen J. Cutler, PhD, Department of Sociology, University of Vermont, Burlington.

Nicholas L. Danigelis, PhD, Department of Sociology, University of Vermont, Burlington.

Kenneth F. Ferraro, PhD, Department of Sociology, Purdue University, West Lafayette, Indiana.

Katherine J. Follett, PhD, College of Arts and Sciences, Elon College, North Carolina.

Gwendoline Y. Fortune, EdD, Freelance writer, Saxapahaw, North Carolina.

Joseph E. Gaugler, PhD, Department of Behavioral Science, The University of Kentucky, Lexington.

Linda K. George, PhD, Center for the Study of Aging and Human Development, Duke University, Durham, North Carolina.

Charlene Harrington, RN, PhD, Department of Social and Behavioral Sciences, University of California, San Francisco.

Marla Harris, PhD, Freelance writer, Winchester, Massachusetts.

Christopher B. Hays, MDiv, Department of Religion, Emory University, Atlanta, Georgia.

Judith C. Hays, PhD, Center for the Study of Aging and Human Development, Duke University, Durham, North Carolina.

Richard B. Hays, PhD, Divinity School, Duke University, Durham, North Carolina.

Robert B. Heller, PhD, Department of Psychology, Athabasca University, Athabasca, Alberta, Canada.

Jon Hendricks, PhD, University Honors College, Oregon State University, Corvallis.

Martha Holstein, PhD, Center for Research on Women and Gender, University of Illinois, Chicago.

Celia F. Hybels, PhD, Center for the Study of Aging and Human Development, Duke University, Durham, North Carolina.

Marshall B. Kapp, JD, MPH, Geriatrics and Gerontology, Wright State University, Dayton, Ohio.

Robert Kastenbaum, PhD, Department of Communication, Arizona State University, Tempe.

Corinne R. Leach, MS, Department of Education and Counseling Psychology, The University of Kentucky, Lexington.

Jack Levin, PhD, Department of Sociology, Northeastern University, Boston, Massachusetts.

Becca R. Levy, PhD, Department of Psychology, Yale University, New Haven, Connecticut.

Denise C. Lewis, MA, Gerontology Doctoral Program, University of Kentucky, Lexington.

Charles F. Longino Jr., PhD, Department of Sociology, Wake Forest University, Winston-Salem, North Carolina.

J. Beth Mabry, PhD, Department of Sociology, Indiana University of Pennsylvania, Indiana, Pennsylvania.

Kara E. MacLeod, MA, Traffic Safety Center, University of California, Berkeley.

Sandra McGuire, EdD, College of Nursing, University of Tennessee, Knoxville.

Meredith Minkler, DrPH, School of Public Health, University of California, Berkeley.

Nancy J. Osgood, PhD, Department of Sociology, Medical College of Virginia, Richmond.

Molly M. Perkins, PhD, Gerontology Center, Georgia State University, Atlanta.

David R. Ragland, PhD, MPH, Traffic Safety Center, University of California, Berkeley.

Kathryn R. Remmes, MPH, University of North Carolina, Chapel Hill.

Stephen Sapp, MDiv, PhD, Department of Religious Studies, University of Miami, Coral Gables, Florida.

William A. Satariano, PhD, MPH, School of Public Health, University of California, Berkeley.

Nancy E. Schoenberg, PhD, Department of Behavioral Science, University of Kentucky, Lexington.

Sheree T. Kwong See, PhD, Department of Psychology, University of Alberta, Edmonton, Alberta, Canada.

Robert Seymour, DD, retired, Chapel Hill, North Carolina.

Kathy M. Shipp, PhD, Center for the Study of Aging and Human Development, Duke University, Durham, North Carolina.

Michael W. Steinhour, MA, Department of Sociology, Purdue University, West Lafayette, Indiana.

James T. Sykes, PhD, School of Medicine, University of Wisconsin, Madison.

Heidi K. White, MD, Center for the Study of Aging and Human Development, Duke University, Durham, North Carolina.

Frank J. Whittington, PhD, Gerontology Center, Georgia State University, Atlanta.

Foreword

I was reared by two active and effective grandparents, so it was not until my professional training that I became aware that old people—especially women—are dehumanized by negative neglect and age discrimination.

I first confronted ageism in medical school. We were not taught much about older people, and, indeed, basic knowledge of human aging was minimal. I was shocked by the medical lexicon concerning older persons, abounding as it did with cruel and pejorative terms, such as crock, which was also used to denigrate any woman who was no longer young.

Ageism, of course, is not isolated within the medical culture. It is pervasive, gross and subtle, and omnipresent. It is found in the reduced delivery of services, time limits to mortgages, depiction in the media and by Madison Avenue, poor nursing homes, passed over promotions, and other prejudices in the workplace. Age discrimination is present in our language and even within families.

The first step to overcoming a socially accepted prejudice is to give it a name, and in 1968 I coined the term *ageism* to identify the stereotypes to which people are subjected when they grow old. The term has made it into *The Oxford Dictionary.* In 1975, my book *Why Survive? Being Old in America* was published. It presented an indictment of ageism in American society and suggested ideas for comprehensive reforms. The book examines the enduring myths that surround growing old—from attributions of dependency and unproductivity to senility and asexuality.

Ageism, of course, is universal and reaches far beyond the United States, although this country, with its youth-oriented culture, may propagate an unusually virulent form. This psychosocial disease, however, exists in both East and West. It was recognized by the French author and philosopher Simone de Beauvoir in her book *The Coming of Age,* and by Japanese director Yasujiro Ozu in the brilliant film *Tokyo Story.*

Freedom from prejudice on the basis of age should be one civil right that is embraced by all, since we all have the potential to grow old. As the number of older persons grows I predict that the baby boomers, with their history of social activism, will be the ones to watch. I envision a grassroots movement that takes examples from the best of other fights for equality, such as the civil rights and women's movements. Human rights activists will borrow a variety of tools, from consciousness raising to class-action suits, and add ageism to their domains of concerns.

Nothing less than a transformation of the culture and experience of aging is necessary. Successful efforts will require more than education. It will require the passage of laws and their strict enforcement, as well as political empowerment. (For example, the Age Discrimination in Employment Act is one legislative step in the right direction, but it has not been strictly enforced.)

From an early age, children need to be taught the concept of the life cycle, provided with positive images of old age, and helped to appreciate the essential unity and continuity of human life.

We must overcome denial, for beneath the devaluation of old people lies the profound fear and dread of aging and a reminder of our own mortality. It is not easy to deal with such powerful forces. Proust wrote, "Old age is one of those realities we retain the longest as an abstract conception."

The *Encyclopedia of Ageism* focuses discussion and provides the necessary background for the work that must be done. Let us do it!

Robert N. Butler, MD
International Longevity Center
New York

Preface

When I was an undergraduate student at Duke University (class of 1952), there was no course offering or research on gerontology on campus, much less any concern with ageism. But there was a growing concern with racism on our then-segregated campus. This stimulated me to make race and ethnic relations one of my specialties in my graduate work at the University of Chicago and Columbia University. Later I became aware that many of the principles of racism also apply to sexism and ageism.

Soon after returning to Duke in 1967 as an associate professor, I became interested in the stereotypes about elders and the inequalities between older and younger people. My first publication on these topics came out one year before Butler first used the term *ageism* in print. Soon after that I published a series of articles dealing with various aspects of ageism which are continuing. These articles culminated in my book, *Ageism: Causes and Consequences* (1999, New York: Springer).

It is remarkable that the field of gerontology, which approximately began thirty years ago, has developed so much interest, discussion, research, printed matter, and legislation. As this book demonstrates, many aspects of ageism are related to specialties within gerontology and to aspects of our beliefs and behaviors, as well as to the major institutions of our society. These many aspects show the need for a comprehensive encyclopedia of ageism.

More than 120 topics by sixty-three different authors are included in this encyclopedia. The topics are arranged in alphabetical order for easy access. Many references are made to related topics in the *See also* sections following the texts. Finally, a detailed index gives page references to the various subjects, concepts, topics, and key words used in this book.

I believe ageism is a kind of psychological and social disease of epidemic proportions in our society and around the world. I hope this encyclopedia will make a contribution toward arresting and reducing this disease—a disease that may afflict all of us if we live long enough.

I am grateful to the many contributors to this book who have made it the comprehensive resource that it is—and especially my co-editors Laurence Branch and Diana Harris. Credit for conceiving of this project and convincing me to undertake it goes to the editors of The Haworth Press.

Erdman B. Palmore

ABUSE IN NURSING HOMES

Diana K. Harris

Although the abuse of patients in nursing homes is widespread, surprisingly few studies are found on this topic. Some of the most useful information to date concerning the mistreatment of nursing home patients is a nationwide series of reports prepared by the Government Reform Committee for members of Congress (Minority Staff of the House Committee on Government Reform, 2001).

These landmark reports document instances in which nursing homes were cited for serious abuse violations. They are considered to be representative of nursing home abuse in the United States for a two-year period from January 1999 through January 2001. These reports document that many patients were subjected to serious physical abuse by the nursing staff. More than 30 percent, or 5,283, of the 17,000 nursing homes in the United States were cited for abuse violations during this period. Although all the violations had the potential to cause more than minimal harm to the patients, 1,345 nursing homes were cited for an abuse violation that actually harmed patients. An additional 256 homes were cited for abuse violations that resulted in death or serious injury or placed patients in immediate jeopardy of death or serious injury. It is likely that the findings in these reports underestimate the incidence of abuse in nursing homes because researchers have found that abuse cases are often undetected and unreported.

The relevance of such abuse to ageism lies in the fact that nearly 90 percent of the patients in nursing homes are age sixty-five and older.

Ageist attitudes among the nursing staff may contribute to the frequency and severity of the abuse of these patients.

Abuse of nursing home patients takes a number of forms. It includes not only physical abuse and neglect but a full range of mistreatment such as psychological abuse and neglect, material abuse, financial exploitation, and the violation of the nursing home patient's rights. Physical abuse refers to acts that cause pain or injury (e.g., pushing, hitting, or pinching). Pillemer and Moore (1989) interviewed 577 nurses and nursing home aides by telephone to assess the nature and extent of patient abuse. They found that 36 percent of their sample said they had seen at least one incident of physical abuse in the last year and as many as 10 percent reported that they had committed one or more abusive acts themselves.

In a mailed questionnaire to forty-seven nursing homes, Harris and Benson (1999) found that 3.5 percent of *all* employees in these nursing homes reported they had shoved or pinched a patient, while 3.4 percent reported they had hit or slapped a patient. Payne and Cikovic (1995) investigated the abuse of nursing home patients by analyzing 488 cases reported to the Medicaid Fraud Control Units throughout the United States. They found physical abuse to be the most frequent type of mistreatment, which occurred in 411 cases (84.2 percent). Although all occupational groups were involved in abusive behavior, the researchers note that nursing aides constituted the largest group of abusers at nearly 62 percent.

Physical abuse may accompany psychological abuse or may eventually lead to it. Psychological abuse is defined as the causing of emotional pain or threat of injury to the patient (e.g., yelling, insulting, or swearing). Pillemer and Moore (1989) found that about 80 percent of the nursing aides and nurses reported that they had seen at least one such incident in the past year and 40 percent said that they had psychologically abused patients. Both physical and psychogical neglect refer to the refusal or failure of nursing home personnel to fulfill their caregiving obligations to patients. It often occurs when there is a shortage of workers as well as the staff not having the time or not wanting to deal with difficult patients.

Another form of mistreatment is material abuse, which is seldom mentioned even though it is a common occurrence in nursing homes. This type of abuse involves the stealing of patients' belongings. Theft of a prized possession that holds precious memories can be psychologically and emotionally devastating.

The prevalence of theft has a harmful effect on the aged; they live in fear that their few possessions will be taken. It is frightening, of course, for them to have to depend for care on those who are stealing their belongings (Kayser-Jones, 1981)

Finally, when the term *exploitation* is used in the context of elder mistreatment in nursing homes, it may be of two types. The first type, financial abuse, includes the embezzlement of patients' funds and improper charges for drugs and services. The second type refers to denying cognitively alert patients the right to make their own decisions.

Due to the vulnerability of aged nursing home patients, they tend to be easy prey for abuse. Society often perceives them as being frail and dependent. They are negatively stereotyped as being useless, nonproductive, and possessing little or no social value. Such ageist attitudes provide the setting for abuse to occur.

Nursing home aides who are responsible for 80 to 90 percent of the care of patients are underpaid and overworked. Their jobs, which are physically demanding and emotionally stressful, can lead to a number of work-related problems, including negative feelings and indifference toward patients. It is not uncommon for nursing aides to report that they were yelled at, scratched, or had something thrown at them by a patient. For some aides, their response to such verbal and physical aggression may be compassion and understanding, whereas for others it may be retaliation such as stealing patients' possessions or physically maltreating them.

See also ABUSE BY ELDERS IN NURSING HOME; NURSING HOMES; STEREOTYPES

REFERENCES

Harris, D. and Benson, M. (1999). Elder abuse in nursing homes: The theft of patients' possessions. *Journal of Elder Abuse and Neglect,* 10, 141-151.

Kayser-Jones, J. (1981). *Old, alone, and neglected.* Berkeley: University of California Press.

Minority Staff of the House Committee on Government Reform (2001). *Abuse of residents is a major problem in U.S. nursing homes.* Washington, DC: U.S. House of Representatives.

Payne, B. and Cikovic, R. (1995). An empirical examination of the characteristics, consequences, and causes of elder abuse in nursing homes. *Journal of Elder Abuse and Neglect,* 7, 61-74.

Pillemer, K. and Moore, D. (1989). Abuse of patients in nursing homes: Findings from a survey of staff. *The Gerontologist,* 29, 314-320.

ABUSE BY ELDERS IN NURSING HOMES

Diana K. Harris

Abuse in nursing homes is a two-way street: caregivers may abuse patients or patients may abuse caregivers. When caregivers abuse patients it may be a form of ageism: the caregivers may vent their frustration and aggression on the patients because the patients are old and vulnerable.

However, patients may also engage in verbal or physical aggression toward their caregivers. A number of studies implicate verbal and physical aggression toward caregivers as a factor increasing the risk of abusive behavior toward patients. When patients violate the expectations of proper patient behavior, this may temporarily release the nursing aides from the restraining power of the norm that prohibits patient abuse (Stannard, 1973). One study found that aggressive patients were four times as likely to be abused than were passive patients (Newbern, 1987).

Goodridge, Johnston, and Thompson (1996) report that most incidents of aggressive behavior by patients in their study occurred while the staff was assisting them with personal care such as bathing, dressing, and grooming. They found that the most common types of physical abuse that nursing aides experienced include being grabbed, shoved, or scratched by the patients. Psychological abuse toward nursing aides such as being insulted or sworn at occurred slightly more frequently than physical abuse. Patients with Alzheimer's disease and other cognitive impairments are especially prone to aggressive behaviors when efforts are made to provide personal care.

Staff training programs in nursing homes are needed to teach strategies and inteventions to help cope with aggressive and violent patients. In this way, nursing homes can prevent or reduce abusive behaviors to their staff and to their patients.

See also ABUSE IN NURSING HOMES; NURSING HOMES

REFERENCES

Goodridge, D., Johnson, P., and Thompson, M. (1996). Conflict and aggression as stressors in the work environment. *Journal of Elder Abuse and Neglect,* 8, 49-67.

Newbern, V. (1987). Caregiver perceptions of human abuse in health care settings. *Holistic Nurse Practitioner,* 1, 64-74.

Stannard, C. (1973). Old folks and dirty work: The social conditions for patient abuse in nursing homes. *Social Problems,* 20, 329-342.

ADVERTISING

Erdman B. Palmore

Ageism in advertising takes several forms. Elders are overrepresented in commercials for over-the-counter remedies for ailments often associated with old age, such as constipation, indigestion, ulcers, skin problems, dentures, osteoporosis, baldness, corns, and other foot problems. This supports the stereotype that most elders are inactive and sick.

Skin creams and other such products are routinely advertised as "antiaging," meaning they reduce wrinkles, dry skin, blemishes, and other skin problems. These advertisements promise that their products can "banish ugly aging skin" and "make you look years younger." These claims imply that old age causes skin problems, rather than excessive exposure to the sun, wind, or other skin stressors.

In contrast, elders tend to be absent from commercials for clothing, appliances, cars, soaps, and cleaning products. This also supports the stereotype that elders are not interested in clothing, appliances, cars, etc. When elders are shown in commercials they are less likely to be physically active and more likely to have health problems than younger people (Harris and Feinberg, 1977). However, because of criticisms by media watch groups such as the Gray Panthers and the Older Women's League (OWL), some commercials have begun to portray older people in more active and positive roles (Bytheway, 1995).

See also ANTIAGING MEDICINE; BOTOX; FACE-LIFTS

REFERENCES

Bytheway, B. (1995). *Ageism.* Philadelphia, PA: Open University Press.
Harris, A. and Feinberg, J. (1977). Television and aging. *The Gerontologist,* 17, 464.

AFRICAN AMERICANS

Gwendoline Y. Fortune

Throughout known human history, until recently, the value of members of the "tribe" with proven experience has been of highest survival value. The longer a member lived, the more respected he or she was. It was recognized that what had enabled the group to survive for eons was to be found in the accumulated wisdom of those who had come before. Securing food, shelter, escape, and protection occurred because of the "old ways."

Americans whose ancestors were captured during the period of slavery and their descendants had particular need to attend to their elders, for there were no written records to provide continuity of their cultures. Whether male or female, the passing of culture was vital to those who were born in lands far from the origins of their people. Those who lived long understood their role and accepted its responsibilities. From childhood, as in the homelands, powers of observation, remembering, and oral transmission were prized abilities. Men and women held these roles, but it was more often the women, under captivity, who were able to exercise their cultural role. Women were less likely to be sold from family and community and, therefore, could exercise their role in storytelling and transmission of rituals and philosophies.

Given the uncertainty of life as a captive, great age was important. The elderly continued the traditions from the African homelands as much as could be remembered. Wrinkles and gray hair denoted experience and wisdom. These, and other signs of age, evoked no stigma for the elders. Actually, they gave the aged dignity and assurance of their own worth.

After 1865, when the descendants of African captives were no longer chattel, the aged remained valued members of the newly developing communities. Although most freed captives remained close to their former plantation homes, migration north and west became a constant among the freed people. Old photographs show the honored place of elder family members sitting atop bundles and chairs in wagons trekking toward hoped for greater freedom and opportunity.

The attitude of respect and honor for the elders continued in the African-American communities of America for more than 100 years after emancipation. Even having dispersed to all parts of the nation, black communities evolved as microcosms of the familiar. The grandmother and grandfather, aged uncle and aunt were gathered around on special occasions: weddings, dinners, reunions. All older people who were not "blood relatives" were offered respect and deference in the community. The visibility of the elders gave a sense of solidity and belonging. Attention conveyed a warmth within these gatherings and the total community as the elders told stories that described both the hardships of the old days and the skills that enabled family and community to survive. Following the tradition of the griots of West Africa the family/tribal tree extended and expanded with a solidity of survival.

As with all Americans, the rapidly changing era that began after World War II accelerated for people of African descent, particularly, following the historical changes of the Civil Rights movement (1954-present). Dislocations in urban areas hastened the disintegration of former mores. The majority/white culture brought pervasive images and ways of being via film and television, and now the Internet, that severed historical lines of communication and attachment among the scattered remnants of a once cohesive culture. Among the casualties of this history are the loss of contact between generations, and dismissal and disdain for "anyone over thirty."

Consequently, people of color have become variously mainstream in regard to aging and ageism. In the cities and towns of America young blacks no longer assist the elderly but have become their predators. In smaller communities and rural areas echoes and reminders of older attitudes, behaviors, and conditions can be noted. Meanwhile, older men and women of color, having lost the respect offered by earlier generations, are, generally, indistinguishable from the dominant culture. Awareness, acceptance, and appreciation for the knowledge of the elders, their role and value to contemporary and future generations have eroded. The most visible observations of the tradition of respect for elders—the opposite of discriminatory ageism—

may be found within communities of fundamentalist religious practices.

Cultures change. Whether the residue of the "old ways" and appreciation of "old folks" emerge as survival aids for the community of people of African descent, and others, is to be seen.

See also AGED AS A MINORITY GROUP; SUBCULTURE THEORY

AGE CONFLICT

Erdman B. Palmore

Age conflict is an extreme form of ageism in which two or more age strata conflict with each other (Foner, 1995). Some age conflict probably occurs in all societies, although it may not be generally recognized and/or may not be organized (Palmore, 1999). It may be the inevitable result of age stratification, which appears to be a universal system that occurs in all societies.

As with other forms of social conflict, age conflicts involve struggles over scarce resources or over values. Age inequalities are a major source of age conflict. Conflict occurs when the disadvantaged age group makes claims for more power or other scarce goods, and the more privileged group seeks to protect their privileges.

However, such conflicts tend to be confined to particular institutions (e.g., the family, workplace, or retirement benefits), rather than becoming society-wide. Several factors tend to check sharp age conflicts: the legitimization of age inequalities by various stereotypes; the fear of retribution by those in power; ties of affection or obligation across age strata; and the social separation of age groups.

The amount of age conflict in our society has been exaggerated. There is little disagreement between the generations about the Social Security system or other programs for elders. Similarly, there is general agreement between generations about our basic value system. There is little difference between generations in voting behavior or party affiliation. The conflict that does occur tends to focus on personal tastes and styles, such as types of music, clothing, hairstyles, tattooing and body piercing, entertainment, and sports.

See also AGE INEQUALITY; AGE NORMS; AGE STRATIFICATION

REFERENCES

Foner, A. (1995). Age conflicts. In G. Maddox (Ed.), *The encyclopedia of aging.* New York: Springer.
Palmore, E. (1999). *Ageism: Negative and positive.* New York: Springer.

AGE DENIAL

Erdman B. Palmore

Age denial is a frequent reaction to ageism. It is similar to the minority group reaction to racism known as "passing." Some minority group members attempt to deny their negative status by passing for members of the dominant racial group: light-skinned African Americans may pass for whites or Jews may change their name and pass for gentiles.

Similarly, many aged refuse to identify themselves as old or aged because of the negative stereotypes and discrimination that elders often face (Drevenstedt, 1976). Only 5 percent of older Minnesota residents thought of themselves as old at sixty-five; more than 40 percent would not consider themselves as old until they were over eighty.

An AARP survey (Speas and Obenshain, 1995) found that half of older people denied that people become "old" in their sixties. One quarter of older persons denied that chronological age determines when a person becomes old.

An earlier AARP survey (Harris, 1975) found that most people sixty-five or older disliked the terms *old man* or *old woman,* or even *aged person.* They preferred to have themselves referred to as *senior citizen* or *mature American.* As Bernard Baruch put it, "Old age is always fifteen years older than I am" (Merriam-Webster, 1992, p. 11).

No one knows how many older people deny their age, but most authorities believe that many do, and that fibbing about one's age is especially common among women. One article asserts, "The majority of women over fifty either feel guilty about their age—and confess to it as if admitting to the Brinks heist—or feel guilty about lying about their age" (Hodge, 1987, p. 40).

In a *Newsweek* article titled "Sometimes Honesty is the Worst Policy: I Never Tried to Hide My Age—Until I Suspected that Telling the Truth May Have Cost Me My Job," Mandel (2002) recounts how she lost her job as a teacher when the headmaster found out that she was fifty years old. She notes that several women friends and relatives deny their age because "no one wants to be with an old lady," and "When younger people know I'm in my mid-fifties, they treat me differently." One relative even tried to change her birth date on her passport.

Age denial is so common that it is usually considered impolite to even ask older people how old they are. However, if you find out the older person's age, the standard compliment is, "You don't look that old." This remark is an encouragement of age denial rather than pride in one's age. Furthermore, it is a dubious compliment because it implies, "You don't look as feeble and decrepit as most people your age."

Age denial is also a common source of jokes about elders. One of Jack Benny's most famous comedy routines was his assertion that he was only thirty-nine. A common joke on coffee mugs and bumper stickers reads, "The secret of staying young is to find an age you really like and stick with it." This is an invitation to lie about one's age.

Lucille Ball said, "The secret of staying young is to live honestly, eat slowly, and lie about your age" (quoted in Adams, 1989, p. 17). Diane de Poitiers said, "The years that a woman subtracts from her age are not lost. They are added to other women's" (Adams, 1989, p. 15).

In my first analysis of jokes about elders, I found that age denial is one of the most common themes, especially in jokes about old women (Palmore, 1971). This finding has since been replicated by several other studies (Palmore, 1986).

Some senior citizen clubs fine their members if they use the word *old*. Before new business, the president calls for "leftover" business, rather than "old" business. It is as if being old is a disgrace (Jacobs and Vinick, 1977).

The attempts to pass for younger or middle-aged persons provide major support for the multibillion-dollar cosmetics industry, as well as the plastic surgery, hair replacement, and Botox industries. Many advertisements for skin cream or lotions and hair dye promise that their products can "make you look young again" and "prevent aging skin."

The denial of "old" as a self-concept may actually be a denial of the negative age stereotypes rather than a denial of chronological age. The denial that one is "old" may simply be an assertion that one still feels as healthy, strong, and vigorous as one did when younger. As Butler (1975) points out, "The problem comes when this good feeling is called 'youth' rather than 'health,' thus tying it to chronological age instead of to physical and mental well-being" (p. 14). This is another aspect of the semantic confusions between the concepts of aging and of deterioration.

Levin and Levin (1980, p. 103) assert, "Given the severe stigma of aging and the negative connotations associated with it, a middle-age self-concept may actually sustain morale and increase satisfaction with life." Considerable evidence supports that elders who continue to consider themselves middle-aged are more healthy, more satisfied with life, and more emotionally well adjusted than those who consider themselves "old" or "elderly" (George, 1985).

However, the question remains whether a younger self-concept sustains better mental health or a younger self-concept is an effect of better mental health and satisfaction. Probably the effects run in both directions because of the strength of ageism in our culture.

If we could eliminate ageism, if we could separate chronological age from the connotations of sickness and deterioration, there would be no benefit from denying one's chronological age. A common joke among mental health workers states: "denial is not a river in Egypt." Age denial is perhaps the most frequent reaction to ageism in our society today.

See also ADVERTISING; BOTOX; FACE-LIFTS; HUMOR; LANGUAGE; SEXISM

REFERENCES

Adams, A. (1989). *An uncommon scold.* New York: Simon & Schuster.

Butler, R. (1975). *Why survive?: Being old in America.* New York: Harper & Row.

Drevenstedt, J. (1976). Perceptions of onsets of young adulthood, middle age, and old age. *Journal of Gerontology, 31,* 53.

George, L. (1985). Socialization to old age. In E. Palmore (Ed.), *Normal aging III.* Durham, NC: Duke University Press.

Harris, L. (1975). *The myth and reality of aging in America.* Washington, DC: The National Council on the Aging.

Hodge, M. (1987). Why women lie about their age. *Fifty Plus,* February.

Jacobs, R. and Vinick, B. (1977). *Re-engagement in later life.* Stamford, CT: Greylock.

Levin, J. and Levin, W. (1980). *Ageism: Prejudice and discrimination against the elderly.* Belmont, CA: Wadsworth.

Mandell, J. (2002). Sometimes honesty is the worst policy. *Newsweek,* October 21, 16.

Merriam-Webster (1992). *Dictionary of quotations.* Springfield, MA: Author.

Palmore, E. (1971). Attitudes toward aging as shown by humor. *The Gerontologist,* 11, 181.

_____(1986). Attitudes toward aging shown by humor. In L. Nahemo (Ed.), *Humor and aging.* San Diego, CA: Academic Press.

Speas, K. and Obenshain, B. (1995). *Images of aging in America.* Washington, DC: AARP.

AGE INEQUALITY

Erdman B. Palmore

Of the three great forms of inequality, which is stronger in our society: race, sex, or age inequality? Civil rights leaders assert that racism results in the most serious inequality, whereas feminist leaders assert that sexism is a more serious problem. Some gerontologists argue that ageism is becoming at least as important as racism and sexism (Levin and Levin, 1980; Naisbitt, 1982).

Conversely, Ventrell-Monsees and McCann (1992) assert that policymakers and the public view age discrimination as less pervasive and less insidious than race or sex discrimination. They say that the courts have been consistently unsympathetic to the view that age discrimination should be legally proscribed.

There have been few attempts to compare quantitatively the relative importance of these three kinds of prejudice and discrimination. Palmore and Manton (1973) first analyzed the race, sex, and age inequalities shown by the U.S. census statistics using the method of the equality index (EI). The EI is the positive complement of the older index of dissimilarity (Duncan and Duncan, 1955). It can be described as the proportion of two groups' percentage distributions that overlap each other. It is the sum over all categories of the smaller of the two percentages in each category. It can be thought of as the percentage of complete equality, because 100 would mean that complete identity exists between the two percentage distributions, 50 would mean that 50 percent of the inferior group would have to move upward to equal the higher group, and 0 would mean that no overlap occurs between the two distributions.

The answer to the question of which type of inequality is greatest depends on which measure of inequality is being examined. Using data from the 1970 census, Palmore and Manton (1973) found that for education, age equality (EI = 63) was less than race (76) and sex (91) equality. In terms of income, age equality (65) was less than race equality (83), but more than sex equality (45). However, in terms of occupation (for those employed), age equality (79) was greater than racial (71) and sex equality (56). This is somewhat misleading because the majority of the aged are not employed. In terms of weeks worked, the aged have the least equality.

When comparisons were made combining two factors, the joint effects were generally additive. This is called *double jeopardy*. The combination of all three types of discrimination (comparing older black women to younger white men) produced the lowest equality in both income (13) and occupation (26). This is called *triple jeopardy*. It is noteworthy that triple jeopardy produces only 13 percent overlap in the two income distributions. This shows that most older black women live in a different world than younger white men.

Changes between 1950 and 1970 showed nonwhites and the aged gained substantially more equality in income, occupation, and education, whereas women barely maintained their generally inferior status (Palmore, 1976).

It is difficult to determine the extent to which these inequalities are directly due to ageism, racism, or sexism, as opposed to biological, cohort, or other differences. However, it is clear that the relative amounts of age, race, or sex inequality vary greatly, depending on which type of inequality is being measured.

See also AFRICAN AMERICANS; SEXISM

REFERENCES

Duncan, O. and Duncan, B. (1955). A methodological analysis of segregation indexes. *American Sociological Review,* 9, 243-246.

Levin, J. and Levin, W. (1980). *Ageism.* Belmont, CA: Wadsworth.

Naisbitt, J. (1982). *Megatrends.* New York: Warner Books.

Palmore, E. (1976). The future status of the aged. *The Gerontologist,* 16, 297.

Palmore, E. and Manton, K. (1973). Ageism compared to racism and sexism. *Journal of Gerontology*, 28, 363.
Ventrell-Monsees, C. and McCann, L. (1992). Ageism: The segregation of a civil right. *Eagle Bulletin* (No. 81-13). Norbury, London: International Federation on Ageing.

AGE NORMS

Diana K. Harris

Our culture defines what is proper and improper behavior, what is right and wrong, and what we are expected to do and not to do. These standards or rules of behavior are called *norms*. Norms help us to predict the behavior of others and, in turn, allow others to know what to expect of us. Our society has expectations about what is considered proper behavior at different ages. These expectations are called *age norms*. The familiar phrase "act your age" reflects the concern for age-appropriate behavior.

Age norms are enforced through various mechanisms of social control, apply to a wide range of behaviors, and are supported by a widespread consensus. Some age norms prescribe how we should behave in particular social situations and others concern our dress and personal appearance. Still others govern our entry and exit from certain roles. For instance, how often have you heard someone ask, "Don't you have any grandchildren yet?" or "Shouldn't you be retired by now?" These phrases are illustrations of age norms that govern the timing of our adult behavior and have been referred to as *social clocks* (Neugarten, Moore, and Lowe, 1965). These clocks operate to speed up as well slow down major life events. Even though these clocks are not as powerful and compelling as they once were, people are still aware of their timing and describe themselves as being early, on time, or late regarding life events.

Age norms refer to chronological time and many of our laws and policies are based on assumptions about chronological age and structure rights and responsibilities on that basis. Some of these assumptions regarding the capacities and reactions of older people are unfounded. They are based on erroneous beliefs about what old people *can* do and then they evolve into notions about what they *ought to* do (Riley, Foner, and Waring, 1988). These notions then result in ageist thinking and behavior. For example, the notion that an older man should not make sexual advances toward a younger woman results in accusations of him being "a dirty old man," or the notion that an older person should not engage in any adventurous or dangerous activities results in the accusation, "You are too old for that."

Although age norms are fairly durable, they are becoming less rigid and sometimes are subject to change. For example, on the average, first marriages take place at older ages, retirement occurs at younger ages, and programs for continuing education for the elderly are on the rise (Foner, 1996). This is evidenced by the fact that about 49,000 persons over the age of sixty-five are currently attending college (*Modern Maturity,* 2002). As a result, it no longer surprises us to hear of a seventy-year-old woman pursuing a college degree or a fifty-year-old man deciding to retire.

See also AGEISM SURVEY; ROLE EXPECTATIONS; STEREOTYPES

REFERENCES

American Association of Retired Persons (AARP) (2002), *Modern Maturity,* September/October, 17.
Foner, A. (1996). Age norms and the structure of consciousness. *The Gerontologist,* 36, 221-223.
Neugarten, B., Moore, J., and Lowe, J. (1965). Age norms, age constraints, and adult socialization. *American Journal of Sociology,* 70, 710-717.
Riley, M., Foner, A., and Waring, J. (1988). The sociology of age. In N. Smelser (Ed.), *Handbook of sociology* (pp. 243-290). Newbury Park: Sage Publications.

AGE SEGREGATION

Erdman B. Palmore

Many laws and judicial decisions prohibit racial segregation because of the strong evidence that it breeds suspicion, misunderstanding, stereotyping, and discrimination. However, segregation based on age is rather different and its effects are debatable.

The AARP (2001) noted that geographically, people over sixty-five are somewhat concentrated in Florida (18 percent of the population), some midwestern states such as Arkansas (14 percent) and Iowa (15 percent), and some northeastern states such as Pennsylvania and Rhode Island (16 percent). Conversely, there are less aged in some western states such as Utah (9 percent). Alaska has the least (6 percent).

Within states, older people are more likely than younger people to live outside metropolitan areas, especially in small towns. Those who do live in metropolitan areas are more likely than those younger to live in the central cities. But the differences in these comparisons are relatively small, less than 5 percent.

Such geographical differences are the result mainly of older people voluntarily moving into an area (such as Florida) or from younger people moving out and leaving older people behind (as in small towns and the Midwest). This kind of age concentration is quite different from the kind of forced racial segregation our nation has experienced in the past (and to a lesser extent, in the present).

Therefore, there is little age segregation in terms of large geographical areas. More age segregation occurs on a neighborhood basis where retirement communities have developed or special housing for the aged has been built. In such cases, the segregation results from younger people being kept out, rather than from older people being forced to live there.

Most residents of retirement communities say they prefer to live there because it is easier to make friends, and they like the special facilities and the greater quiet in these communities (Bultena and Wood, 1969). Rosow (1967) found that elders living in age-segregated apartment buildings were more likely to form friendships there than those living in age-integrated housing.

Evidence suggests that some older people do not want and would not benefit from age-segregated housing (Carp, 1975). Furthermore, even if some elders prefer age-segregated housing, it may contribute to ageism nevertheless. When elders feel rejected by the young, they may try to find acceptance only among other elders and thereby segregate themselves from the young—who in turn reject elders more because they have no close contacts with them (Barrows and Smith, 1979).

Conversely, some argue that age-segregated housing may produce feelings of group pride and integration among elders, and therefore, higher self-esteem. This self-esteem may tend to reduce ageism. The net effect of age segregation on ageism is unknown and needs to be studied (Back, 1995).

See also HOUSING

REFERENCES

AARP (2001). *Profile of older Americans.* Washington, DC: Author.
Back, K. (1995). Age segregation. In G. Maddox (Ed.), *The encyclopedia of aging* New York: Springer.
Barrow, G. and Smith, P. (1979). *Aging, ageism, and society.* St. Paul, MN: West Publishing.
Bultena, G. and Wood, V. (1969). The American retirement community. *Journal of Gerontology,* 24, 209.
Carp, F. (1975). Life-style and location within the city. *The Gerontologist,* 15, 27.
Rosow, I. (1967). *Social integration of the aged.* New York: Free Press.

AGE STRATIFICATION

Erdman B. Palmore

Age stratification classifies people by their age (Riley, 1995). All societies also classify their members by sex and socioeconomic status. In all stratification systems there is an explicit or implicit ranking from higher to lower strata.

In gerontocratic societies, the old have the highest status and the youngest have the lowest. In our society, the middle-aged tend to have the most power and prestige and children have the least. The old and young adults tend to be in between, and whether the old or the young are higher than the other depends on which dimension is involved. In terms of income, elders rank higher than the young (Palmore, 1999). In terms of sports and entertainment, the young rank higher. Such ranking on the basis of age is a form of ageism that accompanies age stratification systems.

Age stratification should be distinguished from age norms, which are the expectations about the proper or normal behaviors, obligations, and privileges for the age strata or life stages (Back, 1995). The extent to which such norms are forms of ageism depends on the extent to which the assumptions on which they are based are prejudicial or are realistic and appropriate.

Age stratification may lead to age conflict, but not necessarily. Age conflict is an extreme form of ageism in which two or more age strata conflict with each other (Foner, 1995). At present, little age conflict exists in our society.

See also AGE CONFLICT; AGE NORMS; TYPOLOGIES

REFERENCES

Back, K. (1995). Age norms. In G. Maddox (Ed.), *The encyclopedia of aging.* New York: Springer.
Foner, A. (1995). Age conflicts. In G. Maddox (Ed.), *The encyclopedia of aging.* New York: Springer.
Palmore, E. (1999). *Ageism: Negative and positive.* New York: Springer.
Riley, M (1995). Age stratification. In G. Maddox (Ed.), *The encyclopedia of aging.* New York: Springer.

AGED AS A MINORITY GROUP

Jack Levin

The concept of minority group has long provided a valuable frame of reference for understanding the experiences of groups of people in society who are singled out, based on some physical or cultural characteristic, for discriminatory treatment (Wirth, 1945). Traditionally, the use of the minority concept focused largely on problems encountered by racial and ethnic groups such as blacks, Latinos, and Jews. More recently, the concept has also been applied to the experiences of women, gays, and the disabled (Sagarin, 1971; Davis, 1978; Levin and Levin, 1982).

In the 1960s, some gerontologists argued that the minority group concept can be applied appropriately as well to the experiences of the aged as a group (Breen, 1960; Barron, 1961, Levin and Levin, 1980). Not everyone agreed—most notably Gordon Streib (1965), who suggested instead that the aged should not be regarded as a minority group, because they fail to meet the criteria originally suggested by Wirth. Specifically, Streib argued that they do not constitute a group in any sociological sense, are not stereotyped in a negative manner, and are not discriminated against based on their age. He also suggested that the minority status must cover the entire life cycle. This would exclude the aged, whose minority status by definition does not begin until later in life (Levin and Levin, 1980).

Palmore (1978) was able to narrow, if not resolve, the debate by examining the evidence that indicated how well elders meet the criteria usually associated with the minority status.

1. Elders do share identifying characteristics and status expectations (for example, gray hair, wrinkles, and retirement), but not throughout the life cycle.
2. Research suggests the widespread existence of negative stereotypes about elders. The majority of Americans characterize elders as disabled or sick, senile, ugly, useless, isolated, and impoverished (Levin and Levin, 1980; Palmore, 1999; Kite and Wagner, 2002). At the same time, however, many people also hold positive age stereotypes—they see elders as kind, wise, dependable, wealthy, free from responsibility, politically powerful, and happy (Palmore, 1999).
3. Clearly, elders are the recipients of discrimination, especially in hiring and promotion, government programs, and treatment by other family members; but it is also true that many elders benefit from positive forms of discrimination, including tax exemptions, discounts, low-rent housing, and health care (Palmore, 1990).

Recognizing that elders have some but not all of the attributes of traditional minority groups, Palmore (1978) concludes that the question "Are the aged a minority group?" does not have a simple "yes" or "no" answer. As an alternative, he suggests that Barron's (1961) term *quasi-minority group* might best describe the experiences of today's elders who are both advantaged and disadvantaged by ageism.

See also AGE SEGREGATION; AGEISM SURVEY; BLAMING THE AGED; SOCIETAL AGEISM; SUBCULTURE

REFERENCES

Barron, M. (1961). Minority group characteristics of the aged in American society. *Journal of Gerontology,* 8, 477-482.

Breen, L. (1960). The aging individual. In C. Tibbitts (Ed.), *Handbook of social gerontology* (pp. 145-164). Chicago: University of Chicago Press.

Davis, J. (1978). *Minority-dominant relations.* Arlington Heights, IL: AHM.

Kite, M. and Wagner, L. (2002). Attitudes toward older adults. In D. Todd (Ed.), *Ageism: Stereotyping and prejudice against older persons* (pp. 129-162). Cambridge: MIT Press.

Levin, J. and Levin, W. (1980). *Ageism: Prejudice and discrimination against the elderly.* Belmont CA: Wadsworth.

_____ (1982). *The functions of discrimination and prejudice.* New York: Harper & Row.

Palmore, E. (1978). Are the aged a minority group? *Journal of the American Geriatrics Society, 26,* 214.

_____ (1999). *Ageism: Negative and positive.* New York: Springer.

Sagarin, E. (1971). *The other minorities.* Waltham, MA: Ginn.

Streib, G. (1965). Are the aged a minority group? In B. Neugarten (Ed.), *Middle age and aging* (pp. 36-46). Chicago: University of Chicago Press.

Wirth, L. (1945). The problem of minority groups. In R. Linton (Ed.), *The science of man in the world crisis* (pp. 347-372). New York: Columbia University Press.

AGEISM IN THE BIBLE

Judith C. Hays
Richard B. Hays
Christopher B. Hays

Biblical Terminology for Aging

Old age is a significant interest within the Old Testament/Hebrew Bible canon, and is generally associated with wisdom, health, or blessing. Various terms for old age occur in nearly all of its thirty-nine books (Conrad, 1977; Harris, 1987, 1992). The most common Hebrew term is *zaqen* (old or old man), derived from the term *zaqan* (beard). The old are often contrasted with various terms for younger people ("I have been young, and now am old" [Psalm 37:25]), or combined with such terms ("the young men and the old shall be merry" [Jeremiah 31:13]). The words *yases* and *yasis* each refer to stages of very old age that are associated with decrepitude.

Old Testament authors also used physical characteristics to refer to old age, often describing the hair with terms such as *seba* ("gray hair"): "You shall go to your ancestors in peace; you shall be buried with good old age" (Genesis 15:15). The Aramaic of Daniel 7:9 describes the divine king, the "ancient of days," as having hair "like pure wool."

Finally, biblical Hebrew commonly characterizes the aged simply in terms of their long tenure on the earth. It is generally an image of blessing to lengthen one's days or increase one's days, as when God tells Solomon, "If you will walk in my ways, then I will lengthen your life" (1 Kings 3:14).

In the Greek translation of the New Testament, several different terms refer to aging or to persons of advanced age. The word *presbytes* (old man) is used as a self-description by Zechariah (Luke 1:18) and by Paul (Philemon 9) and referring to old men and old women (presbytides) in the church in Crete, to whom Paul's emissary Titus is to provide instruction (Titus 2:2-3). The closely related term *presbyteros* (elder) is used for those who are recognized as community leaders in the synagogue (e.g., Matthew 21:23) or in the church (e.g., Acts 15:2). This usage presupposes that leadership is linked to seniority in the community. Sometimes, however, the masculine and feminine terms *presbytero* and *presbytera* (elder) refer to older people without reference to any office of leadership, as in 1 Timothy 5:1-2. The noun *geron* (old man, whence our English word gerontology) turns up only once, in Nicodemus's question to Jesus (John 3:4). Related terms are *geras* (old age, Luke 1:36) and the verb *gerasko* (grow old, John 21:18, Hebrews 8:13). This term appears to refer simply to chronological age without carrying any of the connotations of dignity that attach to *presbytes* and *presbyteroi*.

Overall, the terminology used in these ancient sources emphasizes a developmental, wholistic life course perspective on aging. References to frailty are included, but the preponderance of terms connotes positive images of growing older. In this context, the current trends in Western societies toward obsession with youthful appearance (e.g., the widespread use of hair dye for covering gray hair, age discrimination in the workplace, and age segregation in housing), would have been largely unthinkable.

Older Characters in the Old Testament and New Testament

The beginning of the Hebrew Bible suggests that humankind had the potential for immortality. After Adam and Eve transgress against God's order not to eat of the tree of the knowledge of good and evil, God worries aloud: "[Adam] might reach out his hand and take also from the tree of life, and eat, and live forever" (Genesis 3:22). Although God casts the humans out of the garden, the text suggests that there is some seed of immortality in humanity that does not immediately disappear. The life spans recorded for the descendants of Adam and Eve were extremely long, including Methuselah's 969 years (Genesis 5:25-26); his name has become a noun meaning "a very old man." In the rest of the Hebrew Bible, however, only characters of great divine favor live to such an age: Moses (120), Joshua (110), Job (140), and the high priest Jehoiada (130, 2 Chronicles 24:15). The aged are implicitly regarded as the standard for wisdom (Psalm 119:100).

Other texts give a clearer picture of the average life of an ancient Israelite. Psalm 90:10 puts life expectancy at seventy years, "or perhaps eighty, if we are strong." One scholar, working from legal texts that appear to reflect the value of a slave at various stages of life, show a drop-off in value at sixty, which may reflect the expected retirement age (Wenham, 1978). Others have studied the lifespans of kings in Israel's monarchical era (926-597 B.C.E.), concluding that the average king, presumably with the best health care and nutrition of the day, lived only forty-four years (Harris, 1992). Prophetic texts such as Isaiah 65:20 anticipate a day of God's redemption, when "one who dies at a hundred years will be considered a youth, and one who falls short of a hundred will be considered accursed." Thus, longevity is considered desirable and the long-lived to have received a good gift of years.

Old age in the Hebrew Bible may also bring debilitation and susceptibility to abuse. Various leaders of Israel, including the aged Isaac (Genesis 27), Eli (1 Samuel 2:12-17), David (1 Kings 1), and Solomon (1 Kings 11:4), are portrayed as losing their vigor and their ability to guide the people. For common people, the problems seem to have been equally significant: the frequent legal injunctions to honor parents and not to abuse them run from the Ten Commandments throughout the law (Exodus 20:12, 21:15, 21:17, 22:22). Such injunctions probably indicate the necessity of such special protection. Part of one prophet's description of a sinful and broken social order is contempt and contention by children toward their parents (Micah 7:6), suggesting that elder abuse observed in modern societies has ancient roots.

Widows are portrayed as especially vulnerable. In a common formulation, God is the one "who executes justice for the orphan and the widow" (Deuteronomy 10:18, etc.), because the social structures of the day did not. Widows would have had to rely on their children's support, and the situation was particularly desperate for a childless widow such as Naomi in the book of Ruth. Although the account concludes with a happy ending, there lurks the specter of a fearful fate awaiting Ruth had she not remarried and born a son, who would provide for her in her old age (Ruth 4:15). Thus, the ancient texts portray the blessings and honor of old age as balanced by the risks and losses that accompany it.

At the time of the writings of the New Testament, life expectancy at birth was about twenty-five years, due largely to high infant mortality rates; in Roman society, those over the age of sixty years represented between 5 and 10 percent of the total population (Parkin, 1992). Others calculate that in Roman Egypt, female life expectancy at birth was between twenty and twenty-five years, but that females who survived to age ten enjoyed a life expectancy ranging from 34.5 to 37.5 years (Bagnall and Frier, 1994). About half of the populace died before reaching the age of forty-four (Patlagean, 1977). Only a few aged persons appear in the New Testament.

Older characters play a significant role, however, in the opening chapters of Luke's Gospel. The first characters who appear in Luke's story are the priest Zechariah and his wife Elizabeth, who were both "getting on in years" (Luke 1:7) and remained, to their dismay, childless (1:6-7). The angel Gabriel appears to Zechariah in the Temple and promises that Elizabeth will bear a son named John, who is to play the role of Elijah in calling Israel to repentance (1:13-17). Zechariah and Elizabeth are the first two figures in Luke's story who are said to be "filled with the Holy Spirit" (1:41, 67).

As Luke's story of the birth and infancy of Jesus continues, two more aged characters serve as prophetic voices: Simeon and Anna become the prophetic chorus welcoming the child Jesus on the occasion of his purification in the Temple (Luke 2:22-38). The old man Simeon, who has long been hoping for Israel's deliverance from oppression, had been promised by the Holy Spirit that he would not die before he has seen the Lord's Messiah. Anna, an eighty-four-year-old prophetess who frequented the Temple to worship and pray night and day, recognizes Jesus, gives thanks to God, and declares the news about him "to all who were looking for the redemption of Jerusalem" (Luke 2:38).

In John's Gospel, Nicodemus represents an aged character who exemplifies a more ambiguous reception within Israel for Jesus. Nicodemus, a "leader of the Jews," seeks out Jesus by night to question him (John 3:1-21). We are not told his age, but his response to Jesus' mysterious declaration about the necessity of being born again suggests that he may be well advanced in years: "How can anyone be born after having grown old?" (John 3:4). In the last chapter of John's Gospel, the risen Jesus prophesies Peter's eventual death as an old man and implies that both he and John ("the Beloved Disciple"), despite their different manners of death, will continue into their old age as key leaders of the early Christian movement.

In the Pauline Epistles, Paul highlights Abraham's advanced age when casting him as an exemplar of faith (Romans 4). Elsewhere, Paul refers to himself as an "old man" who is now a "prisoner of Christ Jesus" (Philemon 9), a self-description likely intended to elicit sympathetic respect from the letter's addressees.

The respect due to older members of the community is also emphasized in the Pastoral Epistles. See, for example, 1 Timothy 5:1: "Do not speak harshly to an older man, but speak to him as to a father." Here we find also specific directives that the community should provide assistance to widows over the age of sixty, and that women recognized by the church as widows should devote their energies to prayer, hospitality, and service to the afflicted (1 Timothy 5:3-16). The letter to Titus adds that older women should be instructed "to be reverent in behavior, not to be slanderers or slaves to drink," and that they should train the younger women in their domestic duties, so that "the word of God may not be discredited" (Titus 2:3-5). The older men, on the other hand, are to be instructed, in a more general way, to be "temperate, serious, prudent, and sound in faith, in love, and in endurance" (Titus 2:2). These unexceptional moral teachings for older persons are part of a larger concern in the Pastorals that the church community be respectable in the eyes of the wider culture.

Overall, the biblical writers deem elders worthy of honor, respect, and special care. When elders are alone and in need, the religious community is called to provide for their care, and those who fail to provide for their own older family members are harshly condemned (1 Timothy 5:8). In turn, older persons bear a particular responsibility. They are to be paradigms of faith, role models exemplifying reverence and temperance (Titus 2:2-5). They are to exercise leadership in the community, especially in teaching and counseling. Their example of faith continues beyond their deaths as a witness to later generations (Hebrews 11).

Finally, the older biblical characters signal the possibility of unanticipated fruitfulness at the end of the life span. As in the prophecy of Joel, quoted by Peter in his Pentecost sermon, "Your young men shall see visions, and your old men shall dream dreams" (Acts 2:17). They are the righteous people described in Psalm 92:14: "In old age they still produce fruit; they are always green and full of sap." Although the Bible refers to the struggles and vulnerabilities of old age, more characteristic are stories of older persons receiving blessing or a new vocation.

See also CHURCHES

REFERENCES

Bagnall, R. and Frier, B. (1994). *The demography of Roman Egypt.* Cambridge: Cambridge University Press.

Conrad, E.W. (1977). Zaqen. In *Theological dictionary of the Old Testament,* Volume 4 (pp. 122-131). Grand Rapids, MI: Eerdmans.

Harris, J.G. (1987). *Biblical perspectives on aging: God and the elderly.* Philadelphia: Fortress Press.

_____ (1992). Old age. In *Anchor Bible dictionary,* Volume 5 (pp. 10-12). New York: Doubleday.

Parkin, T.G. (1992). *Roman demography and society.* Baltimore: Johns Hopkins University Press.

Patlagean, E. (1977). *Pauvreté économique et pauvreté social á Byzance, 4e-7e siecles.* Paris: Mouton.

Wenham, G.J. (1978). Leviticus 27:28 and the price of slaves. *Zeitschrift für die Alttestamentliche Wissenschaft,* 90, 264-265.

AGEISM SURVEY

Erdman B. Palmore

Until recently, nobody knew how much ageism there was, nor how prevalent the various forms of ageism are in different societies and groups. This is because no one had developed a way to measure ageism. In order to develop such a measure, I designed and tested an ageism survey with twenty items and questions about the respondent's age, gender, and education (see page 29).

I have used this survey in the United States and in Canada to explore three basic questions:

- What is the overall prevalence of ageism in Canada and the United States?
- Which types of ageism are more prevalent?
- What are the main differences between Canada and the United States?

Methods

The items in the survey were developed from the literature on ageism (Palmore, 1999), discussions with colleagues, and experiences of older persons. The survey includes examples of negative stereotypes, attitudes, and personal and institutional discrimination.

In the form published in *CARPnews Report on Ageism,* the respondents were invited to "Circle the number that shows how often you have experienced the events described." In the form used in the United States, the respondents were asked to write a number rather than circle one.

In the United States, the survey was administered to a convenience sample of 152 persons over age sixty in local senior centers and a church group, and who responded to the survey published in the Duke University *Center Report* and in *Fifty Plus.* In Canada, the survey was published in the *CARPnews Report on Ageism,* December 2001. Surveys were filled in and returned by 375 readers who were age fifty or over.

The two samples were fairly similar in terms of gender and education (no statistically significant differences), but the Canadian sample was somewhat younger (44 percent under age seventy) than the U.S. sample (31 percent under age seventy). This was partly due to the fact that 5 percent of the Canadians were in their fifties, compared to only one of the Americans.

The reliability and validity of the survey has been tested in the United States and found to have satisfactory characteristics for an inventory of types of ageism experienced (Palmore, 2001).

Prevalence

The surveys show that ageism is perceived as widespread and frequent by most respondents in both countries. Ninety-one percent of Canadian respondents and 84 percent of U.S. respondents reported one or more incidents of ageism; and more than half of the reported incidents were reported to have occurred "more than once." Each item in the surveys was reported as having been experienced by several persons in both countries. The average item was reported by about one-third of the respondents in Canada and about one-fifth of the respondents in the United States. Thus, ageism was reported more often in Canada than in the United States.

Frequent Types

The most frequent type of ageism, reported by 72 percent of Canadians and 68 percent of Americans, was Item 1: "I was told a joke that pokes fun at old people." A similar type, reported by 55 percent of Canadians and 37 percent of Americans, was Item 2: "I was sent a birthday card that pokes fun at old people." In fact, several respondents wrote notes on their form questioning whether these items were really examples of ageism. This is a debatable question, but such jokes and cards are based on negative stereotypes about old people and therefore fit the definition of ageism. Other frequent types showing disrespect were Items 3 ("ignored"); 4 ("insulting name"); 5 ("patronized"); and 10 ("less dignity").

Another set of frequently reported items dealt with assumptions about ailments or frailty being caused by age: Item 12 ("A doctor or nurse assumed my ailments were caused by age") and Item 18 ("Someone told me I was too old for that"). Both were reported by almost half in both countries. Some respondents indicated on their forms that they agreed that their ailments were due to age—but in fact chronological age does not "cause" anything. Similarly, Item 18 assumes that age causes frailty and/or it reflects a stereotype about "age-appropriate behavior."

Other frequent assumptions about age causing disability are reflected in Item 16 ("Someone assumed I could not hear well because of my age") and Item 17 ("Someone assumed I could not understand because of my age"). Both of these items were reported by over one-third of the respondents in both countries.

The less-frequent items had to do with specific and severe discrimination, such as Items 6 ("refused rental housing"), 7 ("difficulty getting a loan"), 13 ("denied medical treatment"), 19 ("house was vandalized"), and 20 ("victimized by a criminal"). It is somewhat reassuring to find that the more severe forms of ageism as also the less-frequent forms.

Main Differences

The main difference between the Canadian and American samples was that the Canadians reported more incidents of ageism. Canadians reported incidents of ageism that had occurred "more than once" twice as often as Americans. Specifically, the first five items were reported to have occurred "more than once" by a much higher proportion of Canadians than Americans.

There are several alternative explanations of these differences. One explanation would be that ageism is actually more common in Canada than in the United States. Or it may be that Canadians are more aware of ageism than Americans; or more Canadians may be willing to admit these experiences while more Americans deny ageism. I suspect that the 16 percent of Americans and 9 percent of Canadians who claimed that they have never experienced *any* form of ageism were denying it because they did not want to admit being in the category of "old people" who suffer from ageism.

Future Research

More research is needed on larger and more representative samples of Canadians, Americans, and others to test these findings. We also need to find out which types of persons are more vulnerable to experiencing ageism, so that we can target efforts to reduce it.

Hopefully this ageism survey will be widely used so that we can develop an "epidemiology of ageism."

See also: TYPOLOGIES

AGEISM SURVEY

Please put a number in the blank that shows how often you have experienced that event: never = 0; once = 1; more than once = 2. ("Age" means old age.)

____ 1. I was told a joke that pokes fun at old people.

____ 2. I was sent a birthday card that pokes fun at old people.

____ 3. I was ignored or not taken seriously because of my age.

____ 4. I was called an insulting name related to my age.

____ 5. I was patronized or "talked down to" because of my age.

____ 6. I was refused rental housing because of my age.

____ 7. I had difficulty getting a loan because of my age.

____ 8. I was denied a position of leadership because of my age.

____ 9. I was rejected as unattractive because of my age.

____10. I was treated with less dignity and respect because of my age.

____11. A waiter or waitress ignored me because of my age.

____12. A doctor or nurse assumed my ailments were caused by my age.

____13. I was denied medical treatment because of my age.

____14. I was denied employment because of my age.

____15. I was denied a promotion because of my age.

____16. Someone assumed I could not hear well because of my age.

____17. Someone assumed I could not understand because of my age.

____18. Someone told me, "You're too old for that."

____19. My house was vandalized because of my age.

____20. I was victimized by a criminal because of my age.

Please write in your age: _____
Please check: Male _____ or Female _____
What is the highest grade in school that you completed? _____

REFERENCES

Palmore, E. (1999). *Ageism: Negative and positive.* (Second edition). New York: Springer Publishing Co.

_____ (2001). The ageism survey: First findings. *The Gerontologist,* 41(5), 1-3.

AGE-SPECIFIC PUBLIC PROGRAMS

Marshall B. Kapp

In the United States in the twentieth century, Congress created a number of programs that provide special, preferential benefits to which older persons are entitled solely by virtue of having achieved a specified chronological age (Hudson, 1997). This legislative trend, especially active from the 1930s through the 1970s, is exemplified by laws establishing the Social Security retirement system and other public pension programs, Medicare, Supplemental Security Income, various services under the Older Americans Act, and federal housing subsidies for the elderly.

The continuation of *age-based public benefit programs* has become controversial in recent years. One line of argument against preferential treatment in public programs on the basis of age alone is made by *generational equity* proponents, who contend that age-based public programs represent an unfair and unwise redistribution of wealth from one generational cohort (working young and middle-aged adults) to another (the present elderly). In addition, these proponents suggest that, since only limited resources can be devoted to public benefit programs, the process of distributing public funds creates a zero-sum situation, in which a public dollar spent on the elderly is a dollar that is unavailable to be spent on services (e.g., education or health care) for the next generation (Howe, 1995). Under this model, older persons are stigmatized as "greedy geezers."

Another line of argument attacking age-based public programs is that, given the reality of limited resources, it would be better to have program eligibility criteria predicated on each individual applicant's showing of a financial need for assistance rather than mere membership in a group defined by chronological age. This position in favor of *means testing* public programs rejects the ageist assumptions that caused policymakers in the past to build public programs around the idea of age as an automatic proxy for negative characteristics such as poverty, dependency, vulnerability, illness, and disability (Skinner, 1997). As noted by Robert Binstock (1983), the "compassionate ageism" that undergirded the creation of today's age-based public benefit programs actually "set the stage for tabloid thinking about older persons by obscuring the individual and subgroup differences among them." This is the essence of ageism: "the attribution [by public policymakers] of the same characteristics, status, and just deserts to a heterogeneous group that has been artificially homogenized, packaged, labeled, and marked as 'the aged' " (Binstock, 1991). Richard Kalish (1979) referred to the equation of old age with failure, and hence need for public benefits, as the *New Ageism.*

Moreover, an important part of the perspective on old age as almost inevitably a time of decline and decrepitude, such that older persons cannot survive and thrive without government assistance, is that the elderly represent a group of "deserving" program beneficiaries because their sorry condition occurs through no fault of their own. This attitude that older persons are almost always helpless and not personally responsible for their adverse individual circumstances is, arguably, paternalistic and ageist in itself.

Ageism also is evident in the design of certain age-based public programs. Specifically, under Medicare, the Older Americans Act, and federal housing support programs, the federal government pays service providers or property owners directly for covered services provided to older program beneficiaries, rather than giving money or a voucher directly to the older person to purchase desired medical, housing, and social services personally. *Vendor payment* programs such as these are ageist and disrespectful of older persons' autonomy and independence because they assume that older program beneficiaries are incapable of managing money and need the benevolent intervention of government to protect them from exploitation. This paternalistic approach toward the elderly is especially inconsistent with the direct cash-to-beneficiary approach embodied in the same government's Social Security retirement and disability programs. In public programs that are not aged-based but that have many older beneficiaries, Medicaid represents the paternalistic vendor payment philosophy, while the Food Stamp Program, by supplying beneficiaries with a voucher to spend, exemplifies trust in beneficiaries—including the elderly—to manage their own affairs.

See also AGE STRATIFICATION; BENEFITS OF AGING; SCAPEGOATING; SOCIAL SECURITY

REFERENCES

Binstock, R.H. (1983). The aged as scapegoat. *The Gerontologist,* 23, 136-143.

_____ (1991). Aging, politics, and public policy. In B.B. Hess and E.W. Markson (Eds.), *Growing old in America* (Fourth edition) (pp. 325-340). New Brunswick, NJ: Transaction.

Howe, N. (1995). Why the graying of the welfare state threatens to flatten the American dream—or worse. *Generations,* 19(fall), 15-19.

Hudson, R.B. (Ed.) (1997). *The future of age-based public policy.* Baltimore: Johns Hopkins University Press.

Kalish, R.A. (1979). The new ageism and the failure models: A polemic. *The Gerontologist,* 19, 398-402.

Skinner, J.H. (1997). Should age be abandoned as a basis for program and service eligibility? Yes. In A.E. Scharlach and L.W. Kaye (Eds.), *Controversial issues in aging* (pp. 59-62). Boston: Allyn & Bacon.

ALCOHOLISM

Celia F. Hybels
Dan G. Blazer

Alcohol use in older adults is a significant public health problem, yet this use often goes undetected and untreated. Alcoholism in older adults is misunderstood in part due to several myths about alcoholism in late life.

Myth #1: Older Adults Do Not Drink Alcohol

Although older adults are less likely than younger adults to consume alcohol, use among older adults is not uncommon. In the United States Health Interview Survey, more than 47 percent of adults ages sixty-five to seventy-four, 33 percent of adults ages seventy-five to eighty-four, and 24 percent of adults age eighty-five or older reported they were current drinkers, and more than 18 percent of those sixty-five or older reported using alcohol daily (Ruchlin, 1997). In addition, up to 10 percent of older adults can be classified as problem drinkers (Adams and Cox, 1995). Although the percentage of problem drinkers is lower in older than younger adults, older adults who are heavy drinkers tend to suffer more medical alcohol related problems than younger adults (Adams and Cox, 1995).

Myth #2: Once a Drinker, Always a Drinker

Adults often decrease their use of alcohol as they grow older. In the Health Interview Survey, more than 15 percent of older adults were former drinkers but not current drinkers (Ruchlin, 1997). In a study of adults seventy or older conducted in New Zealand, 60 percent of men and 30 percent of women said they took less alcohol now than in middle age, while 7 percent of men and 11 percent of women said they took more (Busby et al., 1988). Older adults reduced their drinking because of medical problems, fewer social interactions, and to decrease drug-alcohol interactions (Adams and Cox, 1995; Busby et al., 1988). Reasons for increased use included more money and more time.

Myth #3: Problems with Alcohol Do Not Begin in Late Life

Although many older persons with alcoholism are lifelong drinkers who have survived to old age, approximately one third of older alcoholics in treatment have late-onset problem drinking (Atkinson, Tolson, and Turner, 1990). Late-onset alcoholism may start as a reaction to stresses such as bereavement and retirement (Johnson, 2000), and is generally associated with less family alcoholism and greater psychological stability than younger onset alcoholism (Atkinson, Tolson, and Turner, 1990).

Myth #4: Older Baptists Do Not Drink

Many Southern Baptist churches, especially in the rural South, proscribe the use of alcohol in any form. Nevertheless, a sizable minority of elders who both indicate membership in rural Baptist churches and who attend services regularly drink alcohol occasionally and sometimes regularly (Musick, Blazer, and Hays, 2000). The potential conflict between the behavior of the older adults who drink and the religious teachings of the Baptist churches that they attend does not appear to create either increased psychological nor physical problems to these elders (Blazer, Hays, and Musick, 2002).

Myth #5: Excessive Alcohol Use Can Be Defined the Same for Adults of All Ages

Older adults are particularly sensitive to the effects of alcohol since with increasing age, there are changes in body composition. Specifically, there is a decrease in lean body mass and total body water with increasing age, which leads to higher blood alcohol concentrations per amount consumed than observed in younger adults (Johnson, 2000). Lower limits for excessive alcohol use have been recommended for older adults (Chermack et al., 1996).

Myth #6: Alcoholism Presents Similarly in Older and Younger Patients

Among new admissions to medical service, only 37 percent of elderly patients who screened positive for alcoholism were identified by their house officers, compared to 60 percent of younger patients. Older patients with alcoholism were less likely to be identified if they were white, female, or had completed high school, suggesting these characteristics did not fit the expected profile of the older alcoholic (Curtis et al., 1989). One reason for poor detection is that alcohol problems in this age group may present in different ways with non-specific symptoms (Johnson, 2000). Patients may present with mild cognitive impairment, a history of falls, and other symptoms that may appear to be related to aging. In addition, screening tools to detect alcoholism have generally been used in younger adults and often include criteria that are less applicable for older adults. For example, older adults are less likely to experience problems at work if they are retired, to cause problems at home if they live alone, and to be caught driving while intoxicated if they no longer drive. In addition, a decline in self-care may be attributed to age-related impairment (Adams and Cox, 1995).

Myth #7: Older Adults Cannot Be Successfully Treated for Alcoholism

Even when diagnosed, older patients with alcoholism are less likely to have treatment recommended than younger patients, and if treatment is recommended it is less likely to be initiated (Curtis et al., 1989). Some physicians may feel older alcoholics cannot be successfully treated. However, studies have found older patients with alcoholism can be successfully treated and generally do not require less-intensive treatment (Hurt et al., 1988; Oslin, Pettinati, and Volpicelli, 2002). Older alcoholics, particularly those with late onset, are more likely to stay in treatment and remain sober for longer periods than younger patients (Atkinson, Tolson, and Turner, 1990; Curtis et al., 1989).

These myths are a kind of prejudice, which may lead to discrimination against older alcoholics. Such forms of ageism should be recognized and reduced in order to better treat alcoholism in old age.

See also COSTS OF AGEISM; RESPONSES TO AGEISM

REFERENCES

Adams, W. L. and Cox, N.S. (1995). Epidemiology of problem drinking among elderly people. *The International Journal of the Addictions,* 30, 1693-1716.

Atkinson, R.M., Tolson, R.L., and Turner, J.A. (1990). Late versus early onset problem drinking in older men. *Alcoholism: Clinical and Experimental Research,* 14, 574-579.

Blazer, D.G., Hays, J.C., and Musick, M.A. (2002). Abstinence versus alcohol use among elderly rural Baptists: A test of reference group theory and health outcomes. *Aging and Mental Health,* 6, 47-54.

Busby, W.J., Campbell, A.J., Borrie, M.J., and Spears, G.F.S. (1988). Alcohol use in a community-based sample of subjects aged 70 years and older. *Journal of the American Geriatrics Society,* 36, 301-305.

Chermack, S.T., Blow, F.C., Hill, E.M., and Mudd, S.A. (1996). The relationship between alcohol symptoms and consumption among older drinkers. *Alcoholism: Clinical and Experimental Research,* 20, 1153-1158.

Curtis, J.R., Geller, G., Stokes, E.J., Levine, D.M., and Moore, R.D. (1989). Characteristics, diagnosis, and treatment of alcoholism in elderly patients. *Journal of the American Geriatrics Society,* 37, 310-316.

Hurt, R.D., Finlayson, R.E., Morse, R.M., and Davis, L.J. (1988). Alcoholism in el-
    derly persons: Medical aspects and prognosis of 216 patients. *Mayo Clinic Pro-
    ceedings,* 63, 753-760.
Johnson, I. (2000). Alcohol problems in old age: A review of recent epidemiologic
    research. *International Journal of Geriatric Psychiatry,* 15, 575-581.
Musick, M.A., Blazer, D.G., and Hays, J.C. (2000). Religious activity, alcohol use,
    and depressive symptoms in a sample of elderly Baptists. *Research on Aging,* 22,
    91-116.
Oslin, D.W., Pettinati, H., and Volpicelli, J.R. (2002). Alcoholism treatment adher-
    ence—Older age predicts better adherence and drinking outcomes. *American
    Journal of Geriatric Psychiatry,* 10, 740-747.
Ruchlin, H.S. (1997). Prevalence and correlates of alcohol use among older adults.
    Preventive Medicine, 26, 651-657

ANTIAGING MEDICINE

Erdman B. Palmore

Many "antiaging" potions are touted in advertisements that claim
to reverse or at least stop the aging process. There is even an American Academy of Anti-Aging Medicine (A4M) that has created an al-
leged medical subspecialty and accreditation in antiaging medicine.
The founder of A4M, Ronald Klatz, claims that the organization has
10,500 members and 1,000 doctors and other health professionals in
various stages of certification in antiaging medicine (Pope, 2002).

However, the A4M is not recognized by the American Board of Medical Specialties nor by the American Medical Association. In fact, fifty-
one scientists issued a position paper (quoted in Pope, 2002) to counter the
claims of the A4M. This paper contains the following warning:

> Our language on this matter must be unambiguous: there are no
> lifestyle changes, surgical procedures, vitamins, antioxidants,
> hormones, or techniques of genetic engineering available today
> that have been demonstrated to influence the process of aging.
> We strongly urge the general public to avoid buying or using
> products or other interventions from anyone claiming that they
> will slow, stop, or reverse aging.

As S. Jay Olshansky, a demographer at the University of Illinois at Chicago, said, "Anyone who claims that they can stop or reverse the aging process is lying" (quoted in Pope, 2002).

Such claims for antiaging medicine are forms of ageism in two senses. First, the term *antiaging medicine* implies that aging is a "disease" that can be "cured." Most scientists agree that aging is not a disease and that aging processes cannot be stopped or reversed with any pills, enema regimes, hormones, testosterone, bee pollen, gingko biloba, ginseng, selenium supplements, chelation, gerovital, chromium, comfrey, lobelia or other herbs, growth hormones, or DHEA (dehydroepiandrosterone). Furthermore, many of these so-called antiaging miracle cures may have dangerous side effects, depending on dosage and interactions with medications.

Second, the antiaging medicine advocates imply that the normal signs of old age, such as wrinkles, gray hair, baldness, and hearing and vision changes are shameful and ugly, rather than conditions to be expected and accepted. Some people are even proud of their signs of aging, as indicators of maturity and experience.

See also BOTOX; FACE-LIFTS

REFERENCE

Pope, E. (2002). Fifty-one top scientists blast anti-aging idea. *AARP Bulletin,* 43(6).

ARCHITECTURE

Erdman B. Palmore

Housing designed for older adults has become big business in the United States (Gelwicks, 2001). Government agencies such as the Federal Housing Administration, Public Housing Administration, the Administration on Aging, and the Department of Housing and Urban Development encourage the development and construction of architecture "for the elderly." Also private organizations (e.g., the AARP) support research, training, and demonstration projects for improving the design of housing for the elderly.

Many books have been published in the field such as *Buildings for the Elderly* (Musson and Heusinkveld, 1963) and *Planning Housing Environments for the Elderly* (Gelwicks and Newcomer, 1974). However, this literature does not really deal with architecture for elders in general, but with architecture for the frail or handicapped. Because most elders are neither frail nor handicapped, most elders do not need any such specially designed architecture (Palmore, 1999).

This example of equating *old* or *elderly* with frail or handicapped is a form of ageism because it perpetuates the negative stereotype that most elders are frail or handicapped.

What is the explanation for this form of ageism? Perhaps the architects and planners use elderly as a euphemism for handicapped, because many handicapped people might not want to admit that they are handicapped. Or perhaps the architects mistakenly think that most elders are in fact handicapped.

Whatever the explanation this is more than a semantic quibble. It reinforces negative stereotypes despite the fact that most people are unaware of its effects. This unconscious form of ageism is especially insidious because most people are not aware of it.

See also HOUSING; STEREOTYPES

REFERENCES

Gelwicks, L. (2001). Architecture. In G. Maddox (Ed.), *The encyclopedia of aging.* New York: Springer.

Gelwicks, L. and Newcomer, R. (1974). *Planning housing environments for the elderly.* Washington, DC: National Council on the Aging.

Musson, N. and Heusinkveld, H. (1963). *Buildings for the elderly.* New York: Reinhold.

Palmore, E. (1999). *Ageism.* New York: Springer.

ART

Erdman B. Palmore

Art in the United States has had a variable effect on ageism (Achenbaum and Kusnerz, 1978). Before the Civil War, most elders were given special respect for the contributions to the new nation and as custodians of virtue. This respect was reflected in the art (McKee and Kauppinen, 1987), woodcarvings, and daguerreotypes of the period.

Toward the end of this period, more negative views are reflected in some art, such as the lithographs of "The Life and Age of Man" and "The Life and Age of Woman" by James Caille printed in 1848. These lithographs show both men and women as rapidly declining in health and abilities after age 70 until they are pitiful figures at ages 90 and 100.

After the Civil War, with the growth of mass production, mass education, and medical sciences, more negative images began to predominate. These include images of disease, "the dirty old man," eccentricity, uselessness, loneliness, unemployment, and poverty.

After establishment of Social Security in 1935, images of elders began to be more positive, along with substantial improvement in their economic and physical health. These images include more healthy, productive, useful, happy, prosperous, creative, politically active, and even sexually active elders (Achenbaum and Kuznerz, 1978). Of course, many negative images still persist (Palmore, 1999).

Stolte (1996) found that the effect of a photograph of an older man had a stronger effect on how he was evaluated than the effect of a verbal statement of his age. Thus, visual images may have a stronger influence on people's attitudes than literature does.

The early images in visual arts encouraged positive attitudes toward aging. The later images support negative attitudes. Recently, more positive attitudes are supported.

See also STEREOTYPES

REFERENCES

Achenbaum, W. and Kusnerz, E. (1978). *Images of old age.* Ann Arbor, MI: Institute of Gerontology.

McKee, P. and Kauppinen, H. (1987). *The art of aging.* New York: Human Sciences Press.

Palmore, E. (1999). *Ageism.* New York: Springer.

Stolte, J. (1996). Evaluations of persons of varying ages. *Journal of Social Psychology, 136,* 305.

ARTS

Michael Beckerman

Ageism can affect attitudes toward artists and their art in two oppo-site ways: negative or positive. The negative prejudice assumes that old artists are "past their prime" and can no longer produce great art. The positive prejudice assumes that artists and their art improve with age, so their later art must be greater than their earlier creations. Nei-ther of these ageist assumptions have a basis in fact.

Not all assumptions about growing older are wrong. The forty-year-old outfielder probably does have less chance of getting to the ball than his twenty-year-old counterpart, even if we factor in such things as "cunning." But in the various branches of "the arts" the situ-ation is rather different. Although a potential decline certainly occurs in the output and even quality of any artist in the face of illness and in-capacity, this can happen just as easily when artists are in their thirties (e.g., Keats, Schubert, Mozart) as later in life.

Although some have written about a "late style," it is something of a chimera—simply a natural attempt at constructing an explanation for works written under the shadow of death and sickness. But even in the case of Beethoven, whose Late Style was a model for later discus-sions, there is no straightforward generalization about the relation-ship between style and aging that may be derived.

A purely chronological Late Style, however is more the norm than the exception. Taking music as an example, it is true that several com-posers ceased their activities midcareer (Rossini, Sibelius); but many more have worked on into their seventies and eighties. These include Stravinsky, Janáček, and currently, Elliott Carter.

Physical conditioning is probably a significant element of later life creativity, and many have noted the longevity of orchestral conduc-tors whose "aerobic" activity is thought to prolong their careers well into their seventies and eighties, with famous examples such as Toscanini, Ormandy, and Stokowski. Arguably the most important creative force in modern dance, Martha Graham, danced until she was seventy-six years old, and was still choreographing dances at her death at ninety-seven. Merce Cunningham continues to function as dancer and choreographer at eighty-three. The greatest force in the "other" branch of dance, ballet, George Balanchine, was still arranging concerts and choreographing at the age of seventy-nine.

Famous instances of later-life creativity in painting include Georgia O'Keeffe, Claude Monet, Grandma Moses, Marc Chagall, and Henri Matisse, whose colorful decoupage (cutouts) came about when, confined to a wheelchair, he could no longer paint. The famous, sometimes infamous, Salvador Dali turned to sculpture late in life and created astonishing fluid figures when he was in his eighties.

Writers such as George Bernard Shaw, Mark Twain, and today, Studs Terkel, are just as effective and creative in their seventies as they were thirty years earlier.

In music Czech composer Leos Janáček composed almost all the works for which he is renowned between the ages of sixty-two and seventy-four.

Although infirmity and illness may cause creative decline, this may happen at any age. The examples listed here, and many more not given, show that creative activities do not cease in old age and that creativity in late life is the norm rather than the exception. Thus, both the negative and positive prejudices about older artists are false.

See also ART; STEREOTYPES

ASSISTED LIVING

Frank J. Whittington
Mary M. Ball
Molly M. Perkins

Assisted living is a newer term, now widely accepted, for a type of congregate long-term care that has existed for many years. In assisted living, physically or mentally impaired residents receive help with some of the activities of daily living, but generally no health-related care. Little federal funding is available for such personal care, and facilities are regulated by states, which permit models ranging from small, usually inexpensive "mom and pop" board-and-care homes to large, corporate institutions with many amenities and much higher cost. Nationally, more than thirty different terms are used to refer to this model of care, including *personal care, residential care, board and care,* and *domiciliary care.* Despite their strong preference to remain living in their own homes, elders and their families tend to view assisted living more favorably than nursing homes, especially before entering them.

Although places referred to as assisted living vary greatly, most facilities promote a philosophy emphasizing residents' autonomy, independence, and ability to age in place in a homelike environment. All assisted living constituents—owners, caregivers, residents, and families—seem to derive comfort from the fact that their facilities are *not* nursing homes and take pains to preserve the distinction. This ideology, at least, is certainly antiageist and, to the extent it is practiced, works to reduce the social image of impaired elders as helpless creatures requiring nursing home care.

Despite the many positive features of assisted living and the satisfaction of many older people who live in such facilities, both the image and some of the actual practices of the industry have unintentionally reflected and even reinforced societal ageism. This has occurred in at least five major ways. First, the term itself is a reminder of the common stereotype of old age as a time of impairment, dependency, and need. It is perhaps unavoidable that any public attempt to address the real needs of some elders will make more visible and reinforce the prevailing age stereotype. As with newspaper headlines describing some rare event or deviant behavior, the net effect of increasingly visible care facilities is to create an impression of commonness. To compound this effect, assisted living facilities, at least the larger, newer ones—unlike nursing homes, which have tended to be tucked away from public view—often are situated prominently on busy streets to attract attention and represent their convenience, both for residents and family visitors.

A second manifestation of ageism in assisted living lies in the decision to move there. Very few older persons who move to assisted living have sole control over this decision. In most cases, a family member first decides a move is necessary and initiates the moving, sometimes without even consulting the older person. A common scenario is one in which the family member, usually a child, "scouts out" homes and offers the older person an opportunity to choose from among those deemed suitable or, possibly, only to approve the family's member's choice. In extreme cases, older persons are moved in with no prior warning, the move being presented in the guise of just a "visit."

Although the roles of family members in this decision-making process run the gamut from merely supportive to fully in control, the premise that typically guides their well-meaning—and ageist—behavior is that the older person is not capable of making a rational decision. Granted that cognitive impairment is an increasing reality in assisted living, but it also is quite clear that older persons are being denied the opportunity to participate in this decision to the extent of their capabilities. By focusing their marketing efforts on families or hospital discharge planners, rather than prospective residents, assisted living owners and operators help nourish such ageist attitudes. Residents who have little or no involvement in decision making often feel "put" in the home, and their feelings of powerlessness contribute to reduced self-esteem. This ageist view of self may contribute to loss of continuity with former identities.

Third, in line with the assisted living philosophy previously described, facilities advertise a broad array of personal care and supportive services, such as individualized care plans, special diets, and daily planned recreational activities, aimed at helping frail elders remain as independent as possible in the least restrictive environment. Yet ageism is clearly evident in the care practices of some assisted living facilities. In a misguided attempt to serve their clients—and impress and reassure families—some providers have adopted a philosophy of paternalism and total care. They seem to believe that the elders in their care are really in their charge. Such providers do not train staff to believe residents can improve, and they argue that it is more efficient to "do for" residents than to allow them to "do for themselves." These providers, however, are victims of ageism in their assumption that older, impaired persons have no capacity for rehabilitation and will inevitably decline. It is easy to understand that a well-motivated, caring professional would want to exercise her or his caring powers to the fullest, but our research has shown that older people retain their strong preference for *self-care,* despite multiple, severe disabilities (Ball and Whittington, 1995). Although many need significant staff support to achieve it, care that usurps the possibility of the receiver's own self-care, and even her or his choice, is no service. It leads to what Seligman (1975) has termed *learned helplessness* and reinforces the tendency toward ageism in all concerned—providers, family members, visitors, and residents.

Although most assisted living facilities tout their homelike environment, many are too large and impersonal, or hotel-like, to be like home. Our research (Ball and Whittington, 1995; Ball et al., 2000) and that of others (Baltes and Baltes, 1986; Rodin, 1986) has shown that an important contributor to a resident's—indeed, any care client's—quality of life is her or his autonomy, or sense of control. Though most facilities grant residents some determination over their own daily routines, giving the illusion of control, the reality is that most residents lack real choice. For example, daily recreational activities, which usually include bingo as a mainstay, often are childish in nature and designed to accommodate the least active, least alert residents.

This focus on the lowest common denominator is the fourth manifestation of ageism in assisted living, since it supports several stereotypes about older persons: (1) they are all alike; (2) they behave like children; and (3) they lack intellectual and productive capabilities. Although the assisted living model emphasizes the adjustment of services to meet individual needs and preferences, in planning these services, many providers overlook individual differences, making it harder for residents to adjust to their new lives as receivers of care.

A fifth way in which ageism is linked with assisted living is through our public policies and regulations governing it. Similar to its elder sister, institutional racism, institutional ageism does not depend on personal prejudice but does produce a discriminatory effect on its victims. Public policies that provide general funding, through Medicaid, for nursing home care but not for assisted living are a remnant of our society's reliance on the medical model to judge any sick or disabled person. Medicaid policy fails a fundamental test of fairness by paying for the care of elders with disabilities deemed to require "health care," but limiting support for those who are merely frail and slightly confused, but who nevertheless require "personal care" to live.

Finally, ageism also is fostered through policies and regulations that endeavor to keep residents safe. Balancing resident safety and choice is a significant challenge in assisted living. Although regulations in most states support resident quality of life, regulatory definitions of abuse and neglect have been broadened, and fear of sanctions, public censure, and liability leads providers to give precedence to safety over resident preferences (Kane and Wilson, 2001). The result is that residents often are not allowed to make choices deemed unsafe, with providers deciding for residents what is in their best interests. Some facilities use negotiated risk agreements (documents that identify risks and propose strategies agreed upon by residents and providers to reduce threats to safety) in response to this quandary, but these tools are not legally binding, and little agreement exists on how they should be used (Kapp and Wilson, 1995).

See also ABUSE IN NURSING HOMES; CONSENT TO TREATMENT; HOUSING; NURSING HOMES; PATRONIZING

REFERENCES

Ball, M. M. and Whittington, F. J. (1995). *Surviving dependence: Voices of African American elders.* Amityville, NY: Baywood Publishing Co.

Ball, M. M., Whittington, F. J., Perkins, M. M., Patterson, V. L., Hollingsworth, C., King, S. V., and Combs, B. L. (2000). Quality of life in assisted living facilities: Viewpoints of residents. *Journal of Applied Gerontology,* 19, 304-325.

Baltes, M. and Baltes, P. (Eds.) (1986). *The psychology of control and aging.* Hillsdale, NJ: Lawrence Erlbaum.

Kane, R. and Wilson, K. (2001). *Assisted living at the crossroads: Principles for the future.* Portland, OR: The Jessie F. Richardson Foundation.

Kapp, M. and Wilson, K. (1995). Assisted living and negotiated risk. *Journal of Ethics Law and Aging,* 1, 5-13.

Rodin, J. (1986). Aging and health: Effects of the sense of control. *Science,* 233, 1271-1276.

Seligman, M. (1975). *Helplessness: On depression, development, and death.* San Francisco: W. H. Freeman and Co.

ATTRIBUTION THEORY

Erdman B. Palmore

Attribution theory states that causal beliefs give rise to inferences about personal responsibility and these beliefs ultimately serve to guide behavior (Weiner, 1995). When individuals perceive an event as resulting from an impersonal and/or uncontrollable cause (such as aging), they are less likely to assume responsibility for doing anything about the event.

This theory has been applied to the achievement domain within social psychology, but it is also applicable to various problems associated with aging. Thus, if elders attribute any problem to aging, they are less likely to think that anything can be done about it, and therefore are less likely to try to cure or prevent that problem. If this attribution is unwarranted (i.e., aging does not cause the problem), it is a form of ageism.

A good example of this is the recent study by Locher and colleagues (2002), which found that older women with urinary incontinence, who attributed their problem to aging, avoided seeking treatment. In contrast, those who did not attribute their problem to aging did seek professional evaluations and treatments to cure or manage their incontinence. The consensus among professionals is that incontinence is usually related to some pathology and is often a treatable syndrome. Falsely attributing problems to aging not only is an ageist assumption; it may also prevent action that might alleviate the problem.

See also GERIATRICS

REFERENCES

Locher, J., Burgio, K., Goode, P., Roth, D., and Rodrigues, E. (2002). Effects of age and causal attribution to aging on health-related behaviors associated with urinary incontinence in older women. *The Gerontologist,* 42(4), 515.

Weiner, B. (1995). *Judgements of responsibility.* New York: Guilford Press.

BENEFITS OF AGING

Erdman B. Palmore

It is difficult to think of any benefits of aging. The leading texts and journals in gerontology are filled with the problems of aging but make little or no mention of any advantages of aging. This negative view is a kind of ageism.

The following list of benefits of aging may help reduce this kind of ageism. The list is divided into two types: those that benefit society and those that benefit the older person (Palmore, 1979). These benefits apply to the United States at present, although some apply to the aged in other places and times as well.

Benefits to Society

- *More law-abiding:* Regardless of how it is measured, the elders are the most law-abiding of all age groups (except for young children). For example, persons over sixty-five have about one-tenth their expected arrest rate for all offenses, and about one-twentieth their expected rate for felony offenses, according to the Federal Bureau of Investigation (Palmore, 1999). However, part of this low crime rate is due to positive discrimination in favor of older offenders by the legal system.
- *More political participation:* Elders are better citizens in the sense that they vote more frequently, are more interested and informed about public issues, contact public officials more often, and more often serve in public office.

- *More voluntary organization participation:* Most elders also serve society through maintaining or increasing their participation in voluntary organizations, churches, and other religious organizations. Cross-sectional participation rates are lower in the older-age categories, but this is due to socioeconomic status. Longitudinal studies show that the large majority of persons over forty-five have stable or increasing rates of participation as they grow older.
- *Better workers:* Despite widespread beliefs to the contrary, most studies of older workers agree that in most jobs, older workers perform as well or better than younger workers. The exceptions to this rule involve jobs requiring fast reaction times. In most jobs, accuracy and consistency of output tend to increase with age. In addition, older workers have less job turnover, have less absenteeism, less alcoholism, less drug addition, and less accidents.

Benefits for the Individual

- *Less criminal victimization:* In addition to engaging in less criminal activity, elders are victimized less often. Contrary to popular opinion, persons over sixty-five have substantially lower victimization rates in nearly all categories of personal crime, according to the U.S. Department of Justice (Palmore, 1999). The only category in which the rate for older persons is equal to that of younger persons is "personal larceny with contact," which includes purse snatching and pickpocketing.
- *Fewer accidents:* Elders also have fewer motor vehicle, work, home, and other accidents than any other age group. Their accident rate is less than two-thirds that of all persons according to the National Center for Health Statistics (Palmore, 1999).
- *Social Security and other pensions:* This is the most important economic benefit of aging for most persons. Social Security now covers most workers and widows and provides benefits to more than 90 percent of persons over sixty-five. A special advantage of Social Security benefits is that they are "inflation-proof": the benefits automatically increase with the cost-of-living index. Other pensions now cover the majority of all wage and salary workers. These pensions combined with personal

savings and investments usually allow most elders to retire if they no longer want to work. This "freedom from work" is perhaps the most cherished benefit of aging.

- *Supplemental Security Income (SSI):* The SSI program provides a guaranteed minimum income for all persons over sixty-five (as well as for the blind and disabled). Thus, regardless of eligibility for Social Security, all elders can be sure they will have at least enough to feed, clothe, and house themselves.
- *Lower taxes:* Many elders enjoy tax benefits because of their age, such as reduced property taxes, double personal exemption on income taxes, and reduced taxes on Social Security benefits.
- *Medicare:* Elders are the only age group with national health insurance. In 1997, Medicare paid $207 billion in benefits (Health Care Financing Administration, 1998).
- *Free services and reduced rates:* The various free or reduced-rate programs and services provided specially for older persons by governments, or by private agencies, are too numerous to list here, but they include the following major ones: housing, meals, groceries, drug discounts, transportation, entertainment, education, information, referral, planning, coordination, employment, and research.
- *Freedom from child rearing:* Most elders no longer have any child-rearing responsibilities. This frees them from both the financial drain of supporting children and the physical and psychological drain of caring for them. This freedom releases large amounts of time, money, and energy for whatever the elder wants to do.
- *Grandchildren:* Most grandparents consider their grandchildren to be a benefit of old age. They can usually enjoy being friends and playing with them without the unpleasant duties of discipline and overall care.
- *Wisdom:* Old age does not guarantee wisdom, but it appears to be a prerequisite for the mature and balanced perspective, based on years of experience, which wisdom requires.
- *Fewer addictions:* Elders have a lower rate of alcoholism, drug addiction, smoking, and other chemical dependencies than younger people. This is partly because more elders have managed to free themselves from these addictions, and partly because those

who could not quit these addictions died before reaching old age.

- *Fewer acute illnesses:* Although elders have more chronic diseases, this is partly compensated for by their lower rates of acute illnesses such as whooping cough, chicken pox, appendicitis, tonsillitis, and upper respiratory illnesses.

Hopefully, more awareness of these benefits may help counter the negative views of old age that are part of ageism.

See also DISCOUNTS; SLOGANS; TYPOLOGIES

REFERENCES

Health Care Financing Administration (1998). Medicare and Medicaid statistical supplement, 1998. *Health Care Financing Review.* Washington, DC: US Government Printing Office.

Palmore, E. (1979). Advantages of aging. *The Gerontologist,* 19, 220-223.

_____ (1999). *Ageism: Negative and positive.* New York: Springer.

BIOLOGICAL DEFINITIONS OF AGING

Erdman B. Palmore

From antiquity, biological definitions of aging have been negative. Aristotle defined old age as that period in life when the body's innate heat diminishes; and heat was the essence of life (Cole and Winkler, 1993). Each individual possesses a finite amount of heat that steadily diminishes throughout life, according to this definition.

The Greek physician, Galen, defined aging as a drying out and desiccation of tissues (Grant, 1963). After the decline of Galenic theory, Enlightenment physicians believed that aging consisted of the gradual deterioration of the "vital life force," resulting a decline and souring of the "humors," narrowing of the blood vessels, wearing out of the organs, and accumulation of earthy materials in the body.

With the growing knowledge of cellular biology in the 1830s and of bacteriology in the 1880s, the principle of decline in an unobservable life force was gradually replaced by the a theory of degeneration of tissues and of cells as the primary explanation of aging.

Even today, biologists tend to define aging in terms of decline and degeneration. For example, Crews (1993) writes, "aging may be measured as frailty, loss of vigor, failure to thrive, loss of physiological function, or decreased adaptability." Even the National Institute on Aging (1993) lists the processes of "normal aging" as declines in function of the heart, lungs, brain, kidneys, muscles, sight, and hearing.

Most recently, Hayflick (2002), a leading biological gerontologist, has defined aging on the molecular level as "the systematic random loss of molecular fidelity that occurs . . . after reproductive success." This loss of fidelity leads to loss of function in various tissues and organs.

More neutral definitions of aging are cited by some biologists. For example, Rockstein and Sussman (1979) defined aging as "any time-dependent change, common to all members of a species, which occurs after maturity . . . and which is distinct from daily, seasonal, and other biological rhythms." Theoretically, this includes all postmaturational changes: both declines (senescence) and improvements (such as fewer acute illnesses, reduced allergic reactions, increased strength from resistance training).

However, in practice, biological gerontologists focus on senescence and neglect the study of factors related to improvements or maintenance of function. This emphasis on senescence tends to support the ageist assumption that aging is nothing but decline and deterioration (Palmore, 1999). This gives aging "a bad name."

To prevent the reinforcement of ageism, terms such as *deterioration, debilitation,* or *senescence,* are preferred to "aging" (Palmore, 2000). Aging then could be used in the neutral sense of "any time-dependent change," changes that may be negative, neutral, or positive.

REFERENCES

Cole, T. and Winkler, M. (1993). Development and aging in historical perspective. In R. Kastenbaum (Ed.), *Encyclopedia of adult development*. Phoenix, AZ: Oryx Press.

Crews, D. (1993). Biological aging. *Journal of Cross-Cultural Gerontology, 8,* 281.

Grant, R. (1963). Concepts of aging. *Perspectives in biology and Medicine, 44,* 10.

Hayflick, L. (2002). Anarchy in gerontological terminology. *The Gerontologist,* 42, 407.

National Institute on Aging (1993). *In search of the secrets of aging.* Bethesda, MD: National Institutes of Health.

Palmore, E. (1999). *Ageism.* New York: Springer.

_____ (2000). Ageism in gerontological language. *The Gerontologist,* 40, 645.

Rockstein, M. and Sussman, M. (1979). *Biology of aging.* Belmont, CA: Wadsworth.

BLAMING THE AGED

Jack Levin

Victim blaming is the tendency to attribute a problem to the characteristics of the people who are its victims (Ryan, 1971). In the area of race relations, for example, educational deficits experienced by black American children have been viewed by some as a result of their inferior intellect, their inadequate parenting, or a self-perpetuating black subculture in which academic success is discouraged (for a review, see Levin, 2002). Similarly, the difficulties that older workers often encounter in the area of hiring and promotion have been attributed not to age discrimination but to the stereotypic view that they are disabled, senile, and useless (Levin and Levin, 1980; Palmore, 1999; Kite and Wagner, 2002; McCann and Giles, 2002). This is a common form of ageism.

An important function of victim blaming is that it allows those in the advantaged segment of society to avoid blaming themselves for the problems experienced by a subordinate group. From this viewpoint, little reason exists for the members of a majority group to address issues of inequity, discrimination, or bigotry. For example, victim blaming locates the roots of educational inequality in characteristics of black American youngsters; institutionalized racism is regarded as playing little if any role. If black students are genetically or culturally inferior, then white teachers, principals, and school committee members have no reason to feel responsible.

In a similar way, holding stereotypic characteristics of unproductive older workers helps to justify terminating them rather than their younger (and sometimes lower paid) counterparts. From a victim-blaming point of view, it is not the company that needs to change its ageist policies; it is older workers who need to retire before they embarrass themselves and their supervisors on the job (Levin and Levin, 1980; McCann and Giles, 2002).

Victim blaming, moreover, makes unnecessary, if not counterproductive, expensive policies and programs to reduce external sources of inequity. Because the problem is viewed as residing in the victim, it is the primary responsibility of the victim to make beneficial changes.

For example, if children living in impoverished circumstances are sickened and damaged by lead paint poisoning, then interventions should focus on teaching their parents about the hazards of lead paint, rather than on legal challenges to landlords who do not spend the money needed to eliminate the lead. If students of color disproportionately fail at school, then programs should be designed to change their parents' thinking about the value of education, rather than to hold teachers and principals accountable.

The victim-blaming approach operates against older workers who might want to keep their jobs, but are discouraged at every turn. They are often encouraged to disengage or retire and find alternative activities that keep them busy. In many cases, they are asked in retirement to volunteer to do exactly the same tasks—for example, tutoring in the schools, consulting with small-business owners, baby-sitting—which they were paid to perform when they were younger and still employed (Levin and Levin, 1980).

See also AGE INEQUALITY; AGED AS A MINORITY GROUP; ATTRIBUTION THEORY; SCAPEGOATING; SOCIETAL AGEISM; STEREOTYPES

REFERENCES

Kite, M. and Wagner, L. (2002). Attitudes toward older adults. In D. Todd (Ed.), *Ageism: Stereotyping and prejudice against older persons* (pp. 129-162). Cambridge: The MIT Press.

Levin, J. (2002). *The violence of hate: Confronting racism, anti-semitism and other forms of bigotry.* Boston: Allyn & Bacon.

Levin, J. and Levin, W. (1980). *Ageism: Prejudice and discrimination against the elderly.* Belmont CA: Wadsworth.

McCann, R. and Giles, H. (2002). Ageism in the workplace: A communication perspective. In T. Nelson (Ed.), *Ageism: Stereotyping and prejudice against older persons* (pp. 163-200). Cambridge: The MIT Press.

Palmore, E. (1999). *Ageism: Negative and positive.* New York: Springer.

Ryan, W. (1971). *Blaming the victim.* New York: Vintage.

BOOKS

Erdman B. Palmore

Many books have been published with the word *ageism* in their titles (see this entry's reference section for a short list). Most of these have been published since 1990. This entry will briefly review in chronological order the more important ones.

One book on ageism was published in 1980 by sociologists Jack and William C. Levin. They were pioneers in pointing out that the "focus on decline" among gerontologists leads to "blaming the victim" for the "problems of aging." They also point out that the aged are similar in many ways to other "minority groups." They then analyze three typical reactions to the form of ageism found in "the role of senior citizen": *acceptance, avoidance,* and *aggression.* They close with a discussion of "proposals and prospects for change." One of the major contributions of this book is the discussion of how ageism is similar and different from racism.

Copper (1988) focused on ageism among women. Copper, a lesbian activist, is most critical of the ways in which feminists participate in the general tendency of American society to treat older women as useless and worthless. She asserts that women have internalized ageism, which causes them to fear and hate their bodies as they age, or to seek an idealized mother figure. To break down this fear, loathing, and idealization, Copper calls for a revival of the feminist consciousness-raising groups prevalent in the 1970s.

Shortly after Copper's book, Rosenthal (1990/1994) wrote a collection of essays on ageism from the perspective of older women. She discusses various issues of concern to older women such as menopause, sexuality, social isolation, violence against women, equal opportunity, and the feminization of poverty.

Another collection of essays on ageism and women is Macdonald and colleague's *Look Me in the Eye* (1991). These essays are full of anger against our society in general and younger feminists in particular, who by not looking older women "in the eye" contribute to their invisibility, making them "twice unseen."

Palmore (1990, 1999) wrote the first comprehensive book on ageism. The first part deals with various concepts related to ageism, including *positive ageism,* which is prejudice or discrimination in favor of older people. The second part analyzes the various causes and consequences of ageism. The third describes in detail the institutional patterns of ageism. The final part discusses various ways of reducing ageism.

Bytheway (1994) points out that ageism is a social construct that is institutionalized in the structures, practices, and organization of culture; and then internalized in the attitudes, beliefs, and behaviors of individuals. He includes ageism against younger people (which Palmore would call positive ageism toward older people), but most of the discussion is about ageism against older people. However, Bytheway tends to neglect the intersection of ageism with sexism.

Falk and Falk (1997) wrote a social psychologically oriented text on aging in America, which used ageism as a lens to evaluate various institutions such as the health care system, the economy, the family, religion, literature, government, and the legal system. They prefer to use the term *gerontophobia* when referring to ageism on the individual level.

Glover and Branine (2001) edited a collection of papers on *Ageism in Work and Employment,* most of which were presented at a conference in Great Britain. Most of the material and discussion deals with Great Britain, so it has limited relevance to ageism in the United States. Branine and colleagues also edited and published in the same year (2001) a similar collection of papers on *Ageism in Work and Environment,* which also focuses on ageism in Great Britain as it relates to employment.

One recent book on ageism is a collection of essays edited by Nelson and published in 2002. This compendium is probably the best review and reference source to date for the theory and research on ageism in the areas it covers: mainly psychology, social psychology, sociology, and communication. However, it tends to neglect other important aspects of ageism, such as economics, public policy, legislation, geriatrics, psychiatry, and religion. The book is organized into three sections: origins, effects, and reduction of ageism.

See also THEORIES OF AGING; TYPOLOGIES

REFERENCES

Branine, M. and Glover, I. (2001). *Ageism in work and environment*. Aldershot, UK: Ashgate.

Bytheway, B. (1994). *Ageism*. Buckingham, UK: Open University Press.

Copper, B. (1988). *Over-the-hill: Reflections on ageism between women*. Berkeley, CA: The Crossing Press.

Falk, U. and Falk, G. (1997). *Ageism, the aged, and aging in America: On being old in an alienated society*. Springfield, IL: Charles C Thomas.

Glover, I. and Branine, M. (Eds.) (2001). *Ageism in work and employment*. Aldershot, UK: Ashgate.

Levin, J. and Levin, W. (1980). *Ageism: Prejudice and discrimination against the elderly*. Belmont, CA: Wadsworth Publishing Co.

Macdonald, B. et al. (1991). *Look me in the eye: Old women, aging, and ageism*. Denver, CO: Spinsters Ink Books.

Nelson, T. (2002). *Ageism: Stereotyping and prejudice against older persons*. Cambridge, MA: MIT Press.

Palmore, E. (1990). *Ageism: Negative and positive*. New York: Springer.

_____ (1999). *Ageism: Negative and positive* (Second edition). New York: Springer.

Rosenthal, E. (1990/1994). *Women, aging and ageism*. New York: The Haworth Press.

FURTHER READING

Gaster, L. (2002). *"Past it" at 40? A grassroots view of ageism and discrimination in employment*. Bristol, UK: The Policy Press.

Gibbs, H. (1990). *Representations of old age (DINROO): Notes toward a critique and revision of ageism in nursing practice*. Geelong, Australia: Deakin University.

Gruman, G. et al. (1979). *The "fixed period" controversy: Prelude to modern ageism*. Manchester, NH: Ayer Company Publishers.

Kingston, P. (1999). *Ageism in history*. London, UK: EMAP Healthcare.

BOTOX

Erdman B. Palmore

Botox is a diluted form of botulin, which is a poison causing botulism, an acute form of food poisoning. It is injected under the skin near wrinkles to paralyze the muscles, which may reduce the wrinkles. The paralysis lasts for three to four months, after which the wrinkles return.

Botox is considered a form of ageism, because it is an attempt to look "younger" or "beautiful" by reducing wrinkles, based on a belief that wrinkles and other signs of aging are ugly and youth is beautiful.

Estimates show that there were 1.6 million Botox treatments administered in 2001, and the popularity of the treatment is increasing. Botox is now the most popular surgical procedure in the United States, more popular than face-lifts and other such attempts to look younger.

Botox parties are also gaining in popularity among middle-aged women. Much like the older Tupperware parties, a hostess invites her friends in for refreshments and socializing; then (instead of selling Tupperware) she tries to sell them Botox injections on the spot at a cost of $500 or more. The hostess usually gets a commission for each treatment.

Botox injections pose several dangers: the paralysis may cause lopsided distortion of the face; the paralysis may become permanent; and the injections can cause infections, bleeding, and other complications. The paralysis also tends to produce a masklike appearance, because one cannot move the eyebrows and other facial features in a normal manner.

See also AGE DENIAL; FACE-LIFTS

C

CARDS

Lucille B. Bearon

It is an American tradition to send greeting cards as a gesture of kindness to others. Sociologists study cards as symbols of popular culture, expressions of shared attitudes and beliefs, mediators of interpersonal relationships, and indicators of social change (Mooney and Brabant, 1998). Among the most frequently purchased cards are birthday cards (Greeting Card Association, 2002), sent to celebrate the anniversary of a person's birth, to acknowledge a person as special, and to "transform communication into a gift" (Dodson and Belk, 1996, p. 14). Because birthdays mark one's chronological aging, many contemporary cards include distinctly age-related messages. Two studies published in 1981 estimated that between 27 and 39 percent of humorous birthday cards focus on aging themes, with more than half of those presenting negative portrayals of aging (Demos and Jache, 1981; Dillon and Jones, 1981), as something to be avoided, denied, lied about, or merely tolerated. As with other forms of humor, birthday cards provide a means of expressing and diffusing anxieties about changes linked to age. But unlike other forms of humor, such as magazine cartoons or television shows that are viewed alone, cards are "intensely interpersonal " and "an excellent mode for transmitting messages that may be difficult to deliver face to face" (Huyck and Douchon, 1986, p.139). The messages in humorous birthday cards range from light humor, to mild teasing, to downright insulting.

Huyck and Duchon (1986) found seven categories of coping strategies represented in a sample of 100 birthday cards:

1. Shared fate between sender and receiver
2. Positive reframing of aging
3. Punctured denial
4. Detachment from older adults
5. Making light of aging
6. Laughing at fears
7. Complimenting people on maintaining youthfulness

A more recent, informal examination of the content of more than 100 birthday cards with age-related messages revealed that many characterized the aging process or older people themselves in terms of negative bodily changes (loss of teeth, constipation, mobility limitations); a return to childhood (infantile behavior and clothing, mention of second childhood); obsolescence (using terms such as *rusty* or *over-the-hill*); and social stigma (older people portrayed as having poor taste in clothes, inappropriate sexual expression) (Bearon, 1997). Some cards imply a competition between the sender and the recipient, suggesting that the recipient is older than the sender and thus at greater risk for acquiring the negative accompaniments of aging. Although fewer in number than negative cards, birthday cards with positive messages about aging emphasize increased knowledge and wisdom, maturity and ripening (equating aging with fine wines, violins, and cycles of nature). Several cards feature the idea that how one ages is a matter of attitude, under one's personal control.

Other developments in merchandising of birthday cards are the profusion of milestone cards (to mark one's thirtieth, fortieth, fiftieth birthday—with cards available for every decade through 100), and related products with an aging theme for birthday parties (e.g., napkins, party hats, banners, tablecloths). Some of these are upbeat and celebratory, but others include "gag" gifts such as imitation laxatives, orthopedic bras, and symbols of approaching death (e.g., a skull and crossbones motif).

Fruitful areas for future research include more systematic study of birthday cards for different target audiences, including trends over time, and an examination of ageist messages in other kinds of greeting cards, (e.g., retirement cards and cards designed for grandchildren to give to grandparents, such as those for Grandparents' Day).

To the extent that the negative cards reinforce negative stereotypes about the aged, they are a frequent source of ageism.

See also AGEISM SURVEY; HUMOR; STEREOTYPES

REFERENCES

Bearon, L. B. (1997). American attitudes toward aging: What do birthday cards tell us? Unpublished paper presented at Encore Colloquium, NCSU, Raleigh, NC, April 14.

Demos, V. and Jache, A. (1981). When you care enough: An analysis of attitudes toward aging in humorous birthday cards. *The Gerontologist,* 21, 209-215.

Dillon, K. M. and Jones, B. S. (1981). Attitudes toward aging portrayed by birthday cards. *International Journal of Aging and Human Development,* 13(1), 79-84.

Dodson, K. J. and Belk, R. W. (1996). The birthday card minefield. *Advances in Consumer Research,* 23, 14-20.

Greeting Card Association (2002). Greeting card industry general facts and trends. <http://www.greetingcard.org/gcindustry_generalfacts.html>.

Huyck, M. H. and Duchon, J. (1986). Over the miles: Coping, communicating and commiserating through age-theme greeting cards. In L. Nahemow, K. A. McCluskey-Fawcett, and P. E. McGhee (Eds.), *Humor and aging* (pp. 139-159). Orlando: Academic Press.

Mooney, L. and Brabant, S. (1998). Off the rack: Emotions and the presentation of self. *Electronic Journal of Sociology,* <http://www.sociology.org/content/vol003. 004/mooney.html>.

CHANGE STRATEGIES

Erdman B. Palmore

Strategies for reducing ageism can be divided into individual actions and group actions. The following are some individual actions based on strategies used to reduce prejudice and discrimination of other kinds, such as racism and sexism (Palmore, 1999).

Individual Actions

- Get the facts in order to combat misconceptions and stereotypes.
- Try to eliminate one's own prejudices.

- Inform relatives, friends, and colleagues about the facts, especially when some prejudice is expressed or implied.
- Avoid ageist jokes and refuse to laugh when you hear one. Or change the ageist joke to one that is age neutral by not specifying the subject's age.
- Do not use ageist terms such as *old fogey* or *old maid*.
- Do not use ageist language, such as equating aging with deterioration and dying, or equating youth with health, vigor, and beauty.
- When others use ageist language, point out to them what they are doing.
- Refuse to go along with age discrimination against adults.
- Write letters to editors of newspapers and magazines pointing out and protesting ageism in current events.
- Write letters to local officials, state, and federal representatives and administrators, pointing out and protesting ageism in government.
- Write letters supporting legislation against ageism.
- Boycott products of companies that use ageist advertisements or discriminate against elders in employment.
- Join groups that oppose ageism and work with them.
- Vote for political candidates who oppose ageism.
- Testify before legislative committees and commissions about instances of ageism.
- Become a candidate for office or get appointed to a commission that can reduce ageism.
- If you experience age discrimination in employment, sue your employer through the Equal Employment Opportunity Commission.

Group Actions

Individual actions become more powerful when they are united and organized. The following is a list of actions that organizations can carry out.

- Reduce prejudice against elders by gathering and disseminating information.
- Reduce prejudice by organizing intergenerational projects.

- Inform people about the facts on aging through public meetings with experts, panels, lecturers, audiovisuals, and other media.
- Publish advertisements opposing ageism and supporting equal opportunity.
- Lobby for legislation to oppose ageism.
- Help pay legal fees for individuals suing for equal opportunity.
- Organize a boycott of products from companies with ageist practices or advertisements.
- Organize watchdog activities to ensure that agencies do not discriminate against elders.
- Organize a petition drive to oppose some aspect of ageism.
- Take class-action suits to court to encourage more enforcement of existing laws against ageism.
- Organize demonstrations such as marches, picketing, and public meetings.
- Organize passive resistance and nonviolent confrontation.
- Support political campaigns for candidates who oppose ageism.
- Register nursing home and retirement home residents as absentee voters.
- Conduct voter registration drives among elders in the community.
- Educate elders about political aspects of ageism.
- Raise funds for campaigns against ageism.
- Enlist the cooperation of other organizations, such as churches and unions, to support campaigns against ageism.
- Remember the slogan, "Don't agonize. Organize!"

See also CHANGES IN ATTITUDES; EMPLOYMENT DISCRIMINATION; INTERGENERATIONAL PROJECTS; LEGAL REVIEW PROGRAM; ORGANIZATIONS OPPOSING AGEISM; POLITICS

REFERENCE

Palmore, E. (1999). *Ageism.* New York: Springer.

CHANGES IN ATTITUDES

Stephen J. Cutler
Nicholas L. Danigelis

Perceptions of how attitudes change as people grow older are often based on stereotypical ageist assumptions. Conventional wisdom would have us believe that aging brings with it either increasingly conservative social and political attitudes or a tendency toward attitudinal rigidity. The issue of population aging, for example, seems to be an especially fertile topic for the expression of these ageist assumptions. Demographer Ansley Coale (1964) writes, "A population with the age composition of a health resort is a mildly depressing prospect. Such a population would presumably be cautious, conservative, and full of regard for the past (p. 57)." The Commission on Population Growth and the American Future (1972) sounded a similar cautionary note: "One concern often expressed about an older age structure is that there will be a larger proportion of the population who are less adaptable to social and political change, thus suggesting the possibility of 'social stagnation (p. 69).'" And, more recently, Wolf (2001) suggests, "There will be some loss of social and economic dynamism as a result of [population] ageing seems inevitable. Middle-aged countries are likely to be a bit stodgy" (p. 23).

Academic commentators are not alone in having these notions. The public holds similar views. Data collected in 2000 for the National Council on Aging as part of the Myths and Realities of Aging Survey show that just 10 percent of persons who were age eighteen to sixty-four and only 16 percent of persons sixty-five and older believe that most persons sixty-five and older are "very open-minded and adaptable." Summing up this set of beliefs about aging and about older persons, of course, is the familiar saying, "You can't teach an old dog new tricks."

Is aging truly accompanied by an inevitable tendency toward increasing attitudinal rigidity? Is there a reduction in the propensity of persons to change as they grow older? Or if people do change, do their social and political attitudes invariably become more conservative as they age? Several strands of evidence suggest these common assumptions are unfounded.

In a major study of how social and political attitudes have changed over more than a quarter of a century, we examined the supposition that aging is associated with attitudinal rigidity or with increasingly conservative attitudes. The work is based on data from twenty-two nationally representative surveys of the United States that were conducted between 1972 and 1998. The information available to us in these surveys includes responses from more than 27,000 persons eighteen years of age and older. To illustrate our larger set of conclusions, here we report the results of analyses in two attitudinal domains: (1) attitudes about race relations (Cutler and Danigelis, 2001) and (2) attitudes about women's work and political roles and about divorce laws (Danigelis and Cutler, 2001).

Using an approach called *cohort analysis,* we identified four groups of respondents according to their age at the beginning of the series of surveys in 1972: those who were eighteen to twenty-nine years old (born between 1943 and 1954), thirty to thirty-nine years old (born between 1933 and 1942), forty to forty-nine years old (born between 1923 and 1932), and persons who were fifty years of age and older (born prior to 1923). For each survey year in which replicated measures were available, we traced the responses of members of each of these cohorts to the questions on attitudes about race relations and about family and gender roles. For example, suppose a question on attitudes about race relations has been asked in 1972, 1982, and 1992. If we look at the responses of persons fifty years of age and older in 1972, sixty and older in 1982, and seventy and older in 1992, we can determine if attitude change is occurring for this cohort (thereby testing the rigidity assumption) and, if there is change, the direction of the change (thereby testing the conservatism assumption).

The results are very clear. In the domain of attitudes about race relations, seven of our ten measures showed each of the cohorts shifting their attitudes in a liberal direction at approximately the same rate. Another measure showed shifts in a liberal direction for each of the cohorts, but the rate of change was fastest for the oldest cohort. Still another measure also showed overall shifts, but in a conservative direction. Even though the attitudes of all of the cohorts moved in this direction, the shift toward conservatism was fastest for the youngest cohort, not for the oldest. On the final measure of attitudes about race relations, little change occurred for any of the cohorts in either a conservative or liberal direction, which demonstrates that stability, when it exists, occurs among the younger as well as the older cohorts.

We reached similar conclusions from the analyses of changes in family and gender role attitudes. On the measures of women's work and political roles, overall trends moved in a liberal direction, each of the cohorts has participated in this general liberal shift, and they have all done so at about the same rate. In contrast, attitudes about obtaining a divorce have become more conservative, but all of the cohorts—not just the older ones—were part of that conservative trend. In fact, the most rapid change occurred again among the youngest cohort.

In short, what this research demonstrates is that aging is quite compatible with attitude change. Whether in a liberal or a conservative direction, we found far more evidence of shifts in attitudes than stability or rigidity. And when change does occur with aging, it is neither necessarily nor invariably in a conservative direction. If societal attitudes are changing in a liberal direction, older cohorts participate in those shifts—and, typically, at least to the same extent as younger cohorts.

Looking at these issues in a different way, recall the earlier predictions about "stodginess" and "social stagnation" that were thought to be accompaniments of older societies. At their core, these concerns imply that social change, including attitude change, is likely to slow or cease altogether with population aging. It is important to recognize, however, that population aging is a phenomenon that has already occurred. Between 1970 and 2000 in the United States, a 75 percent increase occurred in the numbers of persons sixty-five years of age and older and a 200 percent increase in the numbers of persons eighty-five and older (U.S. Bureau of the Census, 1994, Table 13; 2001, Table 11). The "graying" of America was well underway, long before the first of the baby-boom generation will have reached old age. But were the last few decades of the twentieth century a period characterized by the absence of social change? One needs only to think of attitudes and policies pertaining to family and gender roles, the environment, race relations and civil rights—to name but a few areas—to recognize that recent decades have been an era of profound social and political change, all occurring during a period of population aging.

Can old dogs learn new tricks? If by this we are asking whether old age can be a time of attitudinal flexibility and change, the answer is clearly yes. People in their later years are as capable of changing their attitudes—and in a liberal direction—as are younger people.

See also STEREOTYPES

REFERENCES

Coale, A. J. (1964). How a population ages or grows younger. In R. Freedman (Ed.), *Population: The vital revolution* (pp. 47-58). Garden City, NY: Doubleday.

Commission on Population Growth and the American Future (1972). *Population and the American future*. New York: New American Library.

Cutler, S. J. and Danigelis, N. L. (2001). Cohort changes in U.S. racial attitudes: 1972-1998. Paper presented at the Seventeenth World Congress of the International Association of Gerontology, Vancouver, BC, July.

Danigelis, N. L. and Cutler, S. J. (2001). Cohort changes in U.S. family and gender role attitudes: 1972-1998. Paper presented at the 2001 Annual Meeting of the Gerontological Society of America, Chicago, IL, November.

U.S. Bureau of the Census (1994). *Statistical abstract of the United States: 1994* (114th edition). Washington, DC: Author.

U.S. Bureau of the Census (2001). *Statistical abstract of the United States: 2001* (121st edition). Washington, DC: Author.

Wolf, M. (2001). Age shall not weary them. *Financial Times,* February 7, 23.

CHILDREN'S ATTITUDES

Erdman B. Palmore

The evidence on children's attitudes toward the aged is mixed. Considerable evidence suggests that many children do have mostly negative attitudes toward old people (Palmore, 1999). For example, Seefeldt and colleagues (1977) found that 60 percent of schoolchildren preferred to be with the youngest man (in a series of drawings), and only 20 percent preferred to be with the oldest.

By the time children enter school some may have already developed negative attitudes toward older adults. McTavish (1971) found that negative perceptions of some adults could result in overall rejection of older adults. He argues that children tend to fear growing old because of their misconception that aging is bad. Children's attitudes and stereotypes develop early and remain fairly constant, guiding their behavior toward others (Klausmeier and Ripple, 1971).

On the other hand, evidence indicates that children usually have mixtures of negative and positive stereotypes about the elderly (Thomas and Yamamoto, 1975). Marks, Newman, and Onawola (1985) used the Children's Views on Aging questionnaire and found that although children's attitudes toward the aging process were often negative, their general attitudes about older adults were positive. Also most children respond more positively when questioned about their own grandparents, and more negatively when questioned about old people in general.

Newman, Faux, and Larimer (1997) found that children's perceptions of the elderly and attitudes toward the aging process were largely positive. Apparently, the method of assessing children's attitudes can make a big difference in the results. For example, Filmer (1984) asked children to react to pictures of young and old people. When a semantic differential scale (based on adjectives that are polar opposites such as strong/weak) was used, children's attitudes tended to be more *positive* toward older adults than toward young people. However, using a Likert scale (agree strongly, agree, agree somewhat, etc.), Fillmer found children's attitudes toward older adults to be more *negative* than toward younger adults.

Kite and Johnson (1986), in their meta-analysis of the literature on the attitudes of children toward older and younger adults, concluded that these attitudes are complex and composed of conceptually different domains. Thus, there is no simple answer to the question of whether children's attitudes toward the aged are negative, neutral, or positive. The answers depend on what dimension is measured and how it is measured.

See also CHILDREN'S LITERATURE; TYPOLOGIES

REFERENCES

Filmer, H. (1984). Children's descriptions of and attitudes toward the elderly. *Educational Gerontology,* 10, 99.

Kite, M. and Johnson, B. (1986). Attitudes toward older and younger adults. *Psychology and Aging,* 3, 233.

Klausmeier, J. and Ripple, R. (1971). *Learning and human abilities.* New York: Harper & Row.

Marks, R., Newman, S., and Onawola, R. (1985). Latency-aged children's views on aging. *Educational Gerontology,* 11, 89.

McTavish, D. (1971). Perceptions of old people: A review of research methodologies and findings. *The Gerontologist,* 11, 90.

Newman, S., Faux, R., and Larimer, B. (1997). Children's views on aging. *The Gerontologist,* 37, 412.

Palmore, E. (1999). *Ageism.* New York: Springer.

Seefeldt, C., Jantz, R., Galper, A., and Serock, K. (1977). Using picture to explore children's attitudes toward the elderly. *The Gerontologist,* 17, 506.

Thomas, E. and Yamamoto, K. (1975). Attitudes toward age: An exploration in school-age children. *The International Journal of Aging and Human Development,* 6, 117.

CHILDREN'S LITERATURE

Sandra McGuire

Ageism is deeply ingrained in our culture and has crept into children's literature. In general, children's literature is ageist in nature, does little to promote positive attitudes about aging, and gives children little to look forward to in relation to growing old.

Ansello's classic study on age and ageism in children's first literature (1977) and his subsequent research (1988) found older characters underrepresented and stereotyped. His research noted that the adjectives *old, sad,* and *poor* were frequently used to describe older people. When older people were portrayed, they often did not have a major role in the story and were not readily noticeable. Ansello reported that the cumulative portrayals of older people showed them as unimportant, unexciting, inarticulate, flat, unidimensional, unimaginative, noncreative, and boring.

Other reviews of the literature largely concur with these findings (Baggett, 1981; Barnum, 1978; Dodson and Hause, 1981; James and Kormanski, 1999; McGuire, 1992, 1993, 2000, 2004; Peterson and Eden, 1977). In their review of children's literature for ageism, Dodson and Hause (1981) found that the adjective *old* was used so frequently that they concluded no other generation was more completely described by the use of a single word!

Peterson and Karnes (1976), in their review of adolescent literature, found that older people were victims of subtle, traditional bias.
Children's literature remains almost void of older people and frequently fails to fully develop older characters or give them meaningful roles. When older people are portrayed, it is usually as grandparents, and older people from outside the family are rarely main
characters. Myths and stereotypes about aging are pervasive in children's literature, and meaningful and realistic characterizations of
older people are scarce. Fairy tales and other literature often portray
older people as wicked characters such as witches, evil-doers, and
villains.

The first comprehensive research on age-related issues in school
textbooks was conducted under the AARP's Andrus Foundation
(Marskon and Pratt, 1996). The results of the study showed that educational materials in use at the secondary level contain little or no
content on aging-related issues (Couper and Pratt, 1999); this is a
form of ageism by omission. If a textbook did deal with aging the information was usually brief, often misleading, and sometimes
erroneous (Couper and Pratt, 1999).

> Similarly, high school history, government, and economics text-
> books basically ignored the aging of the population and its vast
> implications for society. . . . When later life issues are included
> in instructional materials, it is usually with a focus on problems
> that, in effect, equate aging with dependency, disease, disability,
> and dying. (pp. 10-11)

Rarely will you find mention of things as important as the Older
Americans Act, White House Conferences on Aging, the Administration on Aging, the National Institute on Aging, the American Association of Retired Persons, the National Council on the Aging, Senior Olympics, or senior centers.

Consistently, the potentials of aging are overlooked in children's
literature. Instead, it often incorporates illness, disability, or death
into the characterization of the older person. Portrayals of older people rarely include older leaders, elder heroes and role models, older
workers, older volunteers, companionship, famous older people, active older people, intergenerational activities, similarities between

young and old, life-span activities, community resources and events for older people, and planning for old age. Few books exist that actually portray the real lives of older people.

Although ageism is often not an intentional message of the publisher, author, or illustrator, the message is there (Dodson and Hause, 1981). Ageism in children's literature exists because that is how we have been socialized and educated. We can no longer permit ageism in a medium so essential to attitude development!

See also CHILDREN'S ATTITUDES; LITERATURE

REFERENCES

Ansello, E. F. (1977). Age and ageism in children's first literature. *Educational Gerontology,* 2(3), 255-274.

_____ (1988). Early socialization to biases through children's literature. Paper presented at the 34th Annual Conference of the American Society on Aging, San Diego, CA.

Baggett, C. (1981). Ageism in contemporary young adult fiction. *Top of the News,* 37(3), 259-263.

Barnum, P. (1978). Aging in children's books. *Human Nature,* 1, 13.

Couper, D. and Pratt, F. (1999). *Learning for a longer life: A guide for developers of K-12 curriculum and instructional materials.* Denton, TX: National Academy for Teaching and Learning About Aging (NATLA).

Dodson, A. E. and Hause, J. B. (1981). *Ageism in literature. An analysis kit for teachers and librarians.* Acton, MA: Teaching and Learning About Aging Project.

James, J. Y. and Kormanski, L. M. (1999). Positive intergenerational picture books for young children. *Young Children,* 54(3), 32-37.

Markson, E. W. and Pratt, F. (1996). Sins of commission and omission: Aging-related content in high school textbooks: The status of aging in high school textbooks. *Gerontology and Geriatrics Education,* 17(1), 3-32.

McGuire, S. L. (1992). *Non-ageist picture books for young readers.* An annotated bibliography for pre-school to third grade. [ERIC Document Reproduction Service ED 347 515.]

_____ (1993). Promoting positive attitudes toward aging: Literature for young children. *Childhood Education,* 69(4), 204-210.

_____ (2000). *Growing up and growing older: Books for young readers.* An annotated bibliography of non-ageist early children's literature. [ERIC Document Reproduction Service ED 445 344.]

_____ (2004). *Growing up and growing older: Books for young readers.* Childhood Education.

Peterson, D. and Eden, D. Z. (1977). Teenagers and aging: Adolescent literature as an attitude source. *Educational Gerontology,* 2, 311-325.
Peterson, D. A. and Karnes, K. L. (1976). Older people in adolescent literature. *The Gerontologist,* 16, 225-230.

CHURCHES

Robert Seymour

Probably less ageism exists in churches than any other institution in our society, for a number of reasons. First, most faith communities have many older members in the congregation. Also, frequent occasions for intergenerational activities are effective in eradicating stereotypes. Furthermore, the members of the congregation can serve as a foster family for older persons who are isolated.

At one time pulpit search committees of churches deliberately sought out young preachers to "reach the young people," but that obsession seems to have changed. Now congregations are looking for more seasoned and mature pastors with some experience. It is not uncommon for a beloved minister to remain with "a flock" well into his or her senior years.

Most major denominations also do a good job of giving seniors media coverage in their church publications. Older leaders are recognized and appreciated for their contributions.

One area where ageism may surface is the temptation of older leaders to resist change. The church tends to be a very traditional organization, and new ideas may provoke such comments from older members as, "We have never done it this way before."

See also AGEISM IN THE BIBLE

COHORTS

Erdman B. Palmore

A cohort is a category of people born during a certain period. For example, the cohort of people born between 1930 and 1940 were sixty to seventy years old in the year 2000 (Palmore, 1999). The concept of cohort is similar to the concept of *generation;* but generation is a more ambiguous term because it is used in various ways, only one of which is the same as cohort. Therefore, cohort is the generally preferred term in gerontology.

Cohorts are relevant to ageism in at least three ways: value conflict or generation gap, cohort conflict, and changes in cohorts. One might expect value conflict between cohorts for several reasons. The effects of aging makes older cohorts emphasize different values from those of younger cohorts (e.g., not having children of school age). The effects of being socialized in a different historical age might make older cohorts emphasize different values (such as being more concerned with saving because they were brought up during the Great Depression). Changing fashions may affect younger cohorts differently from older cohorts (as in hairstyles). Such value conflict could be a source of ageism.

According to research, little value conflict occurs between cohorts. For example, Rokeach (1973) found that out of thirty-six values, only three showed large cohort differences: people over sixty ranked "a comfortable life" higher than younger people did; and people over seventy ranked "wisdom" and "responsibility" higher than younger people did.

Other researchers, such as Harris (1981), have also found basic agreement between cohorts on such issues as mandatory retirement, government programs for elders, increasing Social Security taxes if necessary, and family support for elders. Similarly, elders tend to have political preferences and voting patterns in about the same proportions as do younger people (Atchley, 1997).

The conflict between cohorts is largely confined to matters of style and personal preference, such as hairstyles, music, and entertainment. Thus, value conflict does not appear to be a major source of ageism.

Cohort conflict, or a "war between generations," could arise if strong competition arises between cohorts for scarce goods such as health care or the amount of Social Security benefits. One widespread fear is that the federal government cannot continue to pay benefits and health care at the current rate because of the increasing numbers of older people. Such a war would be a strong source of ageism. However, evidence indicates little serious conflict or war between generations on these issues (Palmore, 1999). Younger people understand that when they retire they will want adequate Social Security benefits and health care. Therefore, they have a selfish interest in maintaining these programs. Younger cohorts feel a responsibility to take care of their parents and others in the older cohort. Therefore, they realize that unless Social Security and other programs provide this care, they must provide it themselves.

When it becomes widely known that younger cohorts moving into the old-age category tend to be healthier, better educated, and more affluent than previous cohorts, stereotypes that most elders are sick, poorly education, and impoverished will be dispelled (Palmore, 1998).

See also AGE NORMS; AGE STRATIFICATION; SUBCULTURES

REFERENCES

Atchley, R. (1997). *Social forces and aging.* Belmont, CA: Wadsworth.
Harris, L. (1981). *Ageing in the eighties.* Washington, DC: The National Council on the Aging.
Palmore, E. (1998). *The facts on aging quiz.* New York: Springer.
_____ (1999). *Ageism.* New York: Springer.
Rokeach, M. (1973). *The nature of human values.* New York: Free Press.

CONSENT TO TREATMENT

Heidi K. White

The capacity to consent to medical treatment is an example of a specific competency that is at risk in older adults and can be easily compromised further by ageism. Unlike general competency, which entails the capacity to manage all of one's affairs in an adequate manner and is a legal determination, capacity to consent to medical treatment is rarely adjudicated and is usually determined by medical personnel. These assessments of capacity to consent to medical treatment that are made in physician offices, emergency departments, and hospital wards can have as profound an effect as a courtroom determination, because patients may lose their right to make decisions about medical treatment. The physicians who are responsible for determining the decision-making abilities of older patients often lack training and experience in this process. As a result, a variety of pressures and age-related assumptions may unduly influence the assessment and determination.

Dementia is the most common condition that threatens the decision-making capacity of older adults. Dementia is a condition of progressive loss of memory and other cognitive functions that result in the impairment and eventual loss of usual functional abilities, including the capacity to consent to medical treatment. Dementia is prevalent among older adults; approximately one in twenty are affected at age sixty-five, but as many as one in two are affected at age eighty-five (Evans et al., 1989). The most common cause of dementia is a neurodegenerative condition called Alzheimer's disease (AD). Much of the research concerning capacity to consent to medical treatment has been conducted in the context of AD (Marson, 2001). Even early in the course of AD, capacity to consent can be compromised. However, a diagnosis of AD or other neurodegenerative process is not synonymous with a loss of capacity to consent.

The medical-legal doctrine of informed consent requires that a valid consent be informed, voluntary, and competent. From a functional standpoint, consent capacity can be considered an advanced activity of daily living. Numerous instruments exist for the standardized evaluation of consent capacity (Grisso et al., 1995; Marson, 2001). At best, these instruments represent a first step in a two-step process. The second step is the clinical judgment that incorporates the subject's performance with important contextual factors, including the risks and benefits of the treatment decision at hand. Unfortunately, the opinions of even experienced physicians as to the consent capacity of mild AD patients can vary significantly (Marson et al., 1997).

Furthermore, four legal standards for competency can be applied individually or in combination to assess the competency to consent. These standards have not been consistently applied within or across judicial systems (Appelbaum and Grisso, 1988). These include the capacity

1. to evidence a treatment choice,
2. to understand information relevant to a treatment choice,

3. to appreciate the situation and its consequences for the individual, and
4. to manipulate the information rationally in a manner that allows one to make comparisons and weigh options.

These standards may appear to form a hierarchy of rigorousness but when applied to three groups of patients with schizophrenia, depression, and heart disease, different groups of patients were identified as impaired depending on the standard used, although similar percentages of subjects with impaired performance were found for each of the measures (Grisso and Appelbaum, 1995). This may indicate that because different diseases impair different aspects of cognitive function, different aspects of consent capacity may be impaired depending on the disease process.

Despite the element of confusion brought about by these different legal standards of competency, incorporating them into the assessment of capacity can help to standardize judgments. When specific legal standards such as these were used in addition to expert opinion, the decisions made by physicians showed a higher level of agreement and were most consistent with legal standard four, which is often considered the most rigorous (Marson et al., 2000).

Most of the studies of the decision-making capacity assessment of patients with Alzheimer's disease have used hypothetical vignettes to describe a particular medical situation to extract the information and decision necessary to make a competency determination. This interaction is undertaken in ideal circumstances when the patient is not ill or otherwise compromised. Such hypothetical and controlled settings can be far from the typical situations encountered when the question of capacity to consent to medical treatment arises for the older adult patient.

In real-life medical situations, dementia is a formidable obstacle that should be fully assessed and may hinder the clinician's ability to obtain a competent decision regarding medical treatment or may completely preclude a competent decision by the patient. However, many other factors may hinder decision-making capacity in both patients with dementia and older adults who do not suffer from this condition. Between 10 and 40 percent of older adults who enter a hospital will experience some degree of delirium before discharge (Brown and Boyle, 2002). *Delirium* impairs attention, concentration, memory, orientation, and other cognitive functions and often goes unrecognized and undiagnosed. Generally a temporary condition, delirium can easily be mistaken for dementia and its acute, fluctuating nature can make the assessment of competency difficult. Moreover, delirium is often a manifestation of severe medical or surgical illness, associated with an urgent need for treatment.

One study of the informed consent process in eighty-four hospitalized patients with delirium found that of 173 medical and surgical procedures, 19 percent had no documentation of any consent and 20 percent used surrogate consent (Auerswald, Charpentier, and Inouye, 1997). Among the eighty-four patients in the study, there were no documented assessments of decisional capacity, a cognitive assessment was done in 4 percent of cases, and a legal consultation was obtained in 1 percent. This study underscores the present inconsistency in the evaluation and determination of decision-making ability in the very setting in which many medical decisions must be made. Decision-making capacity should not only be assessed but also reassessed at intervals if temporary conditions are likely to influence an individual's abilities. Other medical conditions that may temporarily inhibit decision-making capacity include severe pain, cognitive effects of medication, and sleep deprivation.

Communication barriers can also hinder the assessment of consent capacity. Hearing impairment can hinder the process of providing appropriate information. The sensorial-neural type of hearing loss experienced by older adults is especially problematic in busy hospital environments with high levels of background noise. Alternative forms of communication, such as writing down necessary information can be slow, awkward, and especially difficult if needed eyeglasses are not readily available. Other medical conditions such as strokes can impair the patients' understanding of verbal and written communication and their ability to meaningfully convey their wishes to medical personnel. Slurred speech resulting from a stroke or missing dentures can also create barriers to communication.

Especially for the oldest old, age may inappropriately become a factor in the assessment of capacity to consent. Because of the much higher prevalence of dementia among the oldest old and the greater likelihood of a variety of communication barriers, ageist assumptions and our time-pressured medical environment may lead to inappropriate assessments that the patient has lost decision-making capacity.

Family members who are available and interested may find that clinicians too quickly turn to them for information and decision making. Family members, even a designated health care power of attorney (HCPOA), need to understand their role and advocate for the older adult to retain decision-making functions for as long as possible.

The assessment of decision-making capacity should focus on the patient's ability to make the decision at hand. Most physicians do this, without even recognizing it as they explain a condition and the options for treatment to their patients. Physicians should be alert to medical diagnoses and other conditions that may hinder communication or impair decision-making capacity. When concern arises about decision-making ability, the assessment should start with a general assessment of cognitive abilities, usually a cognitive screening test that will help to quantify the cognitive abilities of the patient. An effort should be made to use simple terminology and to clearly state the options and the decision that is to be made. The physician should give consideration to the complexity and seriousness of the treatment decision at hand and should assess the patient according to appropriate legal standards. In some cases the consultation of a neuropsychologist or psychiatrist may be helpful. Rare cases will be adjudicated; especially when no one can be identified to provide a substitute decision (e.g., when there is no next of kin).

Some patients with impaired decision-making capacity will be capable of making relatively simple decisions but may not be able to fully understand more complicated treatment situations. Patients who are in the early stages of AD and other neurodegenerative diseases should be encouraged to appoint a health care power of attorney. This person can make health care decisions when the patient is deemed incapable of doing so. The patient should discuss his or her preferences with the appointee so that the HCPOA can more accurately make decisions based on what the patient would do if he or she were able to make the decision, a principle known as *substituted judgment.* Even when it is necessary for decisions to be made by the next of kin or a designated HCPOA, clinicians should look for signs of consent from the patient that will help to confirm that an appropriate decision has been made on behalf of the patient. Individuals who express new unusual behaviors, anxiety, or uncooperativeness may be experiencing typical behaviors associated with a dementia or may be expressing to the greatest extent possible their discontent with the treatment plan undertaken. This can be a difficult situation to sort out, but should be considered.

Physicians are often poorly prepared to make competency decisions. This is left to specialists such as psychiatrists, neurologists, and geriatricians. All physicians should have a general education in the process of competency determination. The development of standardized approaches has been a priority in dementia research but the methodology may be more appropriate for the determination of capacity to consent to research experiments and may be difficult to translate into the clinical situations that entail the assessment of capacity to consent to medical treatment. The potential for capacity determinations to be influenced by misconceptions and irrelevant factors such as age should be considered in future research. The best way to alleviate ageism in the assessment of capacity to consent will be to educate physicians and to establish clear standards on which to base these determinations.

See also ABUSE IN NURSING HOMES; GERIATRICS; MENTAL ILLNESS

REFERENCES

Appelbaum P.S. and Grisso, T. (1988). Assessing patients' capacities to consent to treatment. *New England Journal of Medicine,* 319, 1635-1638.

Auerswald, K.B., Charpentier, P.A., and Inouye, S.K. (1997). The informed consent process in older patients who developed delirium: A clinical epidemiologic study. *The American Journal of Medicine,* 103, 410-418.

Brown, T.M. and Boyle, M.F. (2002) Delirium. *British Medical Journal,* 325, 644-647.

Evans, D.A., Funkenstein, S.F., Albers, M.S., et al. (1989). Prevalence of Alzheimer's disease in a community population of older persons: Higher than previously reported. *Journal of the American Medical Association,* 262, 2551-2556.

Grisso, T. and Appelbaum, P.S. (1995). Comparison of standards for assessing patients' capacities to make treatment decisions. *The American Journal of Psychiatry,* 152, 1033-1037.

Grisso, T., Appelbaum, P.S., Mulvey, F., et al. (1995). The MacArthur treatment competency study, II: Measures of abilities related to competence to consent to treatment. *Law and Human Behavior,* 19, 127-148.

Marson, D.C. (2001). Loss or competency in Alzheimer's disease: Conceptual and psychometric approaches. *International Journal of Law and Psychiatry,* 24, 267-283.

Marson, D.C., Earnst, K.S., Jamil, F., et al. (2000). Consistency of physicians' legal standards and personal judgments or competency in patients with Alzheimer's disease. *Journal of the American Geriatrics Society,* 48, 911-918.

Marson, D.C., McInturff, B., Hawkins, L., et al. (1997). Consistency of physician judgments of capacity to consent in mild Alzheimer's disease. *Journal of the American Geriatrics Society,* 45, 453-457.

COST-BENEFIT ANALYSIS

Erdman B. Palmore

In 2002, the White House Office of Management and Budget (OMB) told the Environmental Protection Agency (EPA) to discount the value of saving the life of someone seventy or older to 63 percent as much as saving the life of someone younger (Borenstein, 2002). The EPA was instructed to apply this discount when assessing whether new antipollution regulations would be worth the costs to be imposed on the polluting industries. The idea was to estimate how many dollars would be needed to save an older person's life compared to the cost the polluter would spend to comply with new regulations that would extend the person's life.

"The 63 percent discount on an older person's life is based on the principle that it is fairer to count the number of years of life saved by a government regulation than the number of lives saved," said John D. Graham, regulatory chief at the OMB (Borenstein, 2002, p. 2). The benefits of a potential federal regulation will be less when the discounted standard for the value of older people's lives is applied in a cost-benefit analysis.

Some environmental activists objected to the approach, calling it "morally outrageous" and an example of ageism because it valued older people less than younger people.

See also STEREOTYPES; TYPOLOGIES

REFERENCE

Borenstein, S. (2002). Elderly less valuable in cost-benefit analysis. *Miami Herald,* December 19, p. 2.

COSTS OF AGEISM

Erdman B. Palmore

There are four types of costs of ageism: costs to elders, costs to younger persons, economic costs, and social costs.

Costs to Elders

Many obvious costs to elders result from prejudice and discrimination against them, such as being ignored, rejected, made fun of, denied employment, denied promotion, abused, and victimized. However, a more subtle cost is the cost to one's own self-esteem.

Victims of prejudice and discrimination adopt the dominant group's negative image of the subordinate group and behave in ways that conform to the negative image. This has occurred among African Americans (Simpson and Yinger, 1985) and among women (Friedan, 1963).

Similarly, elders tend to accept many of the negative stereotypes about old age that younger people accept (Palmore, 1998). These include the stereotypes that most aged are asexual, intellectually rigid, unproductive, ineffective, and disengaged. As a result, many aged individuals tend to avoid sexual relations, new ideas, productivity, effective activity, and social engagement (Levin and Levin, 1980). This is an example of the *self-fulfilling prophecy.*

Montague (1977) describes how this works:

> Most old people have a way of acting as if they were older. They're playing a role. This role of elders has not only been imposed by others upon them, but is self-imposed. They think, "I'm this age, so I have to behave this way." They feel they must say, "Oh well, when you're my age . . ." that sort of thing, to emphasize the fact that they're older. (p. 49)

Such conformity with negative stereotypes is a kind of "collaboration with the enemy," that is, the ageists in our society. Such conformity has a cost in the loss of freedom to be sexually active, creative, productive, effective, and engaged. It forms a vicious circle in which the inactivity causes atrophy of abilities, which, in turn, leads to even less activity. Thus, one of the costs of accepting these stereotypes is a more rapid deterioration than would be normal.

Another cost to elders of accepting such stereotypes is usually a loss of self-esteem and happiness. The high rate of suicide among older men may be one effect of such ageism (Kastenbaum, 1995).

Many elders fail to seek proper treatment for various medical and mental ailments because they think such ailments are a normal part of aging and nothing can be done about it. As a result, their ailments tend to get worse and to multiply until it is too late to do much about them (Palmore, 1999).

Costs to Younger Persons

Any program that benefits only older persons (positive ageism) and is supported by taxes represent costs to younger persons. Thus, the billions of dollars spent on elders through Medicare and Medicaid, tax breaks for elders, senior centers, nutrition sites, etc., are mostly paid for by taxes from younger persons.

All these costs are fairly obvious. Less obvious are the costs of prejudice to the prejudiced person. Furthermore, little or no research has examined this area and it is difficult to separate cause from effect. In other words, even if more personality problems exist among ageist persons, is this because the ageism caused the personality problems, or because the personality problems caused the ageism?

However, by definition, prejudice is a categorical prejudgment of persons because they are classified as members of a particular group. To the extent that this prejudice is inaccurate, one of the inevitable effects is a distorted perception of reality. Rationality is contradicted by prejudice, which may furnish an oversimplified or inaccurate explanation of one's difficulties. As a result, the actions that are supposed to solve the difficulties are ineffective and are unable to effect a real cure (Palmore, 1999).

For example, when people use elders as scapegoats for the federal deficit rather than recognizing that the real causes are the tax cuts and the increases in military spending, they are unlikely to favor policies that will actually reduce the federal deficit. When people blame high unemployment on elders who continue to work and "take jobs away from young people," they are unlikely to favor policies that will effectively combat recessions, inefficiencies, negative balance of trade, lack of investment, and other more realistic sources of high unemployment.

In addition to such irrationality, personal cost may occur in terms of guilt, moral ambivalence, and the tension this produces. This tension may not be consciously recognized, but may take its toll through vague feelings of guilt, discomfort, and tendencies toward victim-blaming, projection, and authoritarian personalities. Evidence suggests that people who have more prejudice against elders tend to be prejudiced against other groups as well (Palmore, 1999).

Economic Costs

The economic costs of ageism are difficult to calculate, and the total depends on one's assumptions. I have estimated that the costs of special programs benefiting only older persons, such as Medicare (positive ageism), amount to over $300 billion annually (Palmore, 1999).

It is even more difficult to estimate the costs of negative ageism, such as lost productivity of workers who were forced to retire just because of their age. It has been estimated that 5.4 million Americans age fifty-five or older report that they are willing and able to work, but do not have jobs (Palmore, 1999). If we assumed that at least 4 million of these could contribute to our economy by equal employment opportunity, and we estimated the average value of their productivity at about $15,000 per worker, this would amount to about $60 billion a year in lost productivity.

Social Costs

One of the largest social costs to elders is the social isolation caused by residential segregation, disengagement of organizations, family and friends from elders, unnecessary institutionalization, and other forms of discrimination. Such isolation can be very costly in terms of the mental and physical illness it may produce or encourage.

The costs to younger people would include loss of wisdom and guidance that elders have to offer; loss of personal knowledge of what aging is really like; the development of unrealistic fears and prejudices about aging and death; and the loss of the warm emotional support and enjoyment that can be provided by normal relations with older people.

The social costs would also include the lost volunteer work that elders could provide if they were not discouraged by prejudicial attitudes and discrimination. O'Reilly and Caro (1994) point out several ways that ageism may limit the volunteer contributions of elders:

- Concern about displacement of regular workers by volunteer elders may make the workers resistant to the volunteers.
- Inadequate provision for transportation, reimbursement of expenses, insurance, and training may discourage older volunteers.
- Negative attitudes about the skills of elders reduce their opportunities to volunteer.
- Failure to recognize or respond to the special needs of older volunteers may discourage their participation.

Many different and expensive costs result from ageism. The fact that they are difficult to quantify does not reduce the enormity of such costs.

See also AGEISM SURVEY; AGE-SPECIFIC PUBLIC PROGRAMS; EMPLOYMENT DISCRIMINATION; STEREOTYPES

REFERENCES

Binstock, R. (1983). The aged as scapegoat. *The Gerontologist,* 23, 123.

Friedan, B. (1963). *The feminine mystique.* New York: Norton.

Kastenbaum, R. (1995). Suicide. In G. Maddox (Ed.), *The encyclopedia of aging.* New York: Springer.

Levin, J. and Levin, W. (1980). *Ageism.* Belmont, CA: Wadsworth.

Montague, A. (1977). Don't be adultish! *Psychology Today,* 11, 46.

O'Reilly, P. and Caro, F. (1994). Productive aging. *Journal of Aging and Social Policy,* 6, 39.

Palmore, E. (1998). *The facts on aging quiz.* New York: Springer.

_____ (1999). *Ageism.* New York: Springer.

Simpson, G. and Yinger, J. (1985). *Racial and cultural minorities.* New York: Plenum.

CRIMINAL VICTIMIZATION

Michael L. Benson

Victimization Rates

Violent crimes committed against the elderly provoke strong reactions from politicians and the public, and the high-profile attention given to sensational cases in the news media may leave the impression that the elderly are a major target of violent crime in the United States. Any crime that victimizes the elderly may result from ageism.

However, since 1973, data from the National Crime Victimization Survey (NCVS) indicates that the violent crime victimization rate for persons sixty-five and older is the lowest of any age group (U.S. Department of Justice, 2002). For example, in 2000 the overall victimization rate for crimes of violence for those sixty-five and over was 3.7 per 1,000. This rate is less than one-third that of 13.7 for persons fifty to sixty-four, which is the age group with the next lowest rate. Compared to youths age sixteen to nineteen, who have a victimization rate of 64.3, the elderly live in a much safer world.

With few exceptions, the elderly also are less likely to be victimized by property crime. According to the NCVS, the victimization rate for household burglary, motor vehicle theft, and theft in households headed by someone age sixty-five or over is lower than the rates for all other age groups. Indeed, the NCVS indicates that purse snatching or pickpocketing are the only crimes for which the elderly have a victimization rate that is higher than or close to that experienced by other age groups.

Although the NCVS data suggest that the elderly experience a relatively low level of risk from criminal victimization, these data must be interpreted cautiously. Some scholars argue that the elderly are less exposed to criminal victimization risk factors than are younger people because the elderly take precautions to protect themselves. According to Stafford and Galle (1984), the elderly actually are over-victimized given their exposure to risk. In addition, it is important to note that the NCVS data does not cover some potentially serious forms of elderly victimization. For example, it does not include crimes such as fraud, for which some evidence suggests that the elderly are at higher risk, and it does not pertain to individuals in institutions such as nursing homes who may be assaulted or otherwise victimized by staff members. According to the National Consumers League's National Fraud Information Center, during the first six months of 2002, more than one quarter of all consumers who reported telemarketing fraud were age sixty or older.

Unfortunately, although these data are suggestive, they do not constitute a scientifically valid estimate of fraud victimization rates, as there is no way to determine whether elderly people are more likely to be victimized by telemarketers, or simply more likely to report it, than younger age groups. Ascertaining precise victimization rates among patients in nursing homes is even more difficult, but evidence indicates that instances of physical and psychological abuse are not rare. For example, a survey of 577 nursing home staff members by Pillemer and Moore (1989) found that more than one-third had witnessed at least one instance of physical abuse in the previous year, and 10 percent of the staff members reported engaging in physical abuse of patients themselves.

Consequences of Victimization

Although the elderly are less likely to be victims of violent crime than younger people, research using the NCVS indicates that in some cases the outcomes of the crimes that they do suffer are more serious. Bachman, Dillaway, and Lachs (1998) analyzed three years of NCVS data from the mid-1990s and found that injuries and the need for medical attention resulting from victimizations appear to be more common among older than younger persons. Compared to their younger counterparts, women sixty-five and older were more likely to be injured and to require medical treatment after robbery and assault victimizations. Older men, on the other hand, were less likely to be injured when victimized than younger men were, but more likely to require medical care when injured.

With respect to the financial consequences of victimization, the elderly do not appear to suffer losses that are much greater than those experienced by other adult victims. For example, according to the NCVS, in 2000, persons sixty-five and over who were victimized suffered an average dollar loss of $587 as a result. For persons between twenty and sixty-four, the average dollar losses ranged between $543 and $567.

But these comparisons do not tell the whole story and may over-state the financial consequences of criminal victimization for the el-derly. Many crimes against younger people do not involve any dollar loss, which reduces the average dollar loss from crime for those age groups dramatically. When crimes are restricted only to those involv-ing the loss of at least one dollar, then the mean dollar loss for crime victims age twenty to thirty-four actually exceeds the mean dollar loss for victims age sixty-five and over.

Fear of Crime

Concern for immediate crime victims makes it easy to overlook the broader social consequences of crime. Prominent among these social consequences is fear of crime. As a form of vicarious victimization, fear is potentially important because it can reduce the quality and en-joyment of life. For reasons that are not yet well understood, fear of crime is higher among elderly persons than one would expect given their relatively low level of victimization risk. This *fear-crime para-dox* (Doerner and Lab, 1998) has provoked extensive research and debate. At present, it is not yet settled whether the level of fear ex-pressed by the elderly is significantly more than their level of risk would warrant. Although it is often assumed that the elderly respond to fear by confining themselves to their homes, research to date has not supported this view (Doerner and Lab, 1998).

See also ABUSE IN NURSING HOMES; AGEISM SURVEY; LEGAL SYSTEM

REFERENCES

Bachman, R., Dillaway, H., and Lachs, M.P. (1998). Violence against the elderly. *Research on Aging,* 20, 183-199.

Doerner, W.G. and Lab, S.P. (1998). *Victimology.* Cincinnati: Anderson Publish-ing.

Pillemer, K. and Moore, D.W. (1989). Abuse of patients in nursing homes: Findings from a survey of staff. *The Gerontologist,* 29, 314-320.

Stafford, M. and Galle, O.R. (1984). Victimization rates, exposure to risk, and fear of crime. *Criminology,* 22, 173-185.

U.S. Department of Justice (2002). *Criminal victimization in the United States, 2000 statistical tables.* Washington, DC: Bureau of Justice Statistics.

CROSS-CULTURAL AGEISM

Nancy E. Schoenberg
Denise C. Lewis

Various explanations have been offered for the existence of age-ism, including contemporary value orientations (Palmore, 1999); intergenerational competition over resources (Binstock, 1983); and political/economic organization (Henrard, 1996). Since such explanations for ageism are rooted in and reflect cultural knowledge, a cross-cultural approach provides a useful way to understand how conditions, customs, and institutions contribute to ageism.

Two decades ago, seven anthropologists embarked on a quest to determine "diversity and commonality" in perspectives on well-being, health, and functionality among four distinctive cultural groups (Keith et al., 1994). From their comparative accounts, we are able to better understand social and cultural arrangements that shape the aging experience. For example, dramatic differences emerged among elders from four continents when queried about age-related social distances. For the !Kung of Botswana, there simply was no cultural construct of age-related social distances ("the visual image of !Kung villages . . . was of a coral reef, because people of all ages worked, rested, played, ate together and were in close and almost constant physical contact" Keith et al., 1994, p. 326). On the other hand, the United States and Hong Kong field sites demonstrated highly age-differentiated social networks and household arrangements.

These authors and others who employ cross-cultural approaches (Lock, 1993; Schoenberg and Drungle, 2001; Sokolovsky, 1997) describe the origin of these cultural differences and resultant attitudes toward aging. Understanding how people from a variety of backgrounds think about, behave toward, and structure themselves in the process of growing old, allows us to "unravel universal processes of aging and those features related to culture" (Gattuso and Shadbolt, 2002, p. 100).

As Henrard (1996) states, "any consideration of attitudes, images, and self perceptions of older age needs to examine the context in which these exist, and the social grounds on which they rely (p. 669)." Consistent with this cultural relativistic approach, we examine ageism in three cultural/societal contexts. Rather than constraining our cross-cultural views on ageism to a traditional ethnological focus, we use a broader notion of culture that is understood as a "system of learned and shared codes or standards for perceiving, interpreting, and interacting with others and with the environment" (McElroy and Jezewski, 2000, p. 191). Thus, biomedicine, with its shared and distinct linguistic rules, ritualized practices of achieving status, and hierarchical social network is examined as a cultural milieu replete with ageism.

Biomedicine and Ageism

Ranging from paternalistic medical interactions to the use of demeaning and reductionist slang to describe older adults to medical rationing on the part of National Health Service general practitioners in the United Kingdom, negative attitudes, behaviors, and institutional structures often converge in the culture of biomedicine to offer different and problematic medical care to older adults (*British Medical Journal*, 2000; Butler, 1993). In addition, the financial preoccupation characteristic of many hospitals has made caring for older adults a problematic situation. Declining Medicare reimbursements in conjunction with elders surviving longer with multiple comorbidities has raised considerable concerns among medical institutions about providing services for older patients (Butler, 1993).

As with most culturally embedded policies and practices, ageism is transmitted during multiple exposures. Butler (1993) points to professional training and socialization of health professional students that emphasizes curing the problem, a goal often unobtainable with chronic diseases that frequently afflict older adults. As a consequence of the patients with whom most medical practitioners interact, the older adult population may come to be viewed by biomedical providers as a homogeneous class of physically and cognitively declining bodies (Minkler, 1994). Adjusting this perception requires greater exposure to a wider range of older adults. Indeed, Katz and colleagues (2000) demonstrate that ageism in biomedical encounters can be reduced through greater dialogues between health care providers and "well" elders.

Shifting Perspectives of Asian Filial Piety

A centuries-old notion of hierarchical and reciprocal exchange of care exists within East-Asian cultures, where it is assumed that younger family members readily embrace a "model of obligation" (Holroyd, 2001, p. 1129) to provide care to older family members (Ng, 2002). Recently, however, widespread social and economic shifts in Thailand have created environments that challenge families' abilities to provide such care to elders (Knodel and Saengtienchai, 1999). These trends include smaller family size, increased participation of women in the paid labor force, more frequent migration of younger family members in search of employment, and the spread of Western-style individualism through media and education (Knodel et al., 2000).

To better understand the influence of changing environments on attitudes toward elders, Sharps, Price-Sharps, and Hanson (1998) compared young adults' attitudes about aging in Thailand and in the United States. Young Thais reported continued reverence for elders, as was taught in their homes, schools, and temples. Yet young Thais also reported significantly more negative characterizations of elders than did young Americans (Sharps, Price-Sharps, and Hanson, 1998). Gattuso and Shadbolt (2002, p. 104) similarly conclude that a globalized "focus on youth culture" has led to increased ageist attitudes among young Pacific Islander health professional students, attitudes that can severely hamper provision of appropriate care to elders.

Alterations in Mexican Valuation of Elders

The reality of economic needs associated with changing demographics may preclude family members from fulfilling obligations, even when there is both a normative obligation and a desire to provide care (Parrott, 1998). Sokolovsky's (1997) description of elders in Amatangeo, a rural village outside Mexico City that has witnessed significant economic change, provides a compelling example of how shifting social and economic arrangements may alter the value placed on elders. Specifically, enhanced participation in off-farm employment has provided women with increased financial independence while they continue to maintain traditional reciprocal kinship networks. Conversely, men's value has decreased when they physically become unable to provide reciprocal labor or are not hired for paid labor. Moreover, economic changes have reduced land holdings, resulting in fewer resources to pass onto sons and decreasing economic dependence on fathers and extended families. Although these trends have undermined male status, centuries-old traditional practices still assure older men status and prestige in later life and continue an elder-directed hierarchy of religious and civic service (Sokolovsky, 1997). As in all cases of ageism, a complex picture emerges that belies easy classification of "ageist" or "not ageist" attitudes.

Conclusion

A cross-cultural lens not only places into relief the complexities and subtleties of discriminatory attitudes, behaviors, and institutions, but also requires consideration of the social and cultural origins of ageism. That many health care professionals manifest prejudicial attitudes against older adults is not solely an indictment of this group of individuals; rather, such attitudes and behaviors emerge from generalized negative cultural attitudes about aging that, when placed within a hierarchical, success = cure, and fiscally concerned environment, only perpetuate ageism. The notion of filial piety among many Asians increasingly becomes contested when a globalized youth culture and economic shifts proliferate. On the other hand, older women living outside of Mexico City find their status is enhanced by increased wage-labor participation.

These and other cross-cultural studies encourage consideration of the complex forces that shape the status afforded to elders. Complicating the determination of cultural perspectives on ageism still further is the recognition that no culture is monolithic, that forces such as globalization may further erode the notion of a tightly sealed cultural system, and that important economic and demographic trends foster dramatic shifts in cultural systems (e.g., urbanization in primarily agricultural societies alters extended family arrangements resulting in a realignment of status for elders). Despite these complexities, a cross-cultural perspective on ageism has the potential to reveal the contexts and structures that give rise to attitudes about and behavior toward older adults. Recognition that ageism is created by and through culture provides a first step toward eliminating the constructed category of age as disease, disability, and decline (Minkler, 1994).

See also GERIATRICS; HEALTH CARE

REFERENCES

Binstock, R.H. (1983). The aged as scapegoat. *The Gerontologist,* 23, 136-143.

British Medical Journal (2000). Age concern survey shows ageism in the NHS, 320, 1479.

Butler, R.N. (1993). Dispelling ageism: The cross-cutting intervention. *Generations,* 17, 75-78.

Gattuso, S. and Shadbolt, A. (2002). Attitudes toward aging among Pacific Islander health students in Fiji. *Educational Gerontology,* 28, 99-106.

Henrard, J. C. (1996). Cultural problems of ageing especially regarding gender and intergenerational equity. *Social Science and Medicine,* 43, 667-680.

Holroyd, E. (2001). Hong Kong Chinese daughters' intergenerational caregiving obligations: A cultural model approach. *Social Science and Medicine,* 53, 1125-1134.

Katz, A. M., Conant Jr., L., Inui, T. S., Baron, D., and Bor, D. (2000). A council of elders: Creating a multi-voiced dialogue in a community of care. *Social Science and Medicine,* 50, 851-860.

Keith, J., Fry, C.L., Glascock, A.P., Ikels, C., Dickerson-Putman, J., Harpending, H.C., and Draper, P. (1994). *The aging experience: Diversity and commonality across cultures.* Thousand Oaks, CA: Sage.

Knodel, J., Chayovan, N., Graisurapong, S., and Suraratdecha, C. (2000). Ageing in Thailand: An overview of formal and informal support. In D.R. Phillips (Ed.), *Ageing in the Asia-Pacific region: Issues, policies and future trends* (pp. 243-266). London and New York: Routledge.

Knodel, J. and Saengtienchai, C. (1999). Studying living arrangements of the elderly: Lessons from a quasi-qualitative case study approach in Thailand. *Journal of Cross-Cultural Gerontology,* 14, 197-220.

Lock, M. (1993). *Encounters with aging: Mythologies and menopause in Japan and North America.* Berkeley: University of California Press.

McElroy, A. and Jezewski, M. (2000). Cultural variation in the experience of health and illness. In G.L. Albrecht, R. Fitzpatrick, and S.C. Scrimshaw (Eds.) *The handbook of social studies in health and medicine* (pp. 191-210). Thousand Oaks, CA: Sage.

Minkler, M. (1994). Aging and disability: Behind and beyond the stereotypes. In R. B. Enright Jr. (Ed.), *Perspectives in social gerontology* (pp. 11-23). Needham Heights, MA: Simon and Schuster.

Ng, S. H. (2002). Will families support their elders? Answers from across cultures. In T. D. Nelson (Ed.), *Ageism: Stereotyping and prejudice against older persons* (pp. 295-310). Cambridge, MA: The MIT Press.

Palmore, E.B. (1999). *Ageism: Negative and positive.* New York: Springer.

Parrott, T. M. (1998). Changing family demographics, caregiving demands, and the policy environment. In J. S. Steckenrider and T. M. Parrott (Eds.), *New direc-*

tions in old-age policies (pp. 185-210). Albany: State University of New York Press.

Schoenberg, N.E. and Drungle, S. (2001) Barriers to non-insulin dependent diabetes mellitus (NIDDM) self-care practices among older women. *Journal of Aging and Health,* 13(4), 443-466.

Sharps, M.J., Price-Sharps, J.L., and Hanson, J. (1998). Attitudes of young adults toward older adults: Evidence from the United States and Thailand. *Educational Gerontology,* 24, 655-660.

Sokolovsky, J. (1997). Aging, family and community development in a Mexican peasant village. In J. Sokolovsky (Ed.), *The cultural context of aging: World-wide perspectives* (pp. 191-217). Westport, CT: Bergin and Garvey.

CULTURAL LAG

Erdman B. Palmore

Ageism is partly caused by cultural lag that occurs when one part of a culture (usually the material culture) changes at a faster rate than other parts (usually nonmaterial) of the culture. In this case, the actual health, education, and economic status of elders have changed faster than people's perception of their situation.

Before 1933, most older people fit one or more of the stereotypes about old people: they were sick, senile, poor, isolated, and/or unhappy. Most people did not even live to age sixty-five, and the few who did tended to die soon afterward.

Then came Social Security, Medicare, and the GI Bill (which provided college education to veterans, pensions, and prosperity). As a result, the health, mental abilities, financial security, social activity, and life satisfaction of elders has improved markedly. Most elders no longer fit the old stereotypes (Palmore, 1999).

But most people (even many elders) have not heard the good news. They still assume the old stereotypes are valid. Even when they hear some new facts, old attitudes and stereotypes tend to persist.

So ageism is partly a hangover from a previous era when such negative views of elders were more realistic. Thus, ageism can be reduced by making people aware of the changed status of most elders, so that people's ageist beliefs and attitudes no longer lag behind the changed facts.

See also COHORTS; STEREOTYPES

REFERENCE

Palmore, E. (1999). *Ageism.* New York: Springer.

CULTURAL SOURCES OF AGEISM

Erdman B. Palmore

Our culture encourages ageism through "blaming the victim" with our values, language, humor, songs, art, literature, journalism, television, and cultural lag (Palmore, 1999). Most of these sources of ageism are described in separate entries elsewhere in this book, so they will be described only briefly here.

Blaming the victim is the tendency of dominant groups to blame the victims of oppression for their own plight, thereby absolving the oppressors from guilt for their oppression. Elders are often blamed for the discrimination that is directed toward them. They may be forced to retire because of the stereotype that they are sick, senile, and no longer capable of doing their job.

Ageism is also supported by the perception that older people deviate from basic value orientations in our society such as active mastery, concern for the external world, rationalism, universalism, and concern for horizontal relationships (Williams, 1960).

Language is one of the most pervasive sources of ageism in our culture. Considerable evidence suggests that our language influences our perceptions and prejudices (Berelson and Steiner, 1964). The usual meanings and connotations of "old" and "aged" tend to be negative, such as debilitated, infirm, inactive, deficient, enfeebled, decrepit, exhausted, tired, impaired, anemic, broken down, wasted, doddering, senile, worn, stale, and useless (Laird, 1985). The term *aging* is often used as a code word or euphemism for deterioration or degeneration. Even gerontologists are guilty of this practice (Palmore, 2000). Similarly, the opposites of old, such as "young" and "youthful," tend to have positive connotations such as alert, healthy, vigorous, fresh, innovative, beautiful, and fun-loving.

Most humor and songs about old age tend to be negative. Even those that could be classified as positive tend to depend on negative stereotypes for their humor (Palmore, 1999).

The images of old people portrayed by the visual arts in the United States has shifted from positive and respectful (prior to the Civil War) toward negative and pitiful (Achenbaum and Kusnerz, 1978). More recently after the establishment of Social Security and the improved financial status of elders, these images have shifted toward the more positive. However, many of the old negative images persist and still support ageism.

Literary images of old age also present considerable variety. Classical literature presents ambivalent views of aging. Some show the aged as helpless victims of neglect and indifference; others show the aged as victimizers of youth (Donow, 1994). Analyses of more contemporary novels found that the majority of authors portrayed the older person positively or at least in a neutral light (Sohngen, 1977).

Journalism in the past has supported negative images or stereotypes, but more recently has begun to respond to older subjects more sensitively (Vesperi, 1994).

Television supports ageism in several ways. First, few elder characters are portrayed in prime-time programs (Robinson and Skill, 1995). Second, a sexist bias is evident among the few elders portrayed: most are men (Davis and Davis, 1985). Those few older women who are portrayed are comic or eccentric figures who are treated disrespectfully (Vasil and Wass, 1993). Third, elders in prime-time television are usually "bad guys," prone to failure and unhappiness (Aronoff, 1974). Fourth, televisions's portrayal of elders in news and documentary programming is negative. They usually have some serious problem or have suffered some disaster that is the basis for the human interest (Atchley, 1997). Finally, elders in commercials are more likely to have health problems than younger people (Harris and Feinberg, 1977).

Cultural lag supports ageism because the perceptions of elders lag behind the changes in their actual status. Many of the negative stereotypes have their roots in the situation of elders prior to 1933. These old perceptions persist despite dramatically improved health, education, and economic status (Palmore, 1999).

In general, our culture is so pervaded with negative stereotypes and images that most people are unaware of the many ways in which it supports ageism.

See also AGE CONFLICT; AGE SEGREGATION; CULTURAL LAG; INDIVIDUAL SOURCES OF AGEISM; SELF-FULFILLING PROPHECY; STEREOTYPES

REFERENCES

Achenbaum, W. and Kusnerz, E. (1978). *Images of old age.* Ann Arbor, MI: Institute of Gerontology.

Aronoff, C. (1974). Old age in prime time. *Journal of Communication,* 24, 86.

Atchley, R. (1997). *Social forces and aging.* Belmont, CA: Wadsworth.

Berelson, B. and Steiner, G. (1964). *Human behavior.* New York: Harcourt, Brace.

Davis, R. and Davis, J. (1985). *TV's image of the elderly.* Lexington, MA: Lexington Books.

Donow, H. (1994). The two faces of age and the resolution of generational conflict. *The Gerontologist,* 34, 73.

Harris A. and Feinberg, J. (1977). Television and aging. *The Gerontologist,* 17, 464.

Laird, E. (1985). *Webster's new world thesaurus.* Upper Saddle River, NJ: Prentice Hall.

Palmore, E. (1999). *Ageism.* New York: Springer.

_____ (2000). Ageism in gerontological language. *The Gerontologist,* 40, 645.

Robinson, J. and Skill, T. (1995). The invisible generation. *Communication Reports,* 8, 111.

Sohngen, M. (1977). The experience of old age as depicted in contemporary novels. *The Gerontologist,* 17, 70.

Vasil, L. and Wass, H. (1993). Portrayal of the elderly in the media. *Educational Gerontology,* 19, 71.

Vesperi, M. (1994). Perspectives on aging in print journalism. In D. Shenk and W. Achenbaum (Eds.), *Changing perceptions of aging and the aged.* New York: Springer.

Williams, R. (1960). *American society.* New York: Knopf.

d

DEFINITIONS

Erdman B. Palmore

Definitions of ageism range from simple, one-part definitions to complex ones with up to eight components.

- One-part definitions are "prejudice against an older person" or "the association of negative traits with the aged" (Nelson, 2002).
- Two-part definitions include stereotyping and prejudice against older persons (Nelson, 2002) and "discrimination against, and prejudicial stereotyping of, older people" (*Webster's New World Dictionary*, 1984, p. 25). The latter definition recognizes that ageism may take the form of attitudes (prejudice) or behavior (discrimination).
- Three-part definitions use the traditional components of attitudes: an *affective* component such as a feeling one has toward older individuals; a *cognitive* component such as beliefs or stereotypes about older people; and a *behavioral* component such as discrimination against older people (Nelson, 2002, p. 131).
- Four-part definitions add institutional discrimination to the previous three components (Nelson, 2002, p. 340).
- Eight-part definitions arise when all four of the previous components are recognized as either negative or positive toward elders (Palmore, 1999).

A problem exists regarding separating objective definitions and measures of ageism from evaluative judgments as to whether a given form of differential treatment is good or bad, justified or not. In the area of cognition, ageism clearly refers to those beliefs that are empirically false. But who is to say whether a given age-differentiated behavior or policy is good or bad? The concept of ageism has an implicit evaluative connotation that all ageist beliefs and behaviors are bad.

Is the Social Security system ageist (and bad) because it differentiates between younger and older persons? Most people would probably say no. Similarly, are all negative jokes about old people ageist, or are they just good humor or harmless ways of coping with our anxieties about growing older? Negative jokes about old people are still more socially acceptable than negative jokes about African Americans or women. This probably reflects the lower level of awareness in our society of ageism compared to racism and sexism.

As awareness of ageism increases, definitions of ageism will probably become more inclusive and more complex.

See also AGEISM SURVEY; FACTS ON AGING QUIZ; HUMOR; TYPOLOGIES

REFERENCES

Nelson, T. (Ed.) (2002). *Ageism: Stereotyping and prejudice against older persons.* Cambridge, MA: MIT Press.

Palmore, E. (1999). *Ageism: Negative and positive* (Second edition). New York: Springer.

DEMOGRAPHIC TRENDS

Erdman B. Palmore

Numbers of elderly in the United States have increased rapidly. At the beginning of the twentieth century, only 3.1 million persons were over age sixty-five (U.S. Bureau of Census, 1994). A century later, there are more than ten times this number of older persons. However, the population under age sixty-five has also increased, so the proportions of the population over sixty-five have increased to a lesser extent. Still, that proportion has increased from about 4 percent in 1900 to about 13 percent at present (a threefold increase).

This dramatic increase has had several effects on ageism. The early increase during the first part of the century caused increasing competition with younger workers and therefore of increasing ageism. But the later increase, involving more retirement and less competition with younger workers, resulted in extensive legislation and programs to improve the situation of elders. This has caused a more positive image of elders. The increasing proportions of elders also increases their political power and their attractiveness as a large consumer market, also reducing ageism.

Another demographic trend is the increasing proportion of elders who are women. In 1900, the number of men and women over sixty-five was almost equal; but by 2000 there were about 45 percent more women than men over age sixty-five (AARP, 2000). This proportion is even higher among those older than eighty-five: about two-and-a-half times more women than men are over age eighty-five. The effects of this increasing proportion of elders who are older women increases the stereotype that most aged are frail old women.

On the other hand, a countervailing demographic trend is the increasing health and decreasing disability among elders (Manton, 2001). This reduces the stereotype that older persons are sick or disabled.

See also STEREOTYPES

REFERENCES

AARP (2000). *A profile of older Americans.* Washington, DC: Author.
Manton, K. (2001). The national long term care survey. In G. Maddox (Ed.), *The encyclopedia of aging.* New York: Springer.
U.S. Bureau of the Census (1994). Projections of the population of the United States, by age, sex, and race: 1983 to 2080. *U.S. current population reports.* Washington, DC: U.S. Government Printing Office.

DENTISTRY

David E. Boaz

Age-related misinformation, fears, bias, or prejudice will have a dramatic impact on oral health in the decades ahead. Why? Consider the possibility that most dentists:

- Limit the services offered to aged patients because of misconceptions about their needs and desires
- Fail to accommodate homebound patients because of legal concerns or feelings about incomplete palliative care
- Utilize private care models of delivering dental treatment as the most efficient, knowing that an entire segment of need is being neglected in long-term care facilities

Older patients, on the other side of this relationship, often underestimate the importance of oral health in diet and nutrition and in maintaining their medical health. The elderly may be unaware of the growing evidence showing that, for instance, periodontal (gum) disease is a risk factor in medical conditions that are an important cause of death in the aging population. They may choose to neglect dental care as an unnecessary expense, often facing difficulties with access to affordable dental care. Proven preventive approaches to preserving oral health, often simple and inexpensive to administer, are not receiving the attention they deserve in the care of the elderly.

Of course, teeth and the oral structures that surround and support them are, as with other parts of the mind-body-spirit, subject to changes over time. These changes may result from trauma, wear and tear, and infection. Fortunately, few dental conditions are caused primarily by aging. Indeed, the benefits of age may prevent tooth loss. Knowledge and skills acquired with experience usually reduce the risk of dental problems. Effective use of dental floss, the reduction of dietary sugars and acids, and optimum fluoride exposure help prevent damage to the teeth. An ongoing relationship with a dentist produces confidence that preserving natural teeth is not only possible, but also desirable for reasons of overall health and well-being. In an affluent society that places a premium on preserving natural teeth, dentistry can develop a successful model of partnership with patients, even older adults, to maintain a complete natural dentition (or repair and maintain a partial dentition). An older adult is more likely, in this context, to be motivated and sufficiently experienced to practice preventive self-care skills and habits required to control the disease-causing bacteria, which are primarily responsible for tooth loss. However, for a variety of reasons including fear, access, and affordability, many do not see the dentist regularly.

In older adults, oral health has been linked to quality of life, life satisfaction, psychological well-being (Locker, Clarke, and Payne, 2000), and reduced mortality (Appollonio et al., 1997). The link between a functional dentition and improved dietary quality has been shown to be important, especially for elderly people, in whom nutritional deficiencies may contribute to increased illness and premature death (Marshall et al., 2002). Periodontal disease, which is the leading cause of tooth loss in adults, afflicts more than 86 percent of older Americans. It is now suspected to be a systemic burden of oral infection linked to several important chronic medical problems that affect older adults including diabetes, heart disease, and stroke. Causal relationships are poorly understood and are actively being explored by researchers. The evidence is overwhelming that oral infections also have a profound effect on health care costs and other economic consequences (Mandel, 2002).

Trends in the older population show, not only that a longer life span is expected, but also that a higher proportion of them will have teeth, perhaps 80 percent by 2020 (Steele et al., 2001). In the dentition of people over eighty years of age, tooth damage from either decay or erosion, especially involving root surfaces, may approach 100 percent. At the same time, dentists may demonstrate ageism in treatment planning (Dolan et al., 1992), unnecessarily offering limited services to older patients with resulting less than optimal care. Dentists are not likely to practice in long-term health care facilities where there are built-in limitations on quality of care, treatment options, staffing, facilities, and economic incentives (MacEntee et al., 1992).

In 2002, at The Second World Assembly on Aging sponsored by the United Nations, health promotion and disease prevention for the growing aging population was listed as one of its priority directions (United Nations, 2002). Affordable dental services were included as one of the International Plan of Action on Ageing 2002 list of objectives to prevent and treat disorders that impede eating and cause malnutrition. Universal and equitable access to care was identified as a goal. Dental care can improve the oral health of older adults (Locker, 2001), but they require access to comprehensive dental treatments that can adequately respond to their needs. However, access to affordable dental care is a growing problem that will only get worse unless significant changes are made in our dental delivery system (Dolan and Atchison, 1993).

The complex challenges of ageism in dentistry require urgent attention. Responses to these challenges have been described at four identifiable levels (McNally and Kenny, 1999).

- At the first level, dentists should be sensitive to issues of ageism and support efforts to enhance access to care.
- Second, the dental profession (organized dentistry) must develop age-appropriate standards of care, work to alleviate the marginalization of oral health, and overcome financial and physical obstacles to dental care.
- Third, educators should model a range of practice patterns that include long-term care facilities and home visits. Educators are obviously in a position to promote and review research in the areas critical to the ageing population—-health promotion, disease prevention, and access to care, especially economically viable and effective options to reduce oral disease. Are there public health measures such as fluoridation that can benefit this population? Can an effective and safe vaccine be used to prevent oral diseases? The development and integration of geriatrics in dental school curricula have begun. Is it time to offer specialty training programs for geriatric dentists with board certification and educational accreditation? How can paraprofessionals be utilized to expand the reach of dental care?
- At the fourth level, the public must review policies and practices in long-term care facilities and promote the development of preventive oral health programs for older people. Will governmental intervention be required to provide sufficient dentists to serve the needs of older populations?

In summary, dentistry, as with medical and mental health services, are indispensable to the health and well-being of a rapidly expanding older population. The growing need for dental care for this group will overwhelm responsive resources and leave a predictable legacy of pain, suffering, and indignity if policy attention does not address affordability and access to care. Clearly, the promotion of dental health in the lives of the world's growing elderly population will become one of dentistry's great challenges in the new millennium. Ageism may be one of many obstacles encountered in meeting this challenge.

REFERENCES

Appollino, I., Carabelles, C., Frattola, A., and Trabucci, M. (1997). Dental status, quality of life, and mortality in an older community population: A multivariate approach. *Journal of the American Geriatric Society,* 45, 1315-1323.

Dolan, T.A. and Atchison, K.A. (1993). Implications of access, utilization and need for oral health care by the non-institutionalized and institutionalized elderly on the dental delivery system. *Journal of Dental Education,* 57, 876-887.

Dolan, T.A., McNaughton, C.A., Davidson, S.N., and Mitchell, G.S. (1992). Patient age and general dentists treatment decisions. *Special Care Dentist,* 12, 15-20.

Locker, D. (2001). Does dental care improve the oral health of older adults? *Community Dental Health,* 18, 7-15.

Locker, D., Clarke, M., and Payne, B. (2000). Self-perceived oral health status, psychological well-being, and life satisfaction in an older adult population. *Journal of Dental Research,* 79(4), 970-975.

MacEntee, M.I., Weiss, R.T., Waxler Morrison, N.E., and Morrison, B.J. (1992). Opinions of dentists on the treatment of elderly patients in long-term care facilities. *Journal of Public Health Dentistry,* 52, 239-244.

Mandel, I.D. (2002). Oral infections: Impact on human health, well-being, and health care costs. *Compendium,* 43, 403-413.

Marshall, T.A., Warren, J.J., Hand, J.S., Xie, X.J., and Stumbo, P.J. (2002). Oral health, nutrient intake and dietary quality in the very old. *Journal of the American Dental Association,* 133, 1369-1379.

McNally, M. and Kenny, N. (1999). Ethics in an aging society: Challenges for oral health care. *Journal of the Canadian Dental Society,* 65, 623-626.

Steele, J., Marcienes, W., Sheivham, A., Fay, N., and Walls, A. (2001). Chemical and behavioral risk indicators. *Gerontology,* 19(2): 95-101.

United Nations (2002). International strategy for action on ageing 2002. The Second World Assembly on Ageing. <http://www.un.org/ageing/coverage/action.doc>.

DISABILITY

Elias S. Cohen

This entry contends that the core, the hallmark, and the fundamental notions that constitute ageism are directly connected to the realities and perceptions of disability in late life. Both have emerged as issues involving social justice.

Definitional Issues

Given the historical and cultural experience that embraces disability, the nexus between ageism and disability is logical. Defining disability is somewhat more complex than definitions of other areas comprising issues of social justice—-age, gender, race, national origin, or poverty (Greenwood, 1985). Definitions useful in the vindication of legal rights will differ from those useful in assessing population health. Definitions differ depending on whether they are from the perspective of the person with the disability or the perspective of the nondisabled. In terms of ageism, it makes a difference whether disability is viewed through the medical model lens, i.e., disability is pathology in need of repair (Hahn, 1991), or whether it is viewed in terms of societal and environmental failures to remedy barriers to people with disability.

The definition of *disability* and related terms such as *impairment* and *handicap* for purposes of population health differs from everyday popular usage. The *International Classification of Functioning, Disability and Health* (ICF), published by the World Health Organization (WHO) in 1980 and revised in 2001, defines *disability* as "an umbrella term for impairments, activity limitations or participation restrictions." ICF recognizes, in addition, environmental factors that interact with *functioning,* a term "encompassing . . . all body functions, activities and participation." This broad approach, one based upon "health domains" includes such functions as "seeing, hearing, walking, learning and remembering." It also includes "health related domains such as transportation, education and social interactions." However, it excludes non–health-related circumstances such as gender, race, religion, age, or other socioeconomic characteristics that might restrict participation in a given environment. Nor does it take into account the extent to which societal, environmental, and/or technological modifications may have been made or not made.

This definition represents a break from the earlier classification, which was a consequence of disease classification (i.e., pathology which needs fixing), focusing on the *impact* of disease or other constituent of health.

The current definition is undoubtedly more appropriate from a WHO perspective assessing population health. However, in the context of ageism, the definition, grounded in perceived or actual consequences of disease or other health condition, is more apt to support ageist belief than counteract it.

The earlier ICF definitions (Pope and Tarlov, 1991) that distinguished between and among *impairment, disability,* and *handicap* were no better. *Impairment* referred to an identifiable pathological condition that compromised the ability or capacity of an individual to carry out essential physiological, psychological, or social tasks. *Disability* referred to the actual inability to carry out such tasks. *Handicap* adds the contextual component to the consequences approach, taking into account social attitudes about people that may stigmatize particular impairments (e.g., diminished cognitive functioning, gross physical disfigurement or impairment, or diminished stamina, of strength, gender, and wrinkles).

Greenwood (1985) points out a "central semantic problem: the terms disability and handicapped are intricately bound together in the minds of laymen and professionals alike, but are conceptually distinct" (p. 1242). This distinction lies at the heart of disability-based ageism.

LaPlante (1991), exploring who the potential beneficiaries of the Americans with Disabilities Act might be, suggests three perspectives which yield different results: the perspective of researchers, the perspective of advocates for persons with disabilities, and individual perception of the person with a disability. Complicating the definitional aspects of disability even more is the distinction between impairment and disability contained in the Act. Disability involves action (walking, talking, writing, driving, etc.). Impairment applies to a biological and/or medical characteristic. Activities may be accomplished through alternative actions: a quadriplegic may overcome a mobility impairment through use of a "puff-and-sip" equipped wheelchair; a speech-impaired person may accomplish speech through computer-generated assistive devices; a paraplegic may fulfill all of the activities of the office of president of the United States through a variety of assistive devices, services, and accommodations.

Thus, these definitions begin to address remedial steps for accommodation other than "curing" the disabling condition. This introduces a nuanced view that has not received as much attention in gerontological inquiry as in the independent-living movement.

Putnam (2002) explores the potential impact on theory and programming of increased numbers of individuals with lifelong disabilities reaching old age. She points out that the service programs for people with disabilities compared to those for the elderly differ in significant measure. Aging programs are more apt to follow a medical model. Programs for the physically disabled incorporate consumer direction and self-determination—currently at odds with the medical model. The entry of independent living advocates into old age may force significant changes in both theoretical and programmatic approaches addressing disability in late life.

Views and Attitudes

Both the former and current WHO definitions of disability reinforce ageist attitudes by ascribing to the elderly in general, attributes that form the basis of discrimination against persons with disabilities.

Such discrimination is said to have two aspects: prejudice and barriers. *Prejudice* is an attitude based upon the negative exaggeration of the disability (read "impairment") to the exclusion of other characteristics. This gives rise to myths, stereotypes, and stigma that holds that personhood itself is diminished because of the disability (West, 1991).

Barriers, the second aspect of discrimination against people with disabilities, are "defined as *any aspects of the social or physical environment that prohibit meaningful involvement by persons with disabilities"* (emphasis in original) (West, 1991, p. 7). Examples of such barriers might include stairs confronting someone in a wheelchair, absence of a sound signal at a crossing light (important to the blind), lack of accessibility to public transit for mobility impaired, etc. The notion of barriers leads directly to what has been termed the *accommodation imperative.* The accommodation imperative requires that the experience in the environment must be rendered in a way that makes it available to the person with the disability. Considering disability and the consequent prejudices that have grown up around disability in this way shifts the emphasis away from the "imperfections" and impairments of the individual to the broader society and to the remediation that makes the environment accessible.

Common attitudes about disability encompass both broad-based health policies and everyday interactions between older people and their families, friends, caregivers, providers, and public and private entities giving ageism its pervasive presence.

The emphasis on functional limitations, and disability as a patho-logical condition that needs fixing, affects how we view people with disabilities. This view stresses the inabilities of the person with the disability and ignores the environmental and societal limitations that diminish or block a disabled person's ability to participate and enjoy life as much as nondisabled persons do (Treloar, 1999).

Furthermore, and perhaps most important, this medicalized ap-proach to disability overlooks the significant elements of autonomy. Collopy's (1988) seminal work on the complex aspects of autonomy makes the important distinction between *executional* autonomy and *decisional* autonomy. Physical disabilities inhibit or destroy execu-tional autonomy absent prostheses or other assistive devices. How-ever, decisional autonomy may remain intact, enabling the person with a disability to carry out all sorts of activities of daily living, di-recting other persons or servomechanisms to carry out functions that cannot be otherwise exercised. If these decisions are not frustrated by environmental, social, or economic barriers, the choices made can be perfected. Where autonomy is perceived only in its executional terms, it reduces the possibilities for independence and self-determination (Cohen, 1992).

Historical Antecedents

The prejudice against people with disabilities is one of long stand-ing. People with disabilities have been isolated and often physically removed from the mainstream population (Gellman, 1959; Marshall, 1985).

Almshouses, county homes, and "workhouses" were repositories for what were regarded as the flotsam and jetsam of American soci-ety—the disabled, the mentally retarded, the mentally ill, the inebri-ate, and the aged (Tollen, 1964; Schneider and Deutsch, 1941). Mental hospitals became huge, out-of-the-way facilities, housing at their peak in the late 1950s and early 1960s about 600,000 people, one-third of whom were sixty-five or over (Cohen, 1961). At the time, mental hos-pital beds constituted half of all hospital beds in America (Lerner, 1957).

The Social Security Act sought to alter what was the normal rem-edy for poverty and chronic disability by prohibiting any federal re-imbursement for "indoor relief," care in public or private institutional settings. However, less than a generation later, long-term care facilities, particularly catering to the elderly, began their inexorable growth and now are supported in major proportion by the very act that sought the change.

Today, long-term care facilities house 1.6 million elderly, more than half of whom suffer from a dementing illness—a number greater than the total number of mentally ill *of all ages* in mental hospitals when they were at their peak (Cohen, 1979).

Relatively recent history offers informative examples of how definitions and views of disability, which in the end support ageism, have worked their way into legal benefit structures and programs.

Realities and Social Norms

A reality of age-related changes may occur as people approach old age, however that may be defined. These changes may include changes in sensory acuity, diminution in physical energy, stamina and strength, immune system changes, change in cognitive powers, increased incidence of mobility limiting diseases, and increased incidence of carcinoma and cardiovascular diseases. Not all diseases and changes result in disability.

Indeed, the impact of any change that diminishes or obstructs behavior differs with the perception of the person with the disability, the resources available (including prostheses, assistive devices, environmental modifications, and economic support for personal assistance), and the reaction of society at large to the individual. Impact differs depending upon family composition; economic status; available support systems including transportation, medical, and social service availability; and housing arrangements.

The disability/aging nexus that underlies ageism springs from the medicalized definition of disability. Social age norms appear to incorporate notions of associated disability with advanced age (Lerner, 1957).

Perceived Inherent Biological Inferiority

Old age is a period of life in which the organism's physical and cognitive capabilities may diminish. The conventional formulation equates this diminution with pathology. It holds that those afflicted with pathological conditions are regarded as inherently, in fact biologically, inferior to the dominant reference group. This same logic that spawned racism, sexism, and prejudice against those with physical or cognitive disabilities is applied to the elderly and emerges as ageism (Marshall, 1985).

In an odd twist, scholarly choice of language has supported a view of aging that is ageist. Bearon (1996) traces the history of the concept of successful aging, its evolution in gerontological theory, and its iteration in both the scholarly and popular literature. Although she points out that some gerontologists have opted for other terms such as *adjustment* or *adaptation* to aging, *successful aging* (with its inherent flip side, *failed aging*) retains currency.

An outgrowth of the substantial studies on predictors of successful aging funded by the MacArthur Foundation, *Successful Aging* (Rowe and Kahn, 1998) just by its very title suggests the possibility of failed aging. Although it presents appropriate optimistic and positive views about dealing with the usual changes accompanying late life, the authors adopt the functional criteria of activities of daily living as the measure of successful aging. They point out that "only" 5.1 percent of older Americans reside in nursing homes, that "only" 27 percent between the ages of seventy-five and eighty-four report some disability and that 40 percent of the population over eighty-five is fully functional, leaving, of course, 60 percent who are *not* fully functional. To be blind, to be deaf, to have a disability that limits mobility is, under the theme of this definition, to be designated not fully functional. This is to be less than a real person in a society that values, almost above all, superb functioning, the satisfaction of assigned roles as athletes, workers, captains of industry, stars of film, music, theater, and television. In a culture that most highly values economic success, athletic prowess, stamina, accumulation of political, social, and economic power, people with disabilities are devalued unless they "overcome" their disabilities and succeed in terms of the conventional and cultural measures of success.

The authors are quick to assert, quite appropriately, that successful aging is *not* imitation of youth or the search for immortality. Rather it is comprised of three components: avoiding disease and disability, maintaining mental and physical function, and continuing engagement with life.

In a public health perspective, this view constricts policy goals. A recent review of aging and disability (Guralnik, Fried, and Salive, 1996) explores the measurement of disability, consequences of disability, and potential for preventive intervention almost exclusively in terms of the medical model and impairments definition. The conclusions reached ignore the components of barriers to full participation, the societal and environmental accommodations, and the prosthetic and assistive technologies that admit people with disabilities to full participation. Understandably, the review concludes that the goal of the increased understanding (in its terms) of the impact of disability in the population "must be to reduce the overall prevalence of disability in the population and increase the number of years in which older people lead highly functional, independent lives" (Guralnik, Fried, and Salive, 1996, p. 42). However, this statement is at odds with the recitation of increasing disability with advancing age and the general understatement of disability in most surveys that overlook the disabled population in nursing homes.

These formulations, grounded in a pathology model, are not dissimilar from the "geriactivist" model for successful aging supported and nourished in the past by advocates, program planners, policymakers, and practitioners advancing programs based upon the incompetence model (Minkler, 1990).

If these are the components of successful aging, it appears that the message sent is that failure to do so is failed aging. That is to say, if there is disability (defined in the conventional "failure of function" terms) the older person represents a failed specimen, *by virtue of the undeniable evidence of disability.*

However useful striving for the components of successful aging might be, casting them in a context of avoiding disability unwittingly contributes and in some ways legitimizes the derivative of disability as a parent of ageism. It is one of the substantial ironies of old age in America that definition of success in late life, preventing disease and disability and maintaining engagement with life, ineluctably leads the elderly into the belief that ultimately they will fail.

The Elderly Mystique

Just as women had long accepted their social role as housewife and homemaker (Friedan, 1963), and just as the parents of developmentally disabled had accepted institutionalization of their children, so have the elderly bought into the notion of old age (read "disability") as a period of decline (Cohen, 1988). The phenomenon has been tagged *the elderly mystique.*

The mystique holds that any disability in old age initiates inevitable decline and a dreadful end of mastery, autonomy, and the ability to determine the quality of one's life. The elderly who embark on this path of decline can no longer travel, eat what they enjoy, set their own schedules, go out after 3 p.m., or exercise dominion over a work space or people. There is no hope and there are no risks one can take anymore (Cohen, 1992). The elderly mystique appears to be self-perpetuating and what the elderly want.

Research exploring the elderly mystique is limited. A small study exploring personal attendant care to the elderly in their own homes in California, Maine, and Pennsylvania suggested that "staying out of a nursing home" trumped all other considerations regarding exercising autonomy or consumer control. The elderly subjects gave little thought to how liberating the attendant care programs were or the extent to which self-direction was enhanced. They were resigned to decline, and sought the highly desired, yet narrow goal of remaining at home (Cohen, 1992).

Friedan (1993) writes at some length about the extensive and persistent reporting in the popular press about the "problems of aging," the burdens that a graying America will impose upon the country because of the costs of health care, and the lengths the elderly are going to in order to avoid the appearance of old age—an appearance that equates with negative stereotypes of debilitated late life. These images are absorbed by and influence the elderly in their own view of old age.

A relationship exists between advancing age, the views of the elderly about disability, and the views of the dominant reference group toward the elderly and their perceived disability. Some very early studies suggested that, contrary to expectations, the elderly would be empathetic to people with disabilities. In fact, the more mature respondents to a survey questionnaire tended to be *less* empathetic than younger respondents (Gozali, 1971).

However, as Bearon (1996) points out, the research exploring successful aging has been spotty. Most gerontologists have neglected the impaired and institutionalized populations (citing Austin's reminder [1991] to the gerontological community)

> not to forget those who cannot age well because of factors over the life course (e.g., poverty, rural residence, poor nutrition, substandard housing, limited educational opportunities, abuse or catastrophic losses) that reduce life chances and limit access to an "aging well lifestyle." (p. 75)

Those and others who have been precluded from the formulas to successful aging by illness, trauma, or other cause of impairment, should not be contrasted to the *successful agers,* and even by implication characterized as failures.

See also STEREOTYPES; SUCCESSFUL AGING

REFERENCES

Austin, C.D. (1991), Aging well: What are the odds? *Generations,* 15(1), 73-75.

Bearon, L.B. (1996). Successful aging: What does the "good life" look like? *The Forum,* 1(3), NC State University.

Cohen, E.S. (1961). *Mental illness among older Americans.* Washington, DC: Special Committee on Aging, United States Senate, United States Government Printing Office.

_____ (1979). Nursing homes—The new mental hospitals. *Generations,* 3(4), 9-14.

_____ (1988). The elderly mystique: Constraints on the autonomy of the elderly with disabilities. *The Gerontologist,* 28(Suppl.), 24-31.

_____ (1992). What is independence? In E.F. Ansello and N.N. Eustis (Eds.), *Aging and disabilities: Seeking common ground* (pp. 91-98). Amityville, NY: Baywood Publishing Co. Inc.

Collopy, B.J. (1988). Autonomy in long term care: Some conceptual distinctions. *The Gerontologist,* 28(Suppl.), 10-17.

Friedan, B. (1963). *The feminine mystique.* New York: W.W. Norton.

_____ (1993). *The fountain of age.* New York: Simon & Schuster.

Gellman, W. (1959). Roots of prejudice against the handicapped. *Journal of Rehabilitation,* 40, 115-123.

Gozali, J. (1971). The relationship between age and attitude toward disabled persons. *The Gerontologist,* 11, 289-291.

Greenwood, J.G. (1985). Disability dilemmas and rehabilitation tensions: A twentieth century inheritance. *Social Science Medicine,* 20(12), 1241-1252.

Guralnik, J.M., Fried, L.M., and Salive, M.E. (1996). Disability as a public health outcome in the aging population. In G.S. Omenn, J.E. Fielding, and L.B. Lave (Eds.), *Annual Review of Public Health,* 17, 25-46.

Hahn, H. (1991). Theories and values: Ethics and contrasting perspectives on disability. In R.P. Marinelli and A.E.D. Orto (Eds.), *The psychological and social impact of disability* (Third edition). New York: Springer.

ICF (2001). *International Classification of Functioning, Disability and Health,* endorsed by the fifty-fourth World Health Assembly for international use <www.who.int/classification/icf/intros/ICF-Eng.pdf>.

LaPlante, M. (1991). The demographics of disability. *The Milbank Quarterly,* 69(Suppl.1/2), 55-75.

Lerner, M. (1957). *America as a civilization: Life and thought in the United States today.* New York: Simon & Schuster.

Marshall, T. (1985). Dissenting opinion. *Cleburne v. Cleburne Living Center,* 473 U.S. 432 at 456 et seq.

Minkler, M. (1990). Aging and disability: Behind and beyond the stereotypes. *Journal of Aging Studies,* 3, 245-260.

Pope, A. and Tarlov, A. (Eds.) (1991). *Disability in America: Toward a national agenda for prevention.* Washington, DC: National Academy Press.

Putnam, M. (2002). Linking aging theory and disability models: Increasing the potential to explore aging with physical impairment. *The Gerontologist,* 42, 799-806.

Rowe, J.W. and Kahn, R.L. (1998). *Successful aging.* New York: Pantheon.

Schneider, D. and Deutsch, A. (1941). *The history of public welfare in New York State, 1867-1940.* Chicago: University of Chicago Press.

Tollen, W. (1964). Historical résumé of public welfare in the United States. *Journal of Jewish Communal Service,* 40, 355-364.

Treloar, L.L. (1999). People with disabilities—The same, but different: Implications for health care practice. *Journal of Transcultural Nursing,* 10, 359-364.

West, J. (1991) The social and policy context of the (Americans with Disabilities) Act. *The Milbank Quarterly,* 69(Suppl. 1/2), 3-24.

DISCOUNTS

Erdman B. Palmore

Discounts and free goods or services for elders are examples of positive ageism: discrimination in favor of older persons. The various free or reduced-rate programs and services provided specially for older people by federal or state governments and by private agencies and businesses are too numerous to list here; they include housing, meals, medical care, drug discounts, transportation, entertainment, education, information, referral, planning, coordination, employment counseling, and day care. Some telephone yellow pages and some businesses use a seal or symbol to indicate that they give discounts to seniors.

The rationale for these discounts may partly be the stereotype that the elderly tend to be poor or on fixed incomes and cannot afford to pay full price. More often they may primarily be a way to attract business from elders—especially during times of the day or week when younger people are at their jobs and business is slack.

These discounts have been criticized because they discriminate on the basis of age. However, those who defend these practices argue that they are mainly marketing devices designed to increase business.

See also BENEFITS OF AGING; TYPOLOGIES

DISENGAGEMENT THEORY

J. Beth Mabry
Vern L. Bengtson

The "first generation" of theories in social gerontology (Hendricks, 1992) was dominated by four sociological theories of aging introduced between 1949 and 1969: modernization theory, disengagement theory, subculture theory, and activity theory. Of these early perspectives, disengagement theory was the most conceptually developed. However, it was also most open to charges of ageism (Palmore, 1999).

Based on a structural-functionalist perspective, disengagement theory offers an explanation of aging both at the macrolevel (society and population) and at microlevel (individual, family, group). It also accounts for changes (declines) with aging in physiological (including cognitive) function, psychological activity, and social interaction. However, scholars soon discounted disengagement theory, noting that empirical observations do not support its claims. Indeed, some empirical findings contradict the predictions of disengagement theory (Achenbaum and Bengtson, 1994).

Ambitious in its scope, disengagement theory provoked criticism because it implies that it was "natural" and even beneficial for older adults to disconnect from social life. Disengagement theory claims that aging individuals, in anticipation of death, gradually withdraw from life, physically, psychologically, and socially. Roles link individuals to society by connecting people to social institutions—family, economy, religion, education, government—and roles serve as guides for behavior within those institutions. A person's set of roles, such as student, spouse, parent, and worker, comprise that individual's identity. People enter and exit a host of roles over their lifetimes. Disengagement theory is most concerned with role-exit, especially how role-exits of the elderly serve a positive function for both society and the older individual. At the same time, social networks withdraw from aging individuals, and society limits the roles from elders and curbs investments in them.

In developing disengagement theory, Cumming and Henry (1961) observed that societal renewal and stability depends on an orderly succession of replacement of older generations with younger generations in most social institutions. Older people staying too long in their social roles would threaten this orderly succession and the stability of social organizations. The workplace provides an apt example: Younger workers need to find openings to move up the organizational system, but a system dominated by older workers prevents the replenishment of the organization by younger workers. Disengagement theory, then, predicts that the timely and orderly withdrawal of older workers from the labor market is crucial for the optimal functioning of the economy. If older workers die before they retire, organizations may experience crises related to unpredictable rather than systematic transfers of power.

The idea of disengagement applies to the relationship between elders and all social institutions, including the family. For example, older adults may turn to family roles as a way to compensate for lost work roles. But, people may lose family roles, as well, due to events such as widowhood and the death of friends, or distance and isolation from extended-family members. Thus, disengagement is healthy for the functioning of society because it ensures the continuity in its major social institutions. Death is unavoidable, but the extent of its disruption can be minimized by the orderly withdrawal (even if forced) of older adults from their institutional roles.

Disengagement of older adults is both encouraged and enforced by institutional sanctions. According to disengagement theory, retirement plans, pensions, and old-age economic support policies reward older individual for disengaging from society while also improving elders' quality of life and self-esteem. Furthermore, the theory states that older people should disengage from their social roles before they are no longer able to meet the challenges of those roles due to declines in abilities associated with old age. According to the theory, older individuals' life satisfaction would increase if they went along with social pressures to disengage since they are compensated for their withdrawal by retirement and pension policies such as Social Security.

Critics of disengagement theory point out that elderly individuals and society are not equally powerful actors in the process of disengagement; it is society that compels individuals to disengage. Given the power imbalance between individuals and society, critics suggest disengagement is not a good arrangement for the elderly. Instead, they are part of a system that coerces older people to relinquish valued roles in the interests of societal stability. In questioning whether the process of disengagement is "natural," critiques of disengagement theory suggest that role withdrawals by older people result from a system of rewards and punishments by and for the powerful institutions of society. Detrimental consequences for individuals are viewed as unfortunate but necessary for the continuity of society with minimal disruption. Important questions raised by critics include whether the elderly are being asked to make too much of a sacrifice in this regard, and if older individuals actually are powerless to stop it.

Despite disengagement theory's scope and conceptual clarity, many scholars were intent on discrediting the theory (e.g., Hochschild, 1975). There are several reasons for questioning disengagement theory as a sound explanation for successful aging (Achenbaum and Bengtson, 1994):

- Practitioners who work with the elderly observe quite different patterns than those predicted by disengagement theory. For example, the most socially active older individuals who exited the fewest roles appeared to have the highest life satisfaction, not the least.
- The extent of disengagement among older adults varies considerably. For instance, some older adults retire early while others choose to work until later in life.

- The disenfranchised senior citizen is not a universally shared image of aging. For instance, many older people occupy roles with great prestige and power in business, politics, and education.
- It is far from clear that society benefits from the disengagement of older citizens. Older people are valued resources within the family (caring for grandchildren and supporting adult children), within the community (as volunteers and civic leaders), and within the economy (as workers and consumers).
- Disengagement is socially constructed and a product of our cultural beliefs about the nature of aging. What we define as being disengaged may, from the point of view of the elderly, be very engaged. Are spending time with grandchildren, traveling, volunteering, or even playing bingo passive and empty ways to spend time, or ways of engaging with others around common activities?
- Disengagement theory is a product of historical times in which it arose. In post–World War II America, belief in progress through social order, conformity, and the promise of youth to meet the demands of a post-industrial economy permeated social life. As a historical artifact, disengagement theory reflects the values of a particular historical period that have less relevance in society today.

In summary, disengagement theory proposes that the mutual withdrawal of the elderly from society and of society from the elderly was considered necessary for both the smooth-functioning society and the successful aging of individuals—a mutually beneficial situation. When disengagement theory failed to gain acceptance as an all-encompassing explanation of aging, its demise marked the beginning of the end of attempts to develop comprehensive theories in social gerontology (Bengtson, Burgess, and Parrott, 1997). Nonetheless, disengagement theory still provides an intriguing paradigm for exploring the interplay between individual aging and the societal contexts within which aging occurs.

See also AGE SEGREGATION; BLAMING THE AGED; MODERNIZATION THEORY; SOCIETAL AGEISM; SUBCULTURES; THEORIES OF AGING

REFERENCES

Achenbaum, W.A. and Bengtson, V.L. (1994). Re-engaging the disengagement theory of aging: On the history and assessment of theory development in gerontology. *The Gerontologist,* 34, 756-763.

Bengtson, V.L., Burgess, E.O., and Parrott, T.M. (1997). Theory, explanation, and a third generation of theoretical development in social gerontology. *Journal of Gerontology: Social Sciences,* 52B, S72-S88.

Cumming, E. and Henry, W.E. (1961). *Growing old.* New York: Basic Books.

Hendricks, J. (1992). Generations and the generation of theory in social gerontology. *International Journal of Aging and Human Development,* 35, 31-47.

Hochschild, A. R. (1975). Disengagement theory and the elderly: A critique and a proposal. *American Sociological Review,* 40, 553-569.

Palmore, E. (1999). *Ageism* (Second edition). New York: Springer.

DRIVER'S LICENSE TESTING

David R. Ragland
Kara E. MacLeod
William A. Satariano

There is almost universal consensus that society has a strong interest in ensuring that drivers of motor vehicles have a basic level of ability to perform that task adequately. In the United States, individual states are responsible for addressing that interest through implementation of appropriate testing and licensing. As the population has aged, and with that the number of older adults who drive, a number of states have incorporated chronological age as a component of their testing and/or licensing protocol (IIHS, 2003). Such age-based policies include: (1) accelerated renewal cycles (13 states); (2) requirement for in-person versus mail renewal (five states); and (3) additional testing (for example, road test or vision) (five states). This entry reviews relevant facts regarding aging and driving, discusses ageism and other important factors with respect to the rationale and justification for the policies, and presents recommendations.

Age is associated with decline in functions relevant to driving, particularly vision and cognition. Virtually all dimensions of vision tend to decline with age (Charman, 1997), and these declines can be observed in tests of driving skills and performance (McGwin et al., 2000; Wood, 2002). Though drivers with visual limitations tend to modify their driving (Ragland et al., 2003), vision deficits are associated with increased crash risk (Owsley, Ball, et al., 1998; Owsley, McGwin, et al., 1998; Owsley et al., 2001). Cognitive and psychomotor impairments also increase with age (Morgan and King, 1995; Carr, 2000), which impacts measures of driving performance (Rizzo et al., 2001; Schultheis et al., 2001), and drivers with significant cognitive impairments have higher rates of crashes (Goode et al., 1998; Lundberg et al., 1998; Stutts et al., 1998).

Consensus in the literature suggests that older drivers as a group, especially drivers over the age of seventy-five, have rates of crash involvement per mile driven approaching that of drivers in their teens and early twenties (Evans, 2000). However, the available data to support this consensus are limited in two ways: (1) the data do not fully account for increased susceptibility of older adults, which can render the appearance of high rates of crashes when in fact there is simply a higher rate of injury or fatality per crash (Evans, 2000), and (2) existing studies have not adequately controlled for differences in exposure (types of driving and total miles driven) (Grabowski and Morrisey, 2001). Furthermore, older drivers with functional limitations limit their driving considerably, mitigating the impact of increased risk per mile driven (Ball et al., 1998).

Although further research is needed, declines in function associated with age are related to increased risk for some individual drivers, and this may translate to increased risk for older drivers as a group. However, two additional facts are relevant. First, enormous variability occurs in functional capacity related to driving at every age group, and for some functions this variability increases with age (Christensen, 2001). Second, no evidence suggests increased risk among older drivers in the absence of specific medical conditions of functional declines, i.e., no evidence that age per se is related to increased driving risk (Waller, 1991; Ball et al., 1993).

Given these observations, the only apparent rationale for including chronological age in testing procedures is based on efficiency. Accelerating the renewal cycle, requiring in-person renewal, and requiring additional testing, will all yield a higher proportion of "positives" when limited to an older group than when applied over the entire driving population, that is, limiting testing to older age groups will produce a greater yield per testing dollar spent of functional deficits potentially impacting driving. This increased efficiency may be attractive to states when resources are limited. However, using chronological age to make screening and testing decisions for driver's licensing is arguably a form of ageism, and, from a legal and moral viewpoint, possible gains in screening or testing efficiency need to be weighed carefully against the extra burden placed on individuals above the specified age category.

Furthermore, the popularity of using age as a criterion for screening and testing may be based primarily on negative stereotypes about dangerous older drivers, rather than any factual evidence of the costs and benefits of such policies.

Society has a legitimate interest in driver's testing and licensing for the purpose of public safety. However, other societal consequences must be considered. Losing a driving privilege has potentially adverse consequences, including reduced mobility for meeting basic needs (Harrison and Ragland, 2002). In short, countervailing risks exist. Therefore, we recommend the following steps, which are relevant to drivers of all ages.

First, intensive research needs to be conducted to determine medical conditions and physical functions that are empirically related to driving risk, and screening procedures that are relevant in assessing these conditions and functions. Differences in susceptibility and driving patterns need to be accounted for in such research.

Second, systems of screening and licensure should involve opportunities for rehabilitation and conditional licensure. California, for example, is testing a tiered system for driver assessment and licensure which includes these features (Yanochko, 2002). On the screening and testing side, information from performance tests, medical assessment, and recent driving history are evaluated under this system to produce the most accurate possible profile. On the licensure side, a system of conditional licensure is being developed to allow a graduated rather than an all-or-nothing response.

See also PUBLIC POLICY; STEREOTYPES; TRANSPORTATION

REFERENCES

Ball, K., Owsley, C., et al. (1993). Visual attention problems as a predictor of vehicle crashes in older drivers. *Investigations in Ophthalmological and Vision Science,* 34(11), 3110-3123.

_____ (1998). Driving avoidance and functional impairment in older drivers. *Accident Analysis and Prevention,* 30(3), 313-322.

Carr, D. B. (2000). The older adult driver. *American Family Physician,* 61(1), 141-+.

Charman, W. N. (1997). Vision and driving—A literature review and commentary. *Ophthalmic and Physiological Optics,* 17(5), 371-391.

Christensen, H. (2001). What cognitive changes can be expected with normal ageing? *Australia and New Zealand Journal of Psychiatry,* 35(6), 768-775.

Evans, L. (2000). Risks older drivers face themselves and threats they pose to other road users. *International Journal of Epidemiology,* 29(2), 315-322.

Goode, K. T., Ball, K. K., et al. (1998). Useful field of view and other neurocognitive indicators of crash risk in older adults. *Journal of Clinical Psychology in Medical Settings,* 5(4), 425-440.

Grabowski, D. C. and Morrisey, M. A. (2001). The effect of state regulations on motor vehicle fatalities for younger and older drivers: A review and analysis. *Milbank Q,* 79(4), 517-545, iii-iv.

Harrison, A. and Ragland, D. R. (2002). Consequences of driving reduction or cessation for older adults (unpublished). Berkeley: U.C. Berkeley Traffic Safety Center.

IIHS (2003). U.S. Driver Licensing Renewal Procedures for Older Drivers as of January 2003. New York: IIHS.

Lundberg, C., Hakamies-Blomqvist, L., et al. (1998). Impairments of some cognitive functions are common in crash-involved older drivers. *Accident Analysis and Prevention,* 30(3), 371-377.

McGwin, G. Jr., Chapman, V., et al. (2000). Visual risk factors for driving difficulty among older drivers. *Accident Analysis and Prevention,* 32(6), 735-744.

Morgan, R. and King, D. (1995). The older driver—A review. *Postgraduate Medical Journal,* 71(839), 525-528.

Owsley, C., Ball, K., et al. (1998). Visual processing impairment and risk of motor vehicle crash among older adults. *Jama,* 279(14), 1083-1088.

Owsley, C., McGwin, G. Jr., et al. (1998). Vision impairment, eye disease, and injurious motor vehicle crashes in the elderly. *Ophthalmic Epidemiology,* 5(2), 101-113.

Owsley, C., Stalvey, B. T., et al. (2001). Visual risk factors for crash involvement in older drivers with cataract. *Archives of Ophthalmology,* 119(6), 881-887.

Ragland, D. R., Satariano, W. A., et al. (2003). Reasons given by older people for limitation or avoidance of driving. *Gerontologist,* 44, 237-244.

Rizzo, M., McGehee, D. V., et al. (2001). Simulated car crashes at intersections in drivers with Alzheimer disease. *Alzheimer Disease and Associated Disorders,* 15(1), 10-20.

Schultheis, M. T., Garay, E., et al. (2001). "The influence of cognitive impairment on driving performance in multiple sclerosis. *Neurology,* 56(8), 1089-1094.

Stutts, J. C., Stewart, J. R., et al. (1998). Cognitive test performance and crash risk in an older driver population. *Accident Analysis and Prevention,* 30(3), 337-346.

Waller, P. F. (1991). The Older Driver. *Human Factors,* 33(5), 499-505.

Wood, J. M. (2002). Age and visual impairment decrease driving performance as measured on a closed-road circuit. *Human Factors,* 44(3), 482-494.

Yanochko, P. (2002). Traffic safety among older adults: Recommendations for California. San Diego: California Task Force on Older Adults and Traffic Safety.

e

EDUCATION

Erdman B. Palmore

Education, propaganda, and exhortation have all been used to reduce prejudice and discrimination in the form of racism, sexism, and ageism. These three methods of changing attitudes and behaviors are similar, but useful distinctions can be made between them (Simpson and Yinger, 1985).

- *Education* is the transmission of noncontroversial information or the handling of controversial topics by recognizing them as controversial, using an objective approach, and bringing all relevant facts to bear.
- *Propaganda* is the manipulation of symbols on a controversial topic when the controversial element is disguised as fact, emotional appeals are used, some or all of the relevant facts are left out or distorted, and the motives of the propagandist or the source of propaganda are hidden. Most of advertising uses propaganda techniques.
- *Exhortation* is midway between education and propaganda. It often minimizes the controversial nature of the topic and uses emotional appeals. However, it frequently marshals many facts and makes no effort to disguise its motives or its sources. Education does appear to be effective in reducing misconceptions and ignorance about elders. In many surveys of knowledge about aging using the Facts on Aging Quiz, the one consistent variable associated with greater knowledge has been years of education

(Palmore, 1998). Also, several before-and-after tests of this knowledge have found that classes and workshops on gerontology reduce misconceptions and ignorance in this area. Furthermore, several studies indicate that those with more knowledge about the facts on aging hold fewer negative stereotypes about the aged. Thus, even short-term education in gerontology can reduce prejudice against elders.

Although propaganda and exhortation have been widely used in attempts to reduce racism, they have not been used to a significant extent in attempts to reduce ageism. Whether such methods would be effective in reducing ageism is unknown. Some large-scale experiments would be required to objectively assess their effectiveness.

See also CHANGE STRATEGIES; FACTS ON AGING QUIZ

REFERENCES

Palmore, E. (1998). *The facts on aging quiz.* New York: Springer.
Simpson, G. and Yinger, J. (1985). *Racial and cultural minorities.* New York: Plenum.

EMPLOYMENT DISCRIMINATION

Bruce M. Burchett

Ageism, racism, and sexism are three forms of discrimination that were the focus of attention and protest in the United States during the 1960s. Ageism is distinct from racism and sexism in that while race and gender are determined at birth and remain constant, age evolves over time. In addition, only certain classes of persons may experience race or gender discrimination, yet anyone who lives long enough may be a victim of age discrimination. Racism and sexism represent biases based on who we are; ageism represents a bias against who we become. Ageism takes many forms, ranging from interpersonal attitudes to matters of social policy. One of the most important and visible areas in which age discrimination occurs is with respect to employment.

Age discrimination in employment has existed throughout the twentieth century. Its roots extend to the Civil War, when the United States began its transition from a predominantly rural society with an agricultural economy to a more urban nation with an industrial economic base. In the former, the family was often the primary economic unit, and older persons were not discriminated against because of their age. With the creation of industries and with increased life expectancies, the issue of age discrimination became more relevant. Older workers were often believed deficient in a variety of respects. If the work involved manual labor, they were frequently viewed as weaker than younger workers. On the other hand, if the work was skilled, technical, or intellectual, older workers were often regarded as less likely to possess the requisite training or skills. Age quickly became one of those factors that, similar to race, gender, and social class, profoundly affected one's life prospects.

Whereas race and gender discrimination are widely regarded as irrational, discrimination based on age often reflects legitimate, though competing, moral, social, and economic concerns. On the one hand, as a matter of macroeconomic social policy, it is desirable to keep people working as long as possible. With increasing life expectancies, workers can expect to live many years following retirement. The sooner workers retire, the greater the burden on Social Security and other pension systems. Early retirement also places older workers at risk of exhausting their savings and discovering that their pensions are not sufficient to meet their needs. With increasingly common early retirement, more and more older people must be supported by fewer workers, resulting in a significant transfer of wealth from the young to the old.

On the other hand, it is often felt that the retention of older workers may deprive younger workers of opportunities to succeed, thus raising the specter of reverse age discrimination. Furthermore, older workers tend to be paid more than younger ones; they incur greater health care costs, and they often are viewed by employers as less productive. What some see as age discrimination others see as sound business practice. Nevertheless, age discrimination is pernicious and not consistent with democratic principles of government.

The United States Congress examined the subject of ageism in employment practices during the 1960s. A prohibition against age discrimination was considered for inclusion in the 1964 Civil Rights

Act, but ultimately was rejected. Instead the act directed the secretary of labor to study the problem and report to Congress. In 1965, the Department of Labor issued "The Older American Workers—Age Discrimination in Employment," a report documenting the problem. In 1967 Congress passed the Age Discrimination in Employment Act (29 USC 621; "ADEA"). The ADEA made it unlawful to discriminate against older workers solely on the basis of age with respect to hiring, firing, compensation, hours of employment, or any other term of employment. Originally, the ADEA protected those in the forty- to sixty-five-year-old age range; however, this range was extended to seventy years of age in 1978 by subsequent legislation. The ADEA applies to employers, employment agencies, and to labor unions with twenty or more employees, though certain occupations are not covered by the act (e.g., police, firefighters, the military). The act applies to federal, but not to state employees, though most states have laws against age discrimination.

Since 1979 the enforcement of the ADEA has been assigned to the Equal Employment Opportunity Commission (EEOC). A worker who feels that he or she has been the victim of age discrimination may file a complaint with the EEOC, which will then investigate the allegation. The EEOC is committed to resolving the issue without resorting to lawsuits if possible, but it may bring an action against an employer itself or issue the employee a "right to sue" letter, authorizing a lawsuit under the ADEA. In 2001, 16,000 complaints were filed with the EEOC, making age discrimination complaints the second fastest growing type of complaint filed with the EEOC. Currently nearly one-quarter of all complaints with the EEOC involve allegations of age discrimination.

To establish a valid complaint under the ADEA the employee must produce direct evidence of age discrimination; merely showing that the offending conduct had a "disparate impact" on older workers is not sufficient. Once the standard is satisfied, the burden shifts to the employer to demonstrate that age discrimination did not occur. The major defense for employers is the bona fide occupational qualification (BFOQ) of employment. If the employer can demonstrate a valid business reason, independent of age, for the disputed action, the burden shifts back to the employee to show that the action was a mere pretext for age discrimination.

Even when an older worker experiences age discrimination, he or she may have a very difficult time proving it in court. Increasingly, employers are learning to avoid the obvious errors (i.e., saying "We were looking for someone younger") that had formed the basis of past lawsuits, and they have become more adept in articulating rationales for their actions that appear to be age neutral. Workers must be increasingly vigilant in documenting their cases if they are to prevail in court.

With their reaching employment age in the 1960s, the baby boomers helped to ignite a revolution in retirement policy. Policies were established that made it possible for people to leave the workforce before the age of sixty-five. Now as those same baby boomers are approaching their own retirement years, they are sparking a second revolution in retirement policy, one that permits older workers to remain employed past sixty-five. Mandatory retirement is being challenged in the United States and Canada. The social and medical sciences of gerontology and geriatrics are further pushing back the barriers to employment by older workers, by showing that older workers are capable of performing at high levels and by increasing the functional capacities of older persons.

Creative employment arrangements such as part-time work that can ease the transition from full-time employment to full-time retirement pose future challenges to and opportunities for policymakers. This is especially important as life expectancy, and particularly active life expectancy, are increasing. Part-time employment can ease the burdens on pension systems, help older workers maintain their standard of living, provide opportunities for the young, and ensure that older workers continue to contribute to the economy and to the society. It can also reduce the ageism of employment discrimination.

See also AGE CONFLICT; AGE NORMS; COSTS OF AGEISM; MODERNIZATION THEORY; ROLE EXPECTATIONS; SOCIETAL AGEISM

ETHICAL ISSUES

Jon Hendricks
Stephen J. Cutler

Ethical discussions belong at the forefront of gerontology and of any evaluation of ageism. Whether depicted in terms of predicates of "rightness" or "wrongness" of a given course or consequence insofar as essential human nature is concerned; in terms of implicit "duties" defined by a system of values, presumed moral principles, or professional standards; or in terms of communally accepted norms, ethical frameworks offer a means to interpret appropriate courses of action—ethics provides precepts for what "ought" to take place insofar as aging is concerned (Moody, 1996; Rachels, 1998).

Many discussions of ethics invoke dignity of the individual, self-determination, and rights to autonomy as givens beyond warrant. A second principle revolves around the greater good and well-being of the larger whole. What is oftentimes referred to as *moral reasoning,* and occasionally, after Thompson (1971), as *moral economy,* provides a justification for rationalizing a given course of action in terms of what is called *distributive justice*—that which is deemed fair and appropriate, according to societal norms in a particular place and time. Then, too, *beneficence,* a way of thinking based on principles of doing good and being kind, are sometimes used to justify non-disclosure, even infantilization of dependent persons cloaked as protective of their morale and emotional well-being. Ethical issues are dynamic and multifaceted, depending on circumstances, but cannot be adjudicated by reference to law as they delve deeper into human nature and social judgments than does law (Garrett, Baillie, and Garrett, 1989; Moody, 1996).

Ethical issues are crucial to all facets of gerontology and to emerging advances in one or another subspecialty. With the growth in the numbers of elderly, and in times of scarcity, ethical sensitivity is more critical. Ethicists have looked at allocation and access to health care, long-term care, autonomy, various forms of abuse, use of restraints, end-of-life issues, research protocols, issues of informed consent, capacity and other legal issues, not to mention the portent of breakthroughs in genetics-based innovations; the list goes on and on (Bahr, 1991; Hendricks, Dutton, and Cutler, 2001; Moody, 1996).

This discussion will focus on a few illustrative examples selected to highlight how ageism enters into ethical considerations concerning fundamental concerns in the field of aging. Specifically, issues of genetic innovations, rationing of health care, autonomy and informed consent, and research with older human subjects will be discussed as vehicles to convey the breadth of implications about ageism for ethics.

Genomics: Implications for Ageism

Advances occurring in molecular biology and genomics, especially the mapping of the human genome, provide cases in point of emerging ethical conundrums with tangible implications for ageist points of view. Genetic screening, organ farming, genetic intervention as a means of health care, and the entire panoply of embryonic stem cell research are auguries of ethical dilemmas that prompt strong reactions and need to be sorted out with utmost care as they pertain to older persons. Were the full potential to be realized, how would health insurance or employment practices enter the picture if one knew in advance the prospects of developing Alzheimer's disease or any other deleterious condition? If that information were a factor affecting hiring, continued employment, or health insurance would denial be tantamount to ageism?

Alternatively, when is genetic intervention appropriate and for whom? To illustrate the ethical topography: if geneticists implicitly advocated any form of genetic screening would that also amount to a form of age discrimination? Does testing for conditions known to appear later in life, or assuming that everyone who reaches a certain age is at risk of an actual chronic condition, raise the prospect of ageism? Is germline screening in employment decisions a form of de facto ageism? If tests predict that some individuals will develop a condition over time or at a certain age, is it fair to assume anything about everyone reaching that age? These questions and a host of others are omnipresent in the quest to unravel debilitating and often fatal health conditions.

The ethical permutations proliferate with amazing speed and are rapidly exceeding the understanding of all but the most knowledgeable experts. The resolutions will reach well beyond laboratories and clinics and pose ethical questions for each of us on a daily basis. Along with other specialties, gerontologists are not insulated from the debate about genomic research or intervention, as there are serious ethical elements that relate to ageist attitudes and outcomes. Biomedical ethical deliberations are informed by the same broad principles previously referred to, and three key agencies (Human Genome Project; National Human Genome Research Institue; DOE) are working to fashion usable policy recommendations. A worldwide cooperative group, the Human Genome Organisation (HUGO), has even authored a listing of six ethical parameters that should govern use and manipulation of genetic materials. As potent as their propositions may be, adherence is entirely voluntary and subject to the vagaries of individual interpretation. Along with remarkable biomedical breakthroughs come perplexing ethical quandaries and a prospect of ageist applications not easily resolved (Mehlman and Botkin, 1998).

Health Care Rationing

Calls for setting limits on the access older persons have to health care resources have been a hot-button topic in recent years. The spending pattern has been that a disproportionate fraction of third-party pay health dollars is expended in the final year of life, and as baby boomers near their final days, these costs will escalate. The contention is that age-based rationing, as proposed by Callahan (1987, 1994) and others (Daniels, 1988), is a means of controlling skyrocketing costs of health care, predicated on a presumption that caring and curing are different facets of medical care appropriate at various points in the life course and under different circumstances. Callahan's argument has been that by establishing guidelines in terms of distributive equity for medical entitlements, basic health care, and costly life-extending technologies, resources could be most effectively used for the most appropriate age groups, with ameliorative and respite care concentrated among older persons. In a nutshell: those who favor medical rationing maintain that general levels of medical care might be universal, though society might ration medicine dependent on expensive technologies or procedures on those most likely to continue to make economic contributions to societal well-being in the future (Callahan, 1990, 1994; Conrad and Brown, 1993).

The resulting firestorm is continuing. In an edited collection (Binstock and Post, 1991) in which all contributors rallied against the prospect of health care rationing and constraints on lifesaving technologies, the consensus was that relying on age as a criterion for access is discriminatory and reflects a "what have you done for me lately" mindset. The authors maintain that doing so does not consider lifelong contributions or the great variability that characterizes individuals in any given age category. The arguments are ongoing with proponents and opponents each claiming the moral high ground. Those who enter the fray have to decide whether current age, distributive justice, and "the greater good" are irreconcilable notions. As many commentators point out, allocative rationing already exists in the medical marketplace or by other means of controlling access to medical care. The result may be that only those dependent on third-party payments face a greater prospect of rationing and that a disproportionate share of older persons falls into that category.

Autonomy and Informed Consent

Preservation of personal autonomy is vital when interacting with health and human service providers. Defined as sovereignty, self-determination, or "human agency free of outside intervention and interference" (Collopy, 1988, p. 10), autonomy means that no individual has the authority to decide for another person. In 1990 the U.S. Congress passed the Patient Self-Determination Act (PSDA) to ensure that patients retained the right to self-determination in biomedical decision making, including the right to advance directives and signed durable power of attorney for health care (DPOA-HC) to be exercised in health care arenas (Pietsch and Braun, 2000). By force of both law and ethical argument, principles of autonomy also mandate that people decide for themselves whether or not to participate in medical, social, or behavioral research and those rights are inviolate.

The principle of autonomy and the right to self-determination is assured through the process of *informed consent*. For an individual to engage in autonomous decision making, informed consent presumes four elements. First, information must be provided about one's condition or situation, about alternatives, and about relative risks and benefits of different courses of action. Second, recipients must be able to comprehend information provided. Third, people must be "competent," capable of rationally electing to consent. And, fourth, decisions must be voluntary. If any of these conditions are absent, autonomy is compromised and requirements for informed consent are not met.

In the case of older persons, research suggests ageism can hinder the informed-consent process. For example, Young and Kahana (1989) studied health-promotion information provided by physicians to heart patients over the age of forty-five and found that patients ages sixty or over received significantly less information about cardiac-risk reduction than did younger patients. Attributing this difference to stereotypical perceptions of the willingness of elders to comply with health-promotion regimens, the investigators concluded "older patients are systematically denied the opportunity for lessening the risk of future heart problems by adopting behavioral changes, despite a lack of evidence that aged heart patients will not adhere to medical advice to engage in these changes" (p. 121). Similar results concerning counseling and health-education information given to older patients and how often they are asked to change their health behaviors are reported by Callahan et al. (2000). Minichiello, Browne, and Kendig (2000) point to other instances of ageist treatment by health professionals. For example,

> where there was removal of elder's autonomy when they were not consulted about major decisions regarding their health and lives . . . or where they had minimal access to preventive health initiatives . . . or were not properly informed of the reasons why medical tests were conducted. (p. 271)

Older Persons As Research Subjects

Ethical perspectives and legal regulations govern participation of human subjects in biomedical, social, or behavioral research (Kapp, 2002). In the United States and elsewhere, research ethical concerns revolve around responsibilities researchers have toward those they research, toward one another, and toward society (AGS Ethics and Research Committees, 2001; Good, 2001; Kellehear, 1993). According to the National Commission for the Protection of Human Subjects of Biomedical and Behavioral Research (1978), participation in research should be based on principles of respect, beneficence, and justice, that is,

1. the involvement of human subjects in research requires autonomous decision making and informed consent,
2. the benefits of the research must outweigh possible harms, and
3. the ways research subjects are solicited and selected must be fair and equitable.

It is particularly in regard to the last criterion—justice and equity in the selection of research subjects—where ageism often enters. It is well established that heart disease and cancer are the two leading causes of death, and among the leading causes of hospitalization for the elderly (Anderson, 2002, Table 1; Hall and Owings, 2002, Table 2). Because these conditions are so prevalent among older persons, it would be expected that research intended to develop effective treatments should include appropriate representation of older people as research subjects. Yet the evidence indicates otherwise. One study found people seventy-five and older represented 37 percent of patients with heart attacks in the United States but just 9 percent of patients enrolled in randomized controlled trials dealing with acute coronary syndromes (Lee et al., 2001). Another investigation noted people sixty-five and older accounted for 63 percent of patients with cancer in the United States but only 25 percent of the subjects enrolled in a series of 164 cancer treatment trials (Hutchins et al., 1999). Finally, a British study of upper-age restrictions for participating in biomedical research more generally concluded that over half of the limitations were unjustified and unnecessary (Bayer and Tadd, 2000).

This disproportionately low representation of older persons is due in part to negative stereotypes about competence, reliability, and commitment to and compliance with the requirements for research participation (Bayer and Tadd, 2000; Lee et al., 2001). Undoubtedly, underrepresentation of older people in research on health conditions increasingly prevalent with age makes it problematic to generalize from results of unrepresentative studies to the very persons most affected. As Bayer and Tadd (2000, p. 993) note, "Abolishing ageist practices and attitudes in research, as well as in clinical practice, is important if elderly people are to gain maximum benefit from advances in health care" (p. 993).

Steering an Ethical Course

We need be mindful of two further principles when delving into ethical issues having to do with ageism. The first is the admonition to do no wrong, commit no maleficence. The second is to be beneficent, to do good. Put into the context of the principles alluded to at the beginning of this entry, these principles help establish pragmatic parameters applicable in a great many situations. Ageist tendencies simultaneously violate the first of these and undermine the second. In might well be regarded as a duty of gerontologists to guard against all such tendencies wherever they occur or are encountered.

See also ABUSE IN NURSING HOMES; AGE CONFLICT; AGEISM SURVEY; DEFINITIONS; EMPLOYMENT DISCRIMINATION; FINANCIAL ABUSE; HUMAN RIGHTS OF OLDER PERSONS; LEGAL SYSTEM; TYPOLOGIES

REFERENCES

AGS Ethics and Research Committees (2001). The responsible conduct of research. *Journal of the American Geriatrics Society,* 49, 1120-1122.

Anderson, R. N. (2002). Deaths: Leading causes for 2000 [Advance data from vital health statistics, no. 329]. Hyattsville, MD: National Center for Health Statistics.

Bahr, R. T. (1991). Selected ethical and legal issues in aging. In E. M. Bains (Ed.), *Perspectives on gerontological nursing* (pp. 373-390). Newbury Park, CA: Sage.

Bayer, A. and Tadd, W. (2000). Unjustified exclusion of elderly people from studies submitted to research ethics committee for approval: Descriptive study. *British Medical Journal,* 321, 992-993.

Binstock, R. H. and Post, S. G. (Eds.) (1991). *Too old for health care? Controversies in medicine, law, economics and ethics.* Baltimore, MD: Johns Hopkins University Press.

Callahan, D. (1987). *Setting limits: Medical goals for an aging society.* New York: Simon & Schuster.

_____ (1990). Rationing medical progress: The way to affordable health care. *New England Journal of Medicine,* 322, 1810-1813.

_____ (1994). Setting limits: A response. *The Gerontologist,* 34, 393-398.

Callahan, E. J., Bertakis, K. D., Azari, R., Robbins, J. A., Helms, L. J., and Chang, D. W. (2000). The influence of patient age on primary care resident physician-patient interaction. *Journal of the American Geriatrics Society,* 48, 30-35.

Collopy, B. J. (1988). Autonomy in long term care: Some crucial distinctions. *The Gerontologist,* 28(Suppl.), 10-23.

Conrad, P. and Brown, P. (1993). Rationing medical care: A sociological reflection. In J. J. Kronenfeld and R. Weitz (Eds.), *Research in the sociology of health care* (pp. 3-22). Greenwich, CT: JAI Press.

Daniels, N. (1988). *Am I my parents' keeper? An essay on justice between young and the old.* New York: Oxford University Press.

Garrett, T. M, Baillie, H. W., and Garrett, R. M. (1989). *Health care ethics.* Englewood Cliffs, NJ: Prentice-Hall.

Good, G. A. (2001). Ethics in research with older, disabled individuals. *International Journal of Rehabilitation Research,* 24, 165-170.

Hall, M. J. and Owings, M. F. (2002). *2000 national hospital discharge survey* [Advance data from vital health statistics, no. 329]. Hyattsville, MD: National Center for Health Statistics.

Hendricks, J., Dutton, J. E., and Cutler, S. J. (2001). Will genomics save us? *Contemporary Gerontology,* 8, 10-13.

Hutchins, L. F., Unger, J. M., Crowley, J. J., Coltman, C. A., and Albain, K. S. (1999). Underrepresentation of patients 65 years of age or older in cancer-treatment trials. *The New England Journal of Medicine,* 341, 2061-2067.

Kapp, M. B. (Ed.) (2002). *Ethics, law, and aging review.*Volume 8: *Issues in conducting research with and about older persons.* New York: Springer.

Kellehear, A. (1993). *The unobtrusive researcher: A guide to methods.* St. Leonards, New South Wales, Australia: Allen and Unwin.

Lee, P. Y., Alexander, K. P., Hammill, B. G., Pasquali, S. K., and Peterson, E. D. (2001). Representation of elderly persons and women in published randomized trials of acute coronary syndromes. *Journal of the American Medical Association,* 286, 708-713.

Mehlman, M. J. and Botkin, J. R. (1998). *Access to the genome: The challenge to equality.* Washington, DC: Georgetown University Press.

Minichiello, V., Browne, J., and Kendig, H. (2000). Perceptions and consequences of ageism: Views of older people. *Ageing and Society,* 20, 253-278.

Moody, H. R. (1991) Allocation, yes; age-based rationing, no. In R. H. Binstock and S. G. Post (Eds.), *Too old for health care? Controversies in medicine, law, economics, and ethics* (pp. 180-203). Baltimore, MD: Johns Hopkins University Press.

_____ (1996). *Ethics in an aging society.* Baltimore, MD: Johns Hopkins University Press.

National Commission for the Protection of Human Subjects in Biomedical and Behavioral Research (1978). *The Belmont report.* Washington, DC: Government Printing Office.

Pietsch, J. H. and Braun, K. L. (2000). Autonomy, advance directives, and the Patient Self-Determination Act. In K. L. Braun, J. H. Pietsch, and P. L. Blanchette (Eds.), *Cultural issues in end-of-life decision making* (pp. 37-54). Thousand Oaks, CA: Sage.

Rachels, J. (1998). Introduction. In J. Rachels (Ed.), *Ethical theory* (pp. 1-33). New York: Oxford University Press.

Thompson, E. P. (1971). The moral economy of the English crowd in the eighteenth century. *Past and Present,* 50, 76-136.

Young, R. F. and Kahana, E. (1989). Age, medical advice about cardiac risk reduction, and patient compliance. *Journal of Aging and Health,* 1, 121-134.

EUPHEMISMS

Erdman B. Palmore

A euphemism is the substitution of an agreeable or inoffensive expression for one that may offend or suggest something unpleasant.

Familiar examples of euphemisms are the substitution of "under the weather" for "sick," and "powder room" for "toilet."

Because of ageism in our culture, old age, getting old, and aging are generally considered unpleasant phrases. As a result, many euphemisms have developed for these terms, in order to avoid the unpleasant thing, that is, what we really mean.

Old

The following are common euphemisms for some aspect of aging, along with what is really meant by the term.

- *Of a certain age:* of an old age
- *Over the hill:* past one's prime, abilities declining, frail, senile, or senescent
- *Can't cut the mustard:* unable to function well, impaired
- *Too old for that:* too senile, frail, or impaired to do something
- *You don't look that old:* supposedly a compliment, but actually means, "You don't look as decrepit and impaired as most people your age"
- *Act your age:* when said to an older person, this means do not do any "youthful" things such as loud singing or shouting, playing loud music, wearing loud clothing, getting tattoos, showing off your body, being sexy, engaging in stressful sports, riding motorcycles or bicycles, or doing anything adventurous, dangerous, or even undignified
- *Senior moment:* a moment when you cannot remember a name, word, or what you intended to do
- *Senior citizen:* an old person
- *Old hat:* out-of-date, trite
- *Old-fashioned or old-fangled:* out of date, obsolete, or antiquated
- *Old shoe:* worn out or shabby
- *Old guard or old school:* conservative or old-fashioned
- *Old wives' tale:* a silly story, gossip, or superstitious beliefs
- *He or she is getting old:* deteriorating, becoming senile or senescent
- *Showing signs of aging:* similar to "he or she is getting old." Showing negative changes such as impaired hearing, vision, memory, wrinkles, gray hair. The ageism is implied by the fact

that these are all considered negative things, and the positive changes associated with aging, such as greater experience, wisdom, and maturity; as well as less schizophrenia, less acne, and less childhood diseases, are not considered signs of aging.

Young

The previous uses of old and aging as euphemisms for negative or unpleasant things are fairly obvious. The following uses of young are also ageist euphemisms because they imply that young is good and old is bad.

- *If I were younger:* means "If I were healthier, stronger, or more able" (often used as an excuse for obesity or weakness brought on by overeating and/or lack of exercise)
- *Young blood:* new people with fresh ideas, vigor, and enthusiasm (implies that older people have stale ideas, and lack energy and enthusiasm)
- *Young at heart:* older people with youthful ideas, playful attitudes, vigor, and enthusiasm
- *A young heart:* a healthy, strong heart (implies that aging causes heart disease.)
- *Younger than springtime:* fresh, enthusiastic, and vigorous (implies that older people are the opposite of these positive traits)
- *You're not getting any younger:* means deterioration or showing other negative signs of aging

Most people would like to avoid ageism, just as they would like to avoid racism and sexism. The problem with these ageist euphemisms is that their use tends to reinforce the negative stereotypes and other forms of prejudice against older people. This effect is especially insidious because it is mostly unconscious and unintended. It is difficult to avoid these ageist euphemisms because they are such an accepted and common part of our language; and because we are considered impolite or crude if we say what is really meant by these expressions.

See also LANGUAGE; STEREOTYPES; TERMS PREFERRED BY OLDER PEOPLE

f

FACE-LIFTS

Erdman B. Palmore

Face-lifts, Botox, as well as other kinds of plastic surgery, wigs, hair transplants, and nostrums to prevent balding, are usually attempts to deny one's real age by "looking younger." There is also a multibillion-dollar cosmetics industry devoted to "prevent aging skin" and "make you look young again."

These expensive, often dangerous and desperate, attempts to pass for younger persons show how pervasive and serious prejudice against older people is in our society. Those who claim it is necessary to "look younger" in order to keep their jobs, or make sales, or otherwise succeed in their professions, or to attract mates and even friends, are conceding that strong prejudice and discrimination exists against older persons in these areas. Some people may say that they only want to look good by looking younger, or that wrinkles (baldness, gray hair, etc.) are ugly. These protestations are simply other forms of ageism.

As long as such ageism exists, attempts to deny one's age and pass for a younger person will persist.

See also AGE DENIAL; BOTOX

FACTS ON AGING QUIZ

Erdman B. Palmore

The Facts on Aging Quiz (FAQ) can be used as an indirect measure of both negative and positive ageism (Palmore, 1998). This is based on the assumption that some misconceptions about the aged indicate negative bias and some indicate positive bias. For example, a belief that a majority of old people are senile indicates a negative bias toward the aged. Conversely, denial that the five senses may decline in old age probably indicates a positive bias.

We have classified sixteen of the items in the true/false version of the first FAQ (see Quiz 1, p. 139) as indicating a negative bias if they are marked incorrectly: items 1, 3, 5, 7 through 11, 13,16 through 18, 21, 22, 24, and 25. Conversely, we have classified five items as indicating a positive bias if they are marked incorrectly: 2, 4, 6, 12, and 14.

In the true/false versions of the second FAQ (see Quiz 2, p. 141), the negative-bias items are 3, 4, 5, 9 through 13, 17, 19 through 21, 24, and 25.

Using these items, one can compute three measures of bias: an antiaged bias score, a proaged bias score, and a net bias score. The antiaged bias score is the percentage of the negative-bias items marked wrong (number wrong divided by the number of possible negative-bias items). Similarly, the proaged bias score is the percentage of the positive-bias items marked wrong. The net bias score is the proaged bias score (percent positive errors) minus the antiaged bias score (percent negative errors). If the resulting score is negative, it indicates a net antiaged bias; if it is positive, it indicates a net proaged bias.

For practical purposes, any individual net bias score in the range of +/– 20 percent is probably not significantly different from zero and should be considered a neutral-bias score. Do not count "don't know" responses as incorrect for these purposes because simple ignorance about a fact does not usually indicate a biased attitude. Also note that subtracting percentages of errors (rather than raw numbers) to compute the net bias score controls for the fact that more negative than positive bias items exist.

The two true/false versions are the most common forms because they are shorter and easier to answer than the multiple-choice. However, the multiple-choice versions are more reliable and accurate because they reduce the effect of guessing. If one wishes to use the multiple-choice versions, instructions for computing the bias scores may be found in Palmore (1998, p. 40).

Hundreds of studies using the FAQ have been published (Palmore, 1998). To summarize their results, the average person in the United

States is able to answer only about 55 percent of the items correctly. This shows the general ignorance about aging, because in the true/false version, one would answer 50 percent correctly by chance alone. Also the misconceptions usually err on the negative side: the net bias score ranges from neutral for internists to −25 for the average nurse and other health professionals in North Carolina (Keller, 1986). Furthermore, most of the misconceptions are in the negative direction, such as the belief that 10 percent of those over sixty-five are institutionalized, the belief that the majority have incomes below the poverty line, and that they are often bored.

The main variable consistently related to the antiaged bias is knowledge about aging: those with more knowledge have less negative and more positive attitudes. This suggests that teaching people about the facts on aging would reduce their negative ageism.

See also FACTS ON AGING AND MENTAL HEALTH QUIZ

REFERENCES

Keller, M. (1986). Misconceptions about aging among nurses. Unpublished manuscript.

Palmore, E. (1998). *The facts on aging quiz* (Revised edition). New York: Springer.

FACTS ON AGING AND MENTAL HEALTH QUIZ

Erdman B. Palmore

The Facts on Aging and Mental Health Quiz (FAMHQ) multiple-choice version (see p. 143) can be used as an indirect measure of ageist bias in the area of mental illness, in a similar way that the Facts on Aging Quiz (FAQ) may be used (Palmore, 1998). This is based on the assumption that responses with certain incorrect answers to certain items indicates either a negative or a positive bias. For example, in Item 1, if a person responds that "Severe mental illness among persons over sixty-five afflicts (a) The majority," this indicates a negative bias. Conversely, if the response is "Very few" are afflicted with severe mental illness, a positive bias is indicated.

FACTS ON AGING
QUIZ 1

Mark the statements "T" for true, "F" for false, or "?" for don't know.

____ 1. The majority of old people (age sixty-five+) are senile (have defective memory, are disoriented, or demented).

____ 2. The five senses (sight, hearing, taste, touch, and smell) all weaken in old age.

____ 3. The majority of old people have no interest in, or capacity for, sexual relations.

____ 4. Lung vital capacity tends to decline in old age.

____ 5. The majority of old people feel miserable most of the time.

____ 6. Physical strength tends to decline in old age.

____ 7. At least one-tenth of the aged are living in long-stay institutions (such as nursing homes, mental hospitals, homes for the aged, etc.).

____ 8. Aged drivers have fewer accidents per driver than those under age sixty-five.

____ 9. Older workers usually cannot work as effectively as younger workers.

____ 10. Over three-fourths of the aged are healthy enough to do their normal activities without help.

____ 11. The majority of old people are unable to adapt to change.

____ 12. Old people usually take longer to learn something new.

____ 13. Depression is more frequent among the elderly than among younger people.

____ 14. Older people tend to react more slowly than younger people do.

____ 15. In general, old people tend to be pretty much alike.

____ 16. The majority of old people say they are seldom bored.

____ 17. The majority of old people are socially isolated.

____ 18. Older workers have fewer accidents than younger workers do.

____ 19. Over 20 percent of the population are now age sixty-five or over.

____ 20. The majority of medical practitioners give low priority to the aged.

____ 21. The majority of old people have incomes below the poverty line (as defined by the federal government).

____ 22. The majority of old people are working or would like to have some kind of work to do (including housework and volunteer work).

____ 23. Old people tend to become more religious as they age.

____ 24. The majority of old people say they are seldom irritated or angry.

____ 25. The health and economic status of old people will be about the same or worse in the year 2010 (compared to younger people).

Key: All the odd-numbered items are false and all the even-numbered items are true.

FACTS ON AGING
QUIZ 2

Mark the statements "T" for true, "F" for false, or "?" for don't know.

____ 1. A person's height tends to decline in old age.

____ 2. More older persons (sixty-five or over) have chronic illnesses that limit their activities than do younger persons.

____ 3. Older persons have more acute (short-term) illnesses than do younger persons.

____ 4. Older persons have more injuries in the home than younger persons.

____ 5. Older workers have less absenteeism than do younger workers.

____ 6. Blacks' life expectancy at age sixty-five is about the same as whites'.

____ 7. Men's life expectancy at age sixty-five is about the same as women's.

____ 8. Medicare pays over half of the medical expenses for the aged.

____ 9. Social Security benefits automatically increase with inflation.

____ 10. Supplemental Security Income guarantees a minimum income for needy aged.

____ 11. The aged do not get their proportionate share of the nation's income.

____ 12. The aged have higher rates of criminal victimization than younger persons do.

____ 13. The aged are more fearful of crime than are younger persons.

___ 14. The aged are the most law abiding of all adult age groups.

___ 15. There are about equal numbers of widows and widowers among the aged.

___ 16. More of the aged vote than any other age group.

___ 17. There are proportionately more older persons in public office than in the total population.

___ 18. The proportion of African Americans among the aged is growing.

___ 19. Participation in voluntary organizations (churches and clubs) declines even among the healthy aged.

___ 20. The majority of old people live alone.

___ 21. The aged have a lower rate of poverty than the rest of the population.

___ 22. The rate of poverty among aged African Americans is about three times as high as among aged whites.

___ 23. Older persons who reduce their activity tend to be happier than those who do not.

___ 24. When the last child leaves home, the majority of parents have serious problems adjusting to their "empty nest."

___ 25. The proportion widowed among the aged is decreasing.

Key: Alternating pairs of items are true or false; that is, 1 and 2 are true, 3 and 4 are false, 5 and 6 are true, and so forth, and 25 is true.

FAMHQ MULTIPLE-CHOICE VERSION

Circle the letter of the most accurate answer. If you do not know, you may put a question mark (?) to the left of the answers instead of circling one.

1. Severe mental illness among persons over sixty-five afflicts:
   a. The majority –
   b. About half –
   c. About 15 to 25 percent *
   d. Very few –
2. Cognitive impairment (impairment of memory, disorientation, or confusion):
   a. Is an inevitable part of the aging process –
   b. Increases in old age *
   c. Declines with age +
   d. Does not change with age +
3. If older mental patients make up false stories, it is best to:
   a. Point out to them that they are lying –
   b. Punish them for lying –
   c. Reward them for their imagination –
   d. Ignore or distract them *
4. The prevalence of anxiety disorders and schizophrenia in old age tends to:
   a. Decrease *
   b. Stay about the same –
   c. Increase somewhat –
   d. Increase markedly –
5. Suicide rates among women:
   a. Increase in old age –
   b. Stay about the same *
   c. Decrease somewhat in old age +
   d. Decrease markedly +
6. Suicide rates among men:
   a. Increase markedly *
   b. Increase somewhat +
   c. Stay about the same +
   d. Decrease +
7. When all major types of mental impairment are added together, the elderly have:
   a. Higher rates than younger persons –
   b. About the same rates as younger persons –
   c. Lower rates than younger persons *
   d. Higher rates for ages sixty-five to seventy-four than for those over seventy-five 0

8. The primary mental illness of the elderly is:
   a. Anxiety disorders +
   b. Mood disorders +
   c. Schizophrenia 0
   d. Cognitive impairment *
9. Alzheimer's disease is:
   a. The most common type of cognitive impairment *
   b. An acute illness +
   c. A benign memory disorder +
   d. A form of affective disorder +
10. Alzheimer's disease usually:
    a. Can be cured with psychotherapy +
    b. Can be cured with pharmacology +
    c. Goes into remission among the very old +
    d. Cannot be cured *
11. Most patients with Alzheimer's disease:
    a. Act pretty much the same way −
    b. Have confusion and impaired memory *
    c. Wander during the day or at night −
    d. Repeat the same question or action over and over −
12. Organic brain impairment:
    a. Is easy to distinguish from functional mental illness +
    b. Is difficult to distinguish from functional mental illness *
    c. Tends to be similar to functional mental illness +
    d. Can be reversed with proper therapy +
13. When talking to an older mental patient, it is best:
    a. To avoid looking directly at the patient −
    b. To glance at the patient occasionally −
    c. To ignore the patient's reactions −
    d. To look directly at the patient *
14. Talking with demented older patients:
    a. Tends to increase their confusion −
    b. Is usually pleasurable for the patient *
    c. Should be confined to trivial matters −
    d. Should be avoided as much as possible −
15. When a demented patient talks about his or her past, it usually:
    a. Is enjoyed by the patient *
    b. Depresses the patient −
    c. Increases the patient's confusion −
    d. Has no effect −
16. The prevalence of severe cognitive impairment
    a. Is unrelated to age +
    b. Decreases with age +

    c. Increases after age forty-five *

    d. Increases only after age seventy-five +

17. The primary causes of paranoid disorders in old age are:
    a. Isolation and hearing loss *
    b. Persecution and abuse 0
    c. Near-death experiences 0
    d. None of the above 0

18. Poor nutrition may produce:
    a. Depression 0
    b. Confusion 0
    c. Apathy 0
    d. All of the above *

19. Mental illness in elders is more prevalent among:
    a. The poor *
    b. The rich 0
    c. The middle class 0
    d. None of the above 0

20. The prevalence of mental illness among elderly in long-term care institutions is:
    a. About 10 percent +
    b. About 25 percent +
    c. About 50 percent +
    d. Over 75 percent *

21. Elders tend to have:
    a. Fewer sleep problems +
    b. More sleep problems *
    c. Deeper sleep +
    d. The same sleep patterns as younger persons +

22. Major depression is:
    a. Less prevalent among elders *
    b. More prevalent among elders −
    c. Unrelated to age −
    d. A sign of senility −

23. Widowhood is:
    a. Less stressful among elders *
    b. More stressful among elders −
    c. Similar levels of stress at all ages −
    d. Least stressful among young adults −

24. Elders use mental health facilities:
    a. More often than younger people −
    b. Less often than younger people *
    c. At about the same rate as younger people −
    d. Primarily when they have no family to care for them −

25. Psychotherapy with older patients is:
    a. Usually ineffective –
    b. Often effective *
    c. Effective with Alzheimer's patients 0
    d. A waste of the therapist's time –

In the multiple-choice version of the FAMHQ, the key to whether an incorrect response indicates a negative, positive, or neutral bias is indicated with a negative sign (–), positive sign (+), or a zero (0). The correct answer is indicated with an asterisk.

To calculate the antiaged bias score, divide the number of negative bias options marked by the total number of items with a negative bias option that were answered. Similarly, to compute the proaged score, divide the number of positive bias options marked, by the total number of items answered that have a positive-bias option.

Then to compute the net bias score, proceed the same way as in the true/false versions: subtract the antiaged bias score from the proaged bias score.

See also FACTS ON AGING QUIZ

REFERENCE

Palmore, E. (1998). *The facts on aging quiz* (Revised edition). New York: Springer.

FAMILY

Joseph E. Gaugler
Corinne R. Leach
Keith A. Anderson

Ageism in the family is fostered by negative attitudes and stereotypes. These two concepts are mutually supportive: attitudes help forge stereotypes and stereotypes reinforce negative attitudes (Palmore, 1999). Aggregate results of studies conducted in Western societies indicate that younger generations, and often older people themselves, view the older generation as unattractive, dependent, sexless, and of reduced ability and social worth (Harris, 1975; Korthase and Trenholme, 1982; Levin, 1988; Netz and Ben-Sira, 1993; Rowe and Kahn, 1998). Within the family, some of the most damaging stereotypes are beliefs that older adults are physical and financial burdens and that they are incapable of making autonomous decisions and handling their own affairs. Extreme ageist stereotypes may lead to abuse (physical, sexual, or emotional), financial exploitation, neglect, or abandonment from family members (Wilber and McNeilly, 2002).

The level and quality of intergenerational interaction within the family is an important factor when considering the origins of ageist attitudes and stereotypes. Throughout the Industrial Age, the traditional family structure in Western society has shifted away from the multigenerational household. According to the 2000 U.S. Census, only 3.7 percent of grandparents lived with their adult children and grandchildren (U.S. Census Bureau, 2001). Due to geographic mobility and other factors, children and adults have less in-person contact with older family members, potentially weakening filial bonds and increasing generational gaps. Studies consistently reveal that increased social interaction with older adults can lead to fewer negative attitudes and stereotypes (e.g., Kahana, Kahana, and Kayak, 1979).

Elder mistreatment in the family is due to a number of factors, one of which may be ageism (Wilber and McNeilly, 2002). Stereotypes of older people as useless, sexless, worthless, dependent, and physically repulsive may encourage some family members to vent frustrations on their older relatives, to exploit them based upon perceived weakness, or to prevent older relatives from fulfilling their needs (Palmore, 1999). Physical abuse and neglect, financial exploitation, and discrimination in sexuality and intimacy are the most evident forms of elder mistreatment perpetrated within the family.

Definitions vary, but the Administration on Aging (1998) defines physical abuse as "the use of physical force that may result in bodily injury, physical pain, or impairment" and elderly neglect as "the refusal or failure to fulfill any part of a person's obligations or duties to an elder" (pp. 3-2, 3-3). Some investigators estimate that more than two-thirds of those accused of physical abuse and neglect of older adults are family members, almost half of whom are adult children (Tatara, 1993; Lachs et al., 1997). Data from the National Elder Abuse Incidence Study found that family members perpetrated elder abuse and neglect in almost 90 percent of the cases in which an abuser was identified (Tatara, Thomas, and Cyphers, 1998). Other research findings have emphasized that abusive family members are most likely to live with older victims, with spouses as the most prevalent perpetrators (Pillemer and Finkelhor, 1988; Pittaway and Westhues, 1993).

The actual causes of elder abuse within the family are varied, with the most prominent situations being caregiver stress (particularly in instances in which the older relative has Alzheimer's disease; see Paveza et al., 1992), tension and conflict in prior family relationships, substance abuse on the part of the perpetrator (e.g., see Hwalek et al., 1996), and insufficient support systems (Wilber and McNeilly, 2002). Although the direct role of ageism in the occurrence of physical abuse and neglect is less explored, negative attitudes and stereotypes may facilitate the mind-set that justifies this behavior. By viewing the older family member as a burden, the abuser may be more inclined to abuse or neglect.

Financial exploitation of older people involves the misuse of assets, including funds and property. A recent survey indicated that family members constitute more than 85 percent of the perpetrators of financial exploitation of older people. An overwhelming majority of these perpetrators are adult children (Administration on Aging, 1998). Older adults are often reluctant to report abuse due to feelings of guilt and shame and fears of retaliation and abandonment (Tueth, 2000). Work by Pillemer (1985), as part of a three-state study, found that family members who were financially dependent on older family members were most likely to abuse.

Ageism in the family can also negatively affect the sexual behavior and intimate relationships of the older family member. One common myth is that older adults have no interest or capacity for sexual activity. However, for many healthy individuals, interest and capacity for sexual activity extends into the seventies and eighties. In a recent survey, 67 percent of men and 57 percent of women reported that positive sexual relationships contributed to their quality of life (AARP, 1999). However, many older adults face criticisms from their families who perceive these sexual feelings and relationships as perverse or abnormal (Palmore, 1999).

Negative ageism can also affect the remarriage rates of older people. Studies show that the strongest barrier of remarriage among older adults is the resistance of adult children (Nussbaum, Thompson, and Robinson, 1989). Many adult children feel that the remarriage of widows and widowers is disloyal to the deceased family member. Family members can also negatively influence remarriage decisions based upon financial concerns. Diminished inheritances and the idea that the new spouse is "only in it for the money" are common objections (Walsh, 1988). As a result of this family pressure, older adults may avoid intimate relationships and expressions of sexuality, leaving important needs unfulfilled.

The complex relationships between ageism and family interactions and their potential to lead to elder abuse make future research in this area challenging. Developing comprehensive theoretical frameworks detailing the dimensions, antecedents, and manifestations of ageism in the family will lead to more refined research and potential clinical interventions. If ageism is indeed a key mechanism in the process of elder abuse, future efforts must ensure more effective reporting and investigation; education, training, and collaborative efforts; protective interventions; mental health treatment; and legal solutions to address the potentially devastating impacts of ageism within the family system.

See also ETHICAL ISSUES; FINANCIAL ABUSE; STEREOTYPES

REFERENCES

AARP (1999). Modern maturity sexuality survey. <http://research. aarp.org/health/mmsexsurvey_1.html>. August.

Administration on Aging (1998). The national elder abuse incidence study: Final report. <http://www.aoa.gov/abuse/report/fdesign.htm>. September.

Harris, L. (1975). *The myth and reality of aging in America.* New York: National Council on Aging.

Hwalek, M.A., Neale, A.V., Goodrich, C.S., and Quinn, K. (1996). The association of elder abuse and substance abuse in the Illinois elder abuse system. *The Gerontologist,* 36, 694-700.

Kahana, B., Kahana, E., and Kayak, A. (1979). Perceptions of the aged: Changes are taking place. *Aging: Agenda for the Eighties,* 41-47.

Korthase, K.M. and Trenholme, I. (1982). Perceived age and physical attractiveness. *Perceptual and Motor Skills,* 54, 1251-1258.

Lachs, M.S., Williams, C., O'Brien, S., Hurst, L., and Horowitz, R. (1997). Risk factors for reported elder abuse and neglect: A nine-year observational cohort study. *The Gerontologist,* 37, 469-474.

Levin, W.C. (1988). Age stereotyping. *Research on Aging,* 10(1), 134-138.

Netz, Y. and Ben-Sira, D. (1993). Attitudes of young people, adults, and older adults from three-generation families toward the concepts "ideal person," "youth," "adult," and "old person." *Educational Gerontology,* 19, 607-621.

Nussbaum, J.F., Thompson, T., and Robinson, J.D. (1989). *Communication and aging*. New York: Harper & Row Publishing.

Palmore, E.B. (1999). *Ageism: Negative and positive* (Second edition). New York: Springer.

Paveza, G.J., Cohen, D., Eisdorfer, C., Freels, S., Semla, T., Ashford, J.W., Gorelick, P., Hirschman, R., Luchman, R., Luchins, D., and Levy, P. (1992). Severe family violence and Alzheimer's disease: Prevalence and risk factors. *The Gerontologist, 32,* 493-497.

Pillemer, K. (1985). Domestic violence against the elderly: A case-controlled study. Unpublished doctoral dissertation, Department of Sociology, Brandeis University.

Pillemer, K. and Finkelhor, D. (1988). The prevalence of elder abuse: A random sample survey. *The Gerontologist, 28,* 51-57.

Pittaway, E.D. and Westhues, A. (1993). The prevalence of elder abuse and neglect of older adults who access health and social services in London, Ontario, Canada. *Journal of Elder Abuse and Neglect, 5,* 77-93.

Rowe, J. and Kahn, R. (1998). *Successful aging.* New York: Pantheon Books.

Tatara, T. (1993). *Summaries of the statistical data on elder abuse in domestic settings for FY 90 and 91.* Washington, DC: National Aging Resource Center on Elder Abuse.

Tatara, T., Thomas, C., and Cyphers, G. (1998). *The national elder abuse incidence study: Final report.* Prepared for the Administration for Children and Families and the Administration on Aging. Washington, DC: The National Center on Elder Abuse.

Tueth, M.J. (2000). Exposing financial exploitation of impaired elderly persons. *American Journal of Geriatric Psychiatry, 8,* 104-111.

Walsh, F. (1988). The family in later life. In B. Carter and M. McGo (Eds.), *Changing family life cycle: A framework for family therapy* (pp. 311-332). New York: Garner Press.

Wilber, K.H. and McNeilly, D.P. (2002). Elder abuse and victimization. In J.E. Birren and K.W. Schaie (Eds.), *Handbook of the psychology of aging* (Fifth edition) (pp. 569-591). San Diego, CA: Sage Academic Press.

U.S. Census Bureau (2001). Households and families: 2000. <www.census.gov/population/www/cen2000/briefs.html>.

FINANCIAL ABUSE

Susan J. Aziz

Elder abuse is gaining worldwide recognition as a social, public health, and human rights concern, although too little is known about its nature, magnitude, causes, or consequences, or about effective means of prevention. An estimated one to two million Americans age sixty-five or older have been abused by someone on whom they depended for care or protection (Pillemer and Finkelhor, 1988; Pavlik et al., 2001). As the population ages, there will undoubtedly be an increase in the frequency of occurrence of elder abuse.

Financial exploitation, also referred to as financial, fiduciary, economic, or material abuse, has been defined as the unjust, improper, or illegal use of another's resources, property, or assets (Bonnie and Wallace, 2003). Legal definitions of financial abuse vary considerably from state to state. It is widely recognized that it is difficult to distinguish an unwise but legitimate financial transaction from an exploitative transaction resulting from undue influence, duress, fraud, or a lack of informed consent. Evaluating whether financial abuse has occurred often involves complex and subjective determinations. A question raised in many cases of possible financial abuse is whether the elder had the mental capacity to make a competent decision. Medical and mental health professionals assist the court, law enforcement, prosecutors, and Adult Protective Services by evaluating individuals with questionable mental capacity.

Financial abuse encompasses a broad range of behavior. Examples include an adult son who secures a power of attorney ostensibly to help out with errands and paying bills, and uses it to gain title to his mother's home; a new "friend" who persuades the elder to change his will in her favor; a granddaughter who forges her grandfather's signature on checks; a care attendant who shortchanges her elderly client.

Financial abuse occurs in all socioeconomic, ethnic, and racial groups. Such abuse can be perpetrated by anyone, such as a family member, caregiver, friend, acquaintance, neighbor, landlord, contractor, accountant, lawyer, scam artist, or predatory criminal who specifically targets elderly persons. Financial abuse often occurs in conjunction with other forms of elder abuse. For example, gaining possession of an older person's money and property may be the motive underlying intentional neglect, physical abuse, or psychological abuse.

Are financial abuse and ageism related and, if so, how? Ageism has been defined as "a process of systematic stereotyping of and discrimination against people because they are old" (Butler, 1969, p. 243). A common stereotype about growing old is that "senility" is inevitable; that the older people become, the more likely they are to become forgetful (Butler, 1975). Ageism contributes to elders being targets for financial abuse and to law enforcement and prosecutors not investigating and prosecuting cases of financial abuse. Ageism may influence social policy and government funding patterns, implying that children and young adults are more valued than elders.

Americans over age fifty control 70 percent of the total net worth of U.S. households and own 77 percent of all the financial assets in America (Dychtwald and Flower, 1990). Among numerous reasons cited for older persons being targeted for financial abuse is the abuser's perception that older persons are trusting; are lonely and want someone with whom to talk, particularly if they live alone; and that older persons are likely to be forgetful, senile, frail, disabled, and dependent on others.

Older persons are targets of financial abuse because they may not report and take legal action against their abusers, particularly if the abuser is a family member. If the abuse is reported, the victim may be perceived as lacking credibility as a complainant or witness due to assumptions about the general incompetence of older people.

Ageism may explain why law enforcement and prosecutors discount the victim's description of the abuse in some cases. Law enforcement and prosecutors may believe that cases of elder financial abuse consume more time than may be justified by their limited resources and thus are a low priority for investigation and prosecution. Furthermore, the characterization of victims of financial abuse as incompetent and frail may interfere with the recognition and investigation of financial abuse of competent older persons. Anyone, including not only poor, frail, and vulnerable elders, but also well-educated, healthy, active older persons may be victims of financial abuse.

The proportion of the federal budget allocated to the prevention of elder abuse is less than 1 percent of federal funds spent on abuse prevention. Failure of federal, state, and local governments to fund adequately programs to prevent elder financial abuse may be one consequence of ageism.

See also ABUSE IN NURSING HOMES; CRIMINAL VICTIMIZATION; FAMILY.

REFERENCES

Bonnie, R. J. and Wallace, R. B. (Eds.) (2003). *Elder mistreatment: Abuse, neglect, and exploitation in an aging America. Panel to review risk and prevalence of elder abuse and neglect.* Washington, DC: The National Academies Press.

Butler, R. N. (1969). Ageism: Another form of bigotry. *The Gerontologist,* 9, 243-246.

_____ (1975). *Why survive? Being old in America.* New York: Harper & Row.

Dychtwald, K. and Flower, J. (1990). *Age wave: How the most important trend of our time will change your future.* New York: Bantam Books.

Pavlik, V. N., Hyman, D. J., Festa, N. A., and Dyer, C. B. (2001). Quantifying the problem of abuse and neglect in adults: Analysis of a statewide database. *Journal of the American Geriatrics Society,* 49(1), 45-48.

Pillemer, K. A. and Finkelhor, D. (1988). The prevalence of elder abuse: A random sample survey. *The Gerontologist,* 28(1), 51-57.

FUNCTIONAL AGE

Erdman B. Palmore

Functional age was first used by McFarland (1973) to suggest that the individual's capacity, rather than chronological age, be used as the marker for ability in the workplace. However, as Siegler (1995) points out, the concept of functional age has little practical utility for research.

Furthermore, it is an ageist concept because it equates "older" with more disabled or less functional. It confuses two rather independent dimensions: chronological age and functional ability. Since these two dimensions are independent, it would be better to call the concept "functional ability" or just "ability."

Several other problems arise with this concept. First, many different dimensions are involved in functional ability including physical ability, mental ability, social ability, economic ability, and political ability. Each of these abilities may vary independently of the others. Therefore, no useful way can summarize an individual's many abilities along a single dimension.

It may be possible to specify the major abilities needed for a particular job, to measure an individual's skill in these abilities, and to somehow summarize these skills into a single rating. The resulting functional age would be meaningful only for that job, but not for jobs requiring different abilities and different combinations of abilities.

Due to these problems, the term is rarely used by professional gerontologists. For example, it appeared in the 1995 edition of *The Encyclopedia of Aging* (Siegler, 1995), but not in the 2001 edition (Maddox, 2001). The popular media, such as women's magazines, still use the concept in articles such as "Your Real Age" and "How to Measure Your Functional Age."

See also DISABILITY; SUCCESSFUL AGING

REFERENCES

Maddox, G. (2001). *The Encyclopedia of Aging* (Third edition). New York: Springer.

McFarland, R. (1973). The need for functional age measurements in industrial gerontology. *Industrial Gerontology,* 19, 1.

Siegler, I. (1995). Functional age. In G. Maddox (Ed.), *The Encyclopedia of Aging.* New York: Springer.

FUTURE OF AGEISM

Erdman B. Palmore

Several current trends that (if continued) will reduce ageism in the future: increasing knowledge and research on aging and the aged; increasing health, education, and affluence of elders; and reductions in other forms of prejudice and discrimination (Palmore, 1999).

Increasing Knowledge

Knowledge about aging among the general public has not been measured until recently (Palmore, 1998). However, considerable evidence supports that interest in aging is rapidly increasing. Naisbitt (1982) found that space in the mass media devoted to aging increased rapidly during the 1970s. Legislation and programs for elders have increased rapidly during the past thirty years. Courses on aging in colleges and universities have multiplied during this same period. These increases in interest and information about aging reduce misconceptions and stereotypes about elders.

Increasing Research

The Gerontological Society of America has grown from a few hundred members in the early 1960s to about 6,000 members currently. In the 1960s only two or three journals were devoted to reporting gerontological research. Now more than forty professional journals in gerontology and several dozen books on gerontology are published each year. Gerontological research has been a "growth industry" during the past several decades. This research has reduced ageism in two ways. First, it has revealed the true facts about aging; it has helped to distinguish between aging and disease; and has shown that normal aging is not as bad as the negative stereotypes portray it. Second, it has found ways to treat diseases common in old age; ways to prevent disease in old age; ways to slow the aging process; ways to extend longevity; and, in general, ways to improve the health and happiness of elders. This has made the image of aging less negative.

Improving Health

Elders as a group enjoy better health, as a result of gerontological research, better medical care, and living healthier lifestyles among all age groups (Manton, Corder, and Stallard, 1993; Palmore, 1986). This trend toward better health undermines the stereotype that most elders are sick or disabled.

Increasing Education

Literacy among elders has increased dramatically from a minority in 1900 to more than 98 percent by 1979 (U.S. Bureau of the Census, 1994). Similarly, educational attainment has increased rapidly. In 1959, persons older than age sixty-five had only three-fourths as many years of education as younger adults. However, by 2000, they had almost equal years of education on average. This trend is reducing ageism by narrowing the generational education gap thus chal-

lenging the stereotype the most elders are illiterate or poorly educated. Most important, it contributes to more high-level occupations
and more affluence among elders.

Increasing Affluence

Elders as a group became more affluent each year as a result of
their increasing education, which has resulted in higher-level occupations, and increasing pensions and Social Security benefits. This affluence is a dramatic change from the poverty so common during the
1930s. Before Social Security, poverty or financial dependence was
the usual fate of most elders. Even in 1980, more poverty existed
among elders than among others (Schick, 1986). But now *less* poverty is found among elders than among younger people, and elders receive a disproportionately larger share of the national personal income (Palmore, 1999). This increasing affluence undermines the
stereotype of the pitiful elder depending on charity and handouts,
resulting in more respect for elders in general.

Reductions in Other Forms of Prejudice

Most experts agree that substantial reductions occurred during the
past fifty years in such prejudices as racism and sexism which may
indirectly contribute to reductions in ageism. As people become more
aware of prejudice and discrimination, they become less likely to approve or practice it. Also, legislation designed to reduce racism and
sexism (e.g., as the Equal Employment Opportunity Act) may also reduce ageism. Finally, as racism and sexism wane, some people may
place more attention on reducing ageism because it is a relatively new
and undeveloped concern.

Despite these positive trends, little quantitative evidence suggests
actual reductions in ageism. Furthermore, clouds on the horizon may
indicate some storms in the future. Perhaps the most threatening
cloud is the possibility of intergenerational conflict, even though the
evidence indicates that such conflict is unlikely in the near future.
Current special programs for elders (positive ageism) will require an
increasing share of our government's budget unless such programs
are reduced. Younger people may rebel against this growing burden
and overreact by penalizing elders.

Another cloud on the horizon is the possible environmental destruction resulting from global warming, depletion of the ozone layer,

or pollution of air and water. Such environmental destruction could preoccupy the nation and interfere with attempts to reduce ageism. Elders might even be blamed for such problems because their generation's disregard for the environment would be a major cause of the problems. More recent clouds are the threat of terrorism, AIDS, and a sluggish economy.

The cloud that threatens the most devastation of all is the mushroom cloud: the proliferation of nuclear weapons both within the present nuclear club and by other nations who are developing nuclear weapons. If we have a nuclear war, there will be few elders (and few younger people) left, and ageism will be of little concern to any survivors.

These are only clouds on the horizon at present, and the most likely forecast for the reduction of ageism seems to be "fair and mild."

See also COHORTS; FACTS ON AGING QUIZ; HISTORY

REFERENCES

Manton, K., Corder, L., and Stallard, E. (1993). Estimates of change in chronic disability and institutional incidence and prevalence rates in the U.S. elderly population from the 1982, 1984, and 1989 National Long Term Care Survey. *Journal of Gerontology, Social Sciences,* 47(Suppl.), S153.

Naisbitt, J. (1982). *Megatrends.* New York: Warner Books.

Palmore, E. (1986). Trends in the health of the aged. *The Gerontologist,* 26, 298.

_____ (1998). *Facts on aging quiz.* New York: Springer

_____ (1999). *Ageism.* New York: Springer.

Schick, F. (Ed.) (1986). *Statistical handbook on aging Americans.* Phoenix, AZ: Oryx Press.

U.S. Bureau of the Census (1994). Demographic and socioeconomic aspects of aging in the U.S. *U.S. Current Population Reports* (Series P-23). Washington, DC: U.S. Government Printing Office.

GENERATIONAL EQUITY

Erdman B. Palmore

Generational equity is the term for a campaign to reduce the benefits for elders provided by the government and private organizations. Americans for Generational Equity (AGE) questions the future of the Social Security system and the assumption that the young should support the old. This organization had more that 800 members and a budget of $286,000 in 1987 (Palmore, 1999). However, it folded in 1990.

Binstock (1994) warns that older Americans face increasing hostility in the realm of politics and public programs. He asserts that the campaign for generational equity is based on stereotypes, superficial reasoning, and unrealistic extrapolations of existing policies, as well as diverting attention from more useful issues.

This campaign has led to some hysterical writing about conflict between generations, such as Howe's 1995 article, "Why the Graying of the Welfare State Threatens to Flatten the American Dream—or Worse." He claims that projections indicate catastrophic consequences for after-tax living standards of most working-age Americans because of the increasing numbers of aged and the "untouchable" senior entitlements. Such projections are based on worst-case scenarios and unlikely assumptions, (e.g., nothing will be done to reform Social Security and Medicare).

Pollack (1989) blames the media for the myth of a *generation war* and the call for *generational equity.* He says this myth is based on four false assumptions:

- Elderly poverty has been wiped out.
- Generational equity involves competition for scarce resources.
- The increasing numbers of retirees have created an unsupportable burden for the shrinking workforce.
- The elderly are not paying their share of the federal budget.

Fortunately, most people younger than sixty-five perceive that their own long-term interest is involved in programs for elders. They understand that in the future they will benefit from these programs and that in the meantime they would be required to care for older relatives themselves if these programs did not exist.

See also AGE CONFLICT; AGE INEQUALITY; SOCIAL SECURITY

REFERENCES

Binstock, R. (1994). Transcending intergenerational equity. In T. Marmor, T. Smeeding, and V. Greene (Eds.), *Economic security and intergenerational justice.* Washington, DC: Urban Institute Press.

Howe, N. (1995). Why the graying of the welfare state threatens to flatten the American dream—or worse. *Generations,* 19, 15.

Palmore, E. (1999). *Ageism.* New York: Springer.

Pollack, R. (1989). Granny bashing: New myth recasts elders as victims. *Media and Values,* 45, 2.

GERIATRICS

Erdman B. Palmore

Geriatrics is the study of the medical aspects of old age and the application of knowledge related to the biological, biomedical, behavioral, and social aspects of aging to the prevention, diagnosis, treatment, and care of older persons (Butler, 2001).

Geriatricians and other physicians may be subject to several kinds of ageism. Because they focus on illness and disability, these doctors may forget that health and ability is normal among elders. They may also be tempted to blame any difficult or obscure illness on old age and assume that nothing can be done about it.

Studies of physicians' attitudes toward elders agree that they tend to have the same (or worse) ageist attitudes that the rest of our society shares (Quinn, 1987). Butler (1994) points out that medical students learn to see elderly patients as "vegetables," "gomers" ("get out of my emergency room"), and "gorks" ("God only really knows" the cause of the patient's symptoms).

Apparently extensive professional training does not usually correct these common misconceptions and stereotypes in our culture. Several reasons explain this situation. Health professionals have had little education about normal aging processes. They may know more about pathology and disease among the aged, but not about normal physical, psychological, and social aging (Palmore, 1998). Second, they often share a strong fear of death, which they associate with elders whom they define as "the enemy" (Vickio and Cavanaugh, 1985). Third, they have a biased experience with elders because they see and treat the most frail, sick, and senile aged. After years of such negative experiences, they forget that they rarely see normal healthy elders, and they begin to assume that most elders are similar to their sick patients. Fourth, professionals' feelings about their own parents or older relatives can conflict with their dealings with an elderly patient (Schonfield, 1982).

As a result, physicians label elders as resistant to treatment, rigid in outlook, demanding, and uninteresting. They assess elderly narrowly and prescribe medical solutions for their problems when some of the problems might be better resolved through nonmedical means (such as with a home aide or social worker). Physicians also overlook psychological disorders in elders or misdiagnose them as physical ailments (Waxman and Carner, 1984).

Fineman (1994) interviewed forty-two physicians and nurses and found they shared three stereotypes about old people: disengagement, unproductivity, and inflexibility. Grant (1996) claims that misconceptions about aging have lessened among health care providers, but that ageism still has detrimental effects.

To the extent that physicians use old age as the explanation for ailments and illnesses associated with old age, they assume that nothing can be done about the ailment and that improvement is unlikely. These negative attitudes may also convince their patients that nothing can be done and thus destroy the motivation necessary for patients' recovery.

As a result of these negative attitudes most health professionals would rather not work with older patients. Few specialize in geriatrics and nursing home care, which results in a shortage of qualified professional to care for elders. Despite the availability of dozens of geriatric fellowships, applicants are few, and several medical schools have not been able to fill some of their vacancies.

The International Longevity Center (Fleck, 2002) branded the shortage of geriatricians a national crisis. According to a recent report by the Alliance for Aging Research (2003), at least 20,000 geriatricians are needed to care for the nation's 35 million older people.

Part of the reason for this shortage is that few medical schools promote the teaching of geriatrics: only three have departments of geriatrics and only twelve require their students to take courses in geriatrics (Fleck, 2002). This neglect of geriatrics probably stems from the low reimbursements provided physicians by Medicare, the fact that geriatrics has less prestige than other medical specialties, and the latent ageism among many physicians.

It is tragic that so much ageism prevails among the very professionals who should know better and who are entrusted with the health care of our older population.

See also BIOLOGICAL DEFINITIONS OF AGING; GERONTOLOGY; HEALTH CARE; LANGUAGE; STEREOTYPES

REFERENCES

Alliance for Aging Research (2003). *Ageism: how health care fails the elderly.* Washinton, DC: Author.

Butler, R. (1994). Dispelling ageism. In D. Shenk and W. Achenbaum (Eds.), *Changing perceptions of aging and the aged.* New York: Springer.

_____ (2001). Geriatrics. In G. Maddox (Ed.), *The encyclopedia of aging.* New York: Springer.

Fineman, N. (1994). Health care providers' subjective understandings of old age. *Journal of Aging Studies,* 8, 255.

Fleck, C. (2002). America's "forgotten" patients. *AARP Bulletin,* 43(10), 8.

Grant, L. (1996). Effects of ageism on individual and health care providers' responses to healthy aging. *Health and Social Work,* 21, 9.

Palmore, E. (1998). *The facts on aging quiz.* New York: Springer.

Quinn, J. (1987). Attitude of professionals toward the aged. In G. Maddox (Ed.), *The encyclopedia of aging.* New York: Springer.

Schonfield, D. (1982). Who is stereotyping whom and why? *The Gerontologist, 22,* 267.

Vickio, C. and Cavanaugh, J. (1985). Relationships among death anxiety, attitudes toward aging, and experience with death among nursing home employees. *Journal of Gerontology, 40,* 347.

Waxman, H. and Carner, E. (1984). Physician recognition, diagnosis, and treatment of mental disorders in elderly medical patients. *The Gerontologist, 24,* 593.

GERONTOCRACY

Diana K. Harris

Coined by Jean-Jaques Fazy, the term *gerontocracy* was first used in a pejorative sense to describe the old, conservative French parliament in the 1820s (Achenbaum, 1993). Literally, the term *gerontocracy* means "rule by old men" and may be defined "as a society in which the political system is in the hands of the oldest community members" (Harris, 1988). This is an example of positive ageism in which discrimination occurs in favor of older persons (Palmore, 1999).

Much of the work on gerontocracies has been done by anthropologists studying non-Western societies and cultures. Anthropological investigations of the politics of age and gerontocracy in many African countries reveal that the elders in these places rule by virtue of the superior knowledge they are supposed to possess, which includes knowing the religious and cultural traditions of the group. In addition, their control of society is enhanced by the economic resources they have amassed by living a long time (Aguilar, 1998).

Gerontocracies may also be found in Western societies. The United States may be considered a gerontocracy in the sense that the average age of its political leaders is rather high. For instance, in the case of Congress, the average age is well above sixty years. However, the dominance of older persons in American politics may be largely because it takes time to reach positions of power (Albert, 1996).

Furthermore, Andrew Achenbaum (1993) proposes that the papacy has been a gerontocracy for many centuries. He notes that it is an institution that gives old people the opportunity to exercise power and "raises fresh possibilities for grappling with the psychological, religious, and social dimensions of growing older" (p. 213).

See also CROSS-CULTURAL AGEISM

REFERENCES

Achenbaum, A. (1993). (When) did the papacy become a gerontocracy? In K. Schaie and W. Achenbaum (Eds.), *Societal impact on aging: Historical perspectives* (pp. 204-213). New York: Springer.

Aguilar, M. (1998). Gerontocratic, aesthetic and political models of age. In M. Aguilar (Ed.), *The politics of age and gerontocracy in Africa* (pp. 1-29). Trenton, NJ: Africa World Press.

Albert, S. (1996). Aging. In D. Levinson and M. Ember (Eds.), *Encyclopedia of cultural anthropology,* Volume 1 (p. 28). New York: Henry Holt and Company.

Harris, D. (1988). *Dictionary of gerontology.* Westport, CT: Greenwood Publishing.

Palmore, E. (1999). *Ageism: Negative and positive.* New York: Springer.

GERONTOLOGY

Erdman B. Palmore

Gerontology is the science of aging. It draws on knowledge about aging from many different sciences such as biology, psychology, political science, economics, and sociology. Gerontologists are the scientists who study and teach about aging.

Gerontologists generally agree that ageism is a major problem in our society. Yet many gerontologists use language that implicitly perpetuates ageism through negative images and stereotypes about older people (Palmore, 2000). This negative language is not meant to be ageist and the users are typically not aware of its negative effects. However, the negative effects are insidious and potent, despite their innocent intent.

For example, the term *aging* is a neutral term, referring to *any* process associated with growing older, both positive as well as negative processes. Unfortunately, the usual connotations of aging as used by gerontologists tend to be negative terms such as senility, chronic illness, debilitation, deterioration, and senescence. In a typical example, Crews (1993) writes, "aging may be measured as frailty, loss of vigor, failure to thrive, loss of physiological function, or decreased adaptability" (p. 281).

Even the National Institute on Aging (1993) lists the processes of normal aging as declines in function of the heart, lungs, brain, kidneys, muscles, sight, and hearing. Such usage implies that aging is bad and to be avoided if possible, or at least slowed as much as possible.

Similarly, the term *old* should be a neutral term implying only advanced age. However, gerontologists use the term to refer to persons who are senile, debilitated, infirm, or frail. Other synonyms for *old* include *antiquated, archaic, worn-out,* and *obsolete.* Such usage contributes to ageism by reinforcing the negative stereotypes about old people.

Gerontologists have also been accused of focusing only on the declines of aging and of assuming that the characteristics of the aged are the primary causes of their problems (Levin and Levin, 1980). This subtle form of ageism ignores the possibilities of recovery, restoration, growth, development, and improvement with age.

The assumption that the characteristics of elders are the cause of the problems of elders is another form of ageism, because it ignores the extent to which the ageism embedded in our social structure and culture contributes to the problems of old age.

Some of the widely accepted gerontological theories of aging support negative stereotypes about elders. One of the most famous is disengagement theory. This theory supports the negative stereotype that elders withdraw from social and other activities. It also implies that it is beneficial for society that elders withdraw and that society should encourage this withdrawal. The alternative theories, *activity theory* and *continuity theory,* support a more positive view of aging.

Thus, gerontology should be an objective science, but some of the terms and connotations of terms that gerontologists use, the focus of some of their studies, and some of their theories tend to support ageism.

See also BLAMING THE VICTIM; LANGUAGE; SELF-FULFILLING PROPHECY; THEORIES OF AGING

REFERENCES

Crews, D. (1993). Biological aging. *Journal of Cross-Cultural Gerontology,* 8, 281.
Levin, J. and Levin, W. (1980). *Ageism.* Belmont, CA: Wadsworth.
National Institute on Aging (1993). *In search of the secrets of aging.* Bethesda, MD: National Institutes of Health.
Palmore, E. (2000). Ageism in gerontological language. *The Gerontologist,* 40, 645.

h

HEALTH CARE

Erdman B. Palmore

Both negative and positive forms of ageism are evident in the health care of U.S. elders (Palmore, 1999). Negative ageism is shown in the following:

- A widespread belief (often shared by elders themselves) prevails that most of the illness and ailments of elders are just normal parts of aging and nothing can be done to cure or alleviate them. This prevents the adequate treatment of many conditions that are, in fact, treatable.
- Many, if not most, health professionals are prejudiced against elders and prefer to treat younger people (Palmore, 1998).
- Despite Medicare and Medicaid, formidable barriers still exist to adequate medical care, including financial and transportation barriers, ignorance, and denial among elders (Palmore, 1972).
- Despite the fact that elders have higher rates of medical care than younger people do, these rates are not as high as might be expected on the basis of their much higher rates of illness and chronic conditions. It is probable that many elders would get more adequate care if they were younger.
- Proposals have been made that old age be used as an explicit criteria to ration health care for chronically ill older patients (Callahan, 1995).
- Health care providers are prone to patronize their elderly patients with their speech patterns (Hummert, 1994). These patterns include oversimplification; excessive clarification; simplified sentence structure; demeaning emotional tone; superficiality; and baby talk.

A report released by the Alliance for Aging Research (2003) outlines five key dimensions of the ageist bias in which U.S. health care fails older Americans:

- Health care professionals do not receive enough training in geriatrics to properly care for many older patients.
- Older patients are less likely than younger people to receive preventive care.
- Older patients are less likely to be tested or screened for diseases and other health problems.
- Proven medical interventions for older patients are often ignored, leading to inappropriate or incomplete treatment.
- Older people are consistently excluded from clinical trials, even though they are the largest users of approved drugs.

The report concludes that "medical care shaped by ageism assumptions hurts everyone, because it leads to premature loss of independence, increased mortality and disability, and depression in adults who might otherwise continue to lead productive, satisfying, and healthier lives" (p. 1).

Medicare is an example of positive discrimination in favor of the aged. It is a national health insurance program for elders (and disabled) only, that cost about $210 billion in 2001 (U.S. Social Security Administration, 2002). It should be remembered that affluent elders as well as poor elders benefit from Medicare. For younger people, the government provides health care only to the poor through Medicaid. Many argue that this positive ageism should be eliminated by providing a national health insurance program for all ages.

See also COSTS OF AGEISM; GERIATRICS; MEDICAL STUDENTS

REFERENCES

Alliance for Aging Research (2003). *Ageism: How health care fails the elderly.* Washington, DC: AFAR.

Callahan, D. (1995). *Setting limits.* New York: Simon & Schuster.

Hummert, M. (1994). Stereotypes of the elderly and patronizing speech. In M. Hummert, J. Wieman, and J. Nussbaum (Eds.), *Interpersonal communication in older adulthood.* Thousand Oaks, CA: Sage.

Palmore, E. (1972). Medical care needs of the aged. *Postgraduate Medicine,* May, 194; June, 181.

_____ (1998). *The facts on aging quiz.* New York: Springer.

_____ (1999). *Ageism.* New York: Springer.

U.S. Social Security Administration (2002). *Annual statistical supplement to the Social Security Bulletin.* Washington, DC: Social Security Administration.

HISPANICS

Jacqueline L. Angel

Individuals of Hispanic origin represent a rapidly growing segment of the older minority population in the United States. According to the U.S. Bureau of the Census, in 2000 there were approximately 1,752,000 Hispanics age sixty-five years and over. Under the assumption of the middle-series projections, which are based on moderate estimates for future births, life expectancy, and net international migration, the number of elderly Hispanics (7.8 million) in 2030 is expected to surpass that of African Americans by 1.1 million (U.S. Bureau of the Census, 2001). If current rates of population growth continue, demographers anticipate that Hispanics age sixty-five and over could reach 14 million people by the year 2050, having accounted for 16.4 percent of the total elderly population (Day, 1996). The nation's Hispanic population has dramatically risen not just because of higher rates in past fertility, but also because of huge waves of emigration from Latin America.

Hispanics may suffer from ageism in several ways:

- Their accumulated socioeconomic disadvantages make them vulnerable to many chronic health problems.
- They are less likely to have health insurance than younger Hispanics.
- Language barriers create discrimination against elderly Hispanics.
- They are often forced to live with children because of poverty, lack of long-term care insurance, and discrimination against them by long-term care institutions.
- Elderly Hispanic women suffer from the "triple jeopardy" of ageism, racism, and sexism.

Studies indicate that Hispanics and non-Hispanics differ in terms of numerous characteristics, including educational level, labor force experiences, linguistic fluency, and family living arrangements. These factors persist into old age and translate into a different set of physical and mental health risk factors for Hispanics. Recent evidence suggests that even though Hispanics have favorable mortality rates compared to non-Hispanic whites, their accumulated socioeconomic disadvantages over the life cycle give rise to serious chronic health problems, including diabetes, obesity, and limitations in daily function (Markides and Coreil, 1986). In addition, the data show that the largest subgroup of Hispanic elders—Mexican Americans—report particularly low rates of private health insurance coverage. Approximately eight of every ten elderly Mexican Americans have no supplemental medical insurance (Angel, Angel, and Markides, 2002).

The lack of adequate health insurance coverage among elderly Mexican Americans is directly linked to income disparities earlier in life. Mexican-American workers are much more likely than non-Hispanic whites to work in jobs that do not offer employer-sponsored insurance in retirement. Language barriers also prohibit some Mexican Americans from being involved in government programs that help pay for these extra costs, such as prescription drugs, medical appliances, and physician fees.

The health disparities are largely the result of basic factors in Hispanics' social and economic life that have historically been associated with differential power and, consequently, with differential life chances. For instance, twice as many elderly Mexican Americans than elderly non-Hispanic whites live in poverty (Angel and Angel, 1998). Mexican-American elders have lower household and personal incomes, lower earnings, fewer dividends, and less income from private and Social Security pensions than do elderly non-Hispanic whites (Angel and Angel, 1997). Living alone and being female makes the situation even worse for older Mexican Americans. More than one-third of Mexican-American elderly women report household incomes below the poverty level (Angel et al., 1999).

To compensate for these economic hardships, many unmarried elderly Mexican Americans live with family more often than do non-Hispanic whites (Angel et al., 1996). In the event of poor health, older Mexican Americans also prefer to live with adult children than to enter a nursing home. This is primarily due to importance of the Mexican-American family *(la familia Mexicana)* not viewing nursing homes as a culturally viable alternative for their loved ones, but rather as a place of last resort. Besides the role that culture plays, other reasons account for the lower rates of nursing home use among frail and disabled Mexican-origin elders. They are likely to be poor, and consequently unable to pay for nursing home care; there is a shortage of geographically available nursing facilities within Mexican-American communities; and a greater number of family members are available to help care for infirm parents.

In sum, the differential allocation of social rewards in the aging Hispanic population is partly a result of ageism. Access to education and employment opportunities among recent Hispanic immigrants will be of special importance in anticipating how this ethnic group will age (Mutchler and Angel, 2000). Historically, elderly Hispanics were provided for by their children or other kin, while elderly non-Hispanic whites went to nursing homes. This may change with the projected dramatic increases in the number of elderly Hispanics. Hispanic children are increasingly returning home not to care for aged parents, but to meet their own needs because they are unable to find affordable housing, work, or child care (Goldscheider and Goldscheider, 1993). It is clear that reducing ageism against elderly Hispanics would improve the outlook for their future.

See also CULTURAL SOURCES OF AGEISM

REFERENCES

Angel, R. J. and Angel, J. L. (1997). *Who will care for us? Aging and long-term care in multicultural America.* New York: New York University Press.

———(1998). Aging trends: Mexican-Americans in the southwestern USA. *Journal of Cross-Cultural Gerontology, 13,* 281-290.

Angel, R. J., Angel, J. L., Lee, G., and Markides, K. S. (1999). Age at migration and family dependency among older Mexican immigrants: Recent evidence from the Mexican American EPESE. *The Gerontologist, 39,* 59-65.

Angel, R. J., Angel, J. L., and Markides, K. S. (2002). Stability and change in health insurance among older Mexican Americans: Longitudinal evidence from the Hispanic-EPESE. *American Journal of Public Health, 92,* 1264-1271.

Angel, J. L, Angel, R. J., McClellan, J. L., and Markides, K.S. (1996). Nativity, declining health, and preferences in living arrangements among elderly Mexican Americans: Implications for long-term care. *The Gerontologist, 36,* 464-473.

Day, J. C. (1996). Population projections of the United States by age, sex, race, and Hispanic origin: 1995-2050. *Current Population Reports* [P25-1130]. Washington, DC: U.S. Government Printing Office.

Goldscheider, F. and Goldscheider, C. (1993). *Leaving home before marriage: Ethnicity, familism, and generational relationships.* Madison: University of Wisconsin Press.

Markides, K. and Coreil, J. (1986). The health of Hispanics in the southwestern United States: An epidemiological paradox. *Public Health Reports,* 101, 253-265.

Mutchler, J. E. and Angel, J. L. (2000). Policy development and the older Latino population in the 21st century. *International Journal of Sociology and Social Policy,* 11, 177-188.

U.S. Bureau of the Census (2001). Population by age, sex, race, and Hispanic origin: March 2000. Summary File (SF 1), Table 1. <www.census.gov/population/socdemo/age/pp1-147/tab01.txt>.

HISTORY

Erdman B. Palmore

The history of ageism in the United States shows considerable variation from a tendency toward positive ageism in colonial times, toward negative ageism after the Civil War, to less negative ageism after World War II (Achenbaum, 1978; Palmore, 1999).

During colonial years, the few who survived to old age enjoyed relatively high status in the major institutions of society. In religious institutions, the Bible's traditional respect for elders was expanded into a moral veneration of elders. The ruling body in the local church was often called the board of elders. In agriculture, control of the land gave the elders extensive power. In crafts and trade, the skill and experience of elders gave them more success and power than younger persons.

In Riesman's terminology (1950), colonial America was a *tradition-directed* society in which older people instructed younger people in correct behavior according to traditions. Therefore, older people had higher status because of their age and superior knowledge of the traditions.

After the Revolutionary War, a growing emphasis was placed on equality, individual achievement, secularism, and the free market. All these ideologies undercut the advantages that elders traditionally enjoyed in colonial times. In Riesman's terms, the postrevolutionary United States became an *inner-directed* society in which individuals were guided by internalized norms and values that were adaptable to changing situations rather than by the traditions of the past. Thus, parents were important for instilling these norms in children, but once their children internalized the norms, they no longer needed the detailed guidance of parents and other older persons. This tended to decrease the positive ageism of the colonial era.

After the Civil War, rapid modernization and urbanization took place. According to Cowgill (1974), this modernization reduce the status of elders for several reasons:

- The rapid increase in the proportion of aged in the population makes the supply of older persons exceed the demand.
- The increased use of technology and automation decreases the demand for older workers.
- Increased retirement lowers the income and status of elders.
- Rapid social change makes obsolete much of the knowledge that formerly was a basis for prestige of elders.
- Urbanization often leaves the elderly behind in rural areas.

As science began to replace religion and tradition as sources of knowledge, the average declines in physical functioning and the increases in chronic diseases with aging was documented. These studies were the basis for the ageist view of aging as inevitable decline.

Another factor contributing to the rise of negative ageism around the turn of the century was the increased competition between the older native workers and the younger immigrant workers who would work for lower wages. The incentive to reduce labor costs, and the myth of rapid decline in abilities in old age, combined to increase discrimination against older workers. This, in turn, produced increased poverty among retired workers, which led to the stereotype that most aged are poor.

The advent of Social Security reduced poverty and increased respect for older persons as independent consumers thus undercutting some of the older stereotypes.

During and after World War II, several developments began to improve the image and status of elders.

- The labor shortage during the war increased the demand for older workers.
- Social Security and private pensions made retirement more attractive.
- The increase in numbers of elders increased their political influence and the number of various public and private programs to improve the status of elders.

In the 1960s, three major bills were passed that began to improve the circumstances of elders: the Older Americans Act, the Medicare and Medicaid bill, and the Age Discrimination in Employment Act. This latter bill prohibited the use of age as a criterion for hiring, firing, discriminatory treatment on the job, etc, which had a major effect on reducing ageism in employment.

See also FUTURE OF AGEISM; MODERNIZATION THEORY; SOCIETAL AGEISM; SOCIAL SECURITY

REFERENCES

Achenbaum, W. (1978). *Old age in a new land.* Baltimore, MD: Johns Hopkins University Press.

Cowgill, D. (1974). Aging and modernization. In J. Gubrium (Ed.), *Late life, communities, and environmental policy.* Springfield, IL: Charles C Thomas.

Palmore, E. (1999). *Ageism.* New York: Springer.

Riesman, D. (1950). *The lonely crowd.* New Haven, CT: Yale University Press.

HIV/AIDS

Erdman B. Palmore

Infection with human immunodeficiency virus (HIV) eventually progresses to HIV disease and acquired immunodeficiency syndrome (AIDS). Ageism can affect the epidemiology, diagnosis, reporting, and treatment of this disease in several ways.

Because older persons are assumed to have a low risk of acquiring HIV/AIDS, they have not been targeted for educational and intervention programs. Cross-sectional data indicate that older Americans have less HIV/AIDS-related knowledge than younger persons and have minimal perceptions of their risk for contracting HIV (Zablotsky and Stall, 2001). This actually increases their risk of contracting HIV. For example, among older persons at risk, those age fifty and over are much less likely to use condoms or be tested for HIV infection, compared to their younger counterparts (Stall and Catania, 1994).

Because symptoms of AIDS are often similar to those of age-related diseases (e.g., wasting, dementia, night sweats), older people are often misdiagnosed, especially in the early stages. Consequently, older persons with AIDS often do not get the advantages of early diagnosis and treatment. Early treatment is especially critical for older persons because HIV has been found to progress more rapidly among the elderly than the young.

The majority of cases of HIV transmission involve sexual contact and/or drug abuse. Because of ageism, the elderly are usually assumed to be asexual, or in a stable monogamous relationship, and not engaged in drug abuse. Therefore, family members, physicians, and other health care workers often overlook the possibility that the elder has contracted HIV (Lashley, 2001). This also contributes to late diagnosis. In fact, sexual transmission is the leading mode of HIV acquisition in older adults (Bender, 1997). About half the cases of AIDS in the United States are classified by the Centers for Disease Control and Prevention (CDC) as being due to exposure of men who have sex with men (CDC, 1999).

Because of these effects, the AIDS epidemic has been *invisible* among elders. Such invisibility, resulting from ageism, contributes to the underdiagnosis, undertreatment, and greater mortality from AIDS among elders.

See also HEALTH CARE; SEXUALITY; STEREOTYPES

REFERENCES

Bender, B. (1997). HIV and aging as a model for immunosenescence. *Journal of Gerontology, 52A,* M261-M263.

Centers for Disease Control and Prevention (1999). 1999 USPHS/IDSA guidelines for the prevention of opportunistic infections in persons infected with HIV. *Morbidity and mortality Weekly Report, 48,* 1-66.

Lashley, F. (2001). AIDS/HIV in older adults. In G. Maddox (Ed.), *The encyclope-dia of aging.* New York: Springer.

Stall, R. and Catania, J. (1994). AIDS risk behaviors among late middle-aged and elderly Americans. *Archives of Internal Medicine,* 154, 57-63.

Zablotsky, D. and Stall, R. (2001). AIDS: The epidemiological and social context. In G. Maddox (Ed.), *The encyclopedia of aging.* New York: Springer.

HOLLYWOOD

Erdman B. Palmore

Age discrimination in Hollywood has been charged by more than 150 television writers, who filed twenty-three separate class-action lawsuits in the Los Angeles Superior Court in February 2002 (Gentile, 2002). The lawsuits claim that the major television networks, movie studios, and talent agencies have engaged in a pattern of refusing to hire or represent them because of their age.

In 2002, a group of older entertainment professionals, including actors Ed Asner, Peter Mark Richman, and Kent McCord, have formed a group to lobby producers and networks for more roles for older actors and to support similar legislative efforts. The group, known as the Industry Coalition for Age Equity in the Media (ICAEM), has the backing of the Screen Actors Guild, Women in Film, the American Federation of Television and Radio Artists (AFTRA), and the California Commission on Aging (CCoA). One of the group's main goals is to persuade the entertainment industry that casting actors and actresses over age forty is key to tapping into the buying power of older Americans.

Peter Mark Richman said,

> Ageism is prevalent in our industry and it's like a silent killer, like cancer, and it gets worse every year. The parts are not there. In television, what does a senior do, unless you play a judge? The public and the industry have got to be re-educated. (Gentile, 2002, p. 7E)

The coalition is supporting legislation pending in California that would launch a media campaign to change cultural perceptions of the aging.

See also EMPLOYMENT DISCRIMINATION

REFERENCE

Gentile, G. (2002). Actors fighting against ageism in Hollywood. *News and Observer,* Raleigh, NC, August 9, 7E.

HOUSING

Edna L. Ballard

Housing provides more than security and physical protection against the elements. Housing, whether a mansion by the sea or a mobile home in a trailer park, determines in a number of ways our physical, emotional, and social well-being. Where we live and the kind of housing we live in, help shape our sense of safety, autonomy, pleasure, satisfaction, and well-being. It is the primary repository of possessions and meaningful relationships. It provides the framework for routine interactions with others: family, neighbors, community, and, increasingly, the setting for work.

Housing features may be supportive or barriers to physical or psychological needs of the individual regardless of age. Many features designed to make a home house-friendly (e.g., three-foot-wide doorways, levers that are easier to open than doorknobs, adjustable countertops, grab bars in the bathroom), are helpful to all persons, not to just the older individual who needs wheelchair access, or allowances for limited reach or limited muscle strength.

Sensory and physical changes that may occur in the normal aging process, however, also impact significantly the person's ability to function well in his or her living space. Waning strength, dexterity, or endurance may make tasks such as climbing stairs, performing simple housework, or routine maintenance more difficult. Moreover, the capacity for controlling the environment can be complicated by both a decline in the person's ability to physically or financially make a change for the better, as well as the increasing functional obsolescence of the structural components of the house (e.g., wiring, plumbing, heating or cooling systems). These realities must be acknowledged and given sufficient attention in a manner that does not engender ageism.

Ageism in housing is often the result of policies and practices designed to provide for the special needs of frail or dependent elders.

These policies and practices form the basis of perceptions that define the users of these services as having special needs because of age, rather than because of specific disabilities. These new perceptions thus become the basis of policies regarding elders as requiring special housing because of age-dependent qualifiers. Emerging trends now consider supportive, barrier-free housing that responds to the needs of individuals of all ages.

Ageism, as with discriminations of all kinds, is lessened by the access of the target group to relevant information and resources. Often minor adjustments or changes, ranging from the simple act of making frequently used items most accessible, to help in making simple repairs, can help make aging in place a reality for the individual. Removing clutter (that can lead to debilitating falls), fire hazards, materials that create dirt, bacteria, mold, and other environmental hazards (that can affect one's health and compromise independence) are easily taken steps that benefit the individual in his or her living environment.

Even simple elements can have important consequences in housing for elders. For example, the color of the walls

> can make a home safer and more enjoyable. Light colors reflect light back into the room. Dark colors absorb light. For example, a white wall will reflect 85 percent of the light back into the room, whereas a dark brown wall will reflect only 19 percent back into the room. (NC Cooperative Extension Service, 1992, p. 2)

Does this mean that elders are confined to white walls? No, it means that we must be thoughtful in the use of color in the environment. "When people consider factors adversely affecting their health, they generally focus on influences, such as poor diet or the need for more exercise. Rarely do they consider less traditional factors, such as housing" (Jackson and Kochtitzky, 2001, p. 4).

Discrimination often presents itself in the form of *benign neglect.* We know that many elders live in housing that is old and in need of substantial repairs. Many municipalities have made a gallant effort to give assistance to persons who qualify for financial assistance. The problem, however, is large, costly, and not easily fixed.

The Environmental Protection Agency (EPA) reports that environmental health hazards occur in new and old houses alike and the occupants can experience adverse health effects from, for example, radon gas, carbon monoxide, dust mites, molds, lead, and asbestos (National Institute of Environmental Health Sciences, 1999). Air pollution in our public and private buildings is a another problem: "This is a sobering thought, given that people in the United States spend an average of 90 percent of their time indoors and that many intrinsically associate home with safety and comfort," alludes Manuel in an EPA report (p. A352). Staying indoors in tightly sealed homes may make the house more energy efficient, but may also create air quality that is an ecological hazard. Indoor air pollution is one of the top five risks to public health as ranked by the EPA.

Housing, as it affects elders, should be defined in its broadest sense, including the surrounding environment that can have a substantial impact on the individual. Factors such as inadequate transportation, deterioration of older neighborhoods, fear of crime, and multiple entry ports for services, impact housing satisfaction. Community amenities such as walking and bicycle paths, sidewalks, bus shelters, and controlled traffic patterns are more than safety features; they encourage others to be out and about, thus increasing a sense of safety for elders.

> A study in Houston, Texas, found that three out of five disabled and elderly people do not have sidewalks between residences and the nearest bus stop. The lack of sidewalks, curb cuts, and bus shelters actually make use of transportation systems by these people impossible. (Jackson and Kochtitzky, 2001, p. 12)

The authors add that the lack of physical access to transportation in the community can become a factor leading to illness and even death.

Most older adults prefer to remain in their homes in the community. Some persons, however, by choice or because of illness, disability, or increasing frailty, need more institutional settings that provide help with meals, special diets, personal assistance, shopping, housekeeping, supervision, companionship, or medical care. Options include retirement communities, continuing care (or life care) retirement communities, assisted-living facilities, congregate housing or senior housing including shared housing or group living, foster care, board and care homes, and the traditional nursing home.

Ageism may be involved when elders are forced into these facilities against their wishes simply because of their age, rather than their need. There remains a stigmatizing element to those facilities that serve the more physically and economically dependent. Little has changed in almost three decades since Koncelik (1976) wrote, "The nursing home is a symbol of the meaning of aging to a great many American people. . . . It is for the most part, a negative symbol of aging, the last place anyone wants to be" (p. 2)

See also ABUSE IN NURSING HOMES; AGE SEGREGATION; ARCHITECTURE; ASSISTED LIVING; NURSING HOMES; RETIREMENT COMMUNITIES

REFERENCES

Jackson, R. J. and Kochtitzky, C. (2001). *Creating a healthy environment: The impact of the built environment on public health.* [Sprawl Watch Clearinghouse Monograph series.]Washington, DC: Centers for Disease Control and Prevention.

Koncelik, J. A. (1976). *Designing the open nursing home.* Stroudsburg, PA: Dowden, Hutchinson and Ross, Inc.

National Institute of Environmental Health Sciences, National Institutes of Health (1999). *Environmental Health Perspectives,* 107(7), A352-357.

North Carolina Cooperative Extension Service (1992). *Life-cycle housing: Furnishing a user-friendly home* [brochure]. North Carolina State University College of Agriculture and Life Sciences. 10/92-11.2m-JMG, HE-391.

HUMAN RIGHTS OF OLDER PERSONS

Erdman B. Palmore

Ageism and the denial of human rights of older persons is a worldwide problem (Palmore and Maeda, 1985; Palmore, 1993). This fact was discussed at the first United Nations World Assembly on Aging in 1982. In 2000, Mary Robinson, United Nations Commissioner on Human Rights, emphasized the importance of protecting the human rights of older persons. However, no official United Nations document has ever identified and specified what these rights are and why they are important.

In 2002, the second United Nations World Assembly on Aging was held in Madrid, Spain. At that assembly the International Longevity Center–USA proposed that the following Declaration of the Rights of Older Persons become the basis of action as well as discussion at the assembly and beyond.

Declaration of the Rights of Older Persons

Whereas the recognition of the inherent dignity and of the equal and inalienable rights of all members of the human family is the foundation of freedom, justice, and peace in the world,

Whereas human progress has increased longevity and enabled the human family to encompass several generations within one lifetime, and whereas the older generations have historically served as the creators, elders, guides, and mentors of the generations that followed,

Whereas the older members of society are subject to exploitation that takes the form of physical, sexual, emotional, and financial abuse, occurring in their homes as well as in institutions such as nursing homes, and are often treated in cruel and inaccurate ways in language, images, and actions,

Whereas the older members of society are not provided the same rich opportunities for social, cultural, and productive roles and are subject to selective discrimination in the delivery of services otherwise available to other members of the society and are subject to selective job discrimination in hiring, promotion, and discharge,

Whereas older women live longer than men and experience more poverty, abuse, chronic diseases, institutionalization, and isolation,

Whereas disregard for the basic human rights of any group results in prejudice, marginalization, and abuse, recourse must be sought from all appropriate venues, including the civil, government, and corporate worlds, as well as by advocacy of individuals, families, and older persons,

Whereas older people were once young and the young will one day be old and exist in the context of the unity and continuity of life,

Whereas the United Nations Universal Declaration of Human Rights and other United Nations documents attesting to the inalienable rights of all humankind do not identify and specify older persons as a protected group,

Therefore new laws must be created, and laws that are already in effect must be enforced to combat all forms of discrimination against older people,

Further, the cultural and economic roles of older persons must be expanded to utilize the experience and wisdom that come with age,

Further, to expand the cultural and economic roles of older persons, an official declaration of the rights of older persons must be established, in conjunction with the adoption by nongovernment organizations of a manifesto which advocates that the world's nations commit themselves to protecting the human rights and freedoms of older persons at home, in the workplace, and in institutions, and offers affirmatively the rights to work, a decent retirement, protective services when vulnerable, and end-of-life care with dignity.

This proposal was discussed, but as of 2004 no such declaration has been adopted.

See also ETHICAL ISSUES; PUBLIC POLICY

REFERENCES

Palmore, E. (Ed.) (1993). *Developments and research on aging: An international handbook.* Westport, CT: Greenwood Press.

Palmore, E. and Maeda, D. (1985). *The honorable elders revisited.* Durham, NC: Duke University Press.

HUMOR

Erdman B. Palmore

Several studies have occurred regarding attitudes toward aging shown by humor, using the method of *content analysis* (Davies, 1977; Demos and Jache, 1981; Dillon and Jones, 1981; Nahemow, McCluskey, and McGhee, 1986; Palmore, 1971; Polisar, 1982; Richmond and Tallmer, 1977; Smith, 1979). Most studies analyzed jokes, but some analyzed cartoons or birthday cards about aging. They all reached similar conclusions: most of this humor reflects or supports negative attitudes toward aging, and that positive humor about aging is rare. Even jokes that are judged to be "positive" often depend on a contradiction of negative stereotypes for their humor.

For example, one old lady tells her friend, "I didn't sleep well last night because a man kept pounding on my door."

"Why didn't you open the door?" her friend responds.

"What, and let him out?"

This is funny only because the stereotype that assumes old ladies are not interested in sex. Thus, even "positive" jokes often assume negative stereotypes and may reinforce those stereotypes.

Similarly, an analysis of sheet music related to aging, many of which were humorous, also found that the majority present a negative view of aging and old age (Cohen and Kruschwitz, 1990).

In both the United States and in Canada, being "told a joke that pokes fun at old people" was the most frequent type of ageism reported in the ageism survey (Palmore, 2001, 2002). Being "sent a birthday card that pokes fun at old people" was also one of the most frequent types of ageism reported.

Most people would probably agree that humor about old people is a less serious type of ageism than some more harmful types such as employment discrimination or criminal victimization. However, because negative humor is so frequent and insidious, it may well be a root cause of the more serious forms of ageism.

In summary, most humor about aging supports negative ageism. Just as racist and sexist jokes support negative attitudes about race and sex, most jokes about old people are ageist. Most tellers and listeners are probably unaware of their ageist effects, which may even increase the joke's impact on the listener's unconscious attitudes.

See also AGEISM SURVEY; CARDS

REFERENCES

Cohen, E. and Kruschwitz, A. (1990). Old age in America represented in 19th and 20th century sheet music. *The Gerontolgist,* 30, 345.

Davies, L. (1977). Attitudes toward old age and aging as shown by humor. *The Gerontologist,* 18, 76.

Demos, V. and Jache, A. (1981), Return to sender please. *Women's Day,* September 22, 20.

Dillon, K., and Jones, R. (1981). Attitudes toward aging portrayed by birthday cards. *International Journal of Aging and Human Development,* 13, 79.

Nahemow, L. McCluskey, K., and McGhee, P. (Eds.) (1986). *Humor and Aging.* New York: Academic Press.

Palmore, E. (1971). Attitudes toward aging shown by humor. *The Gerontologist,* 11, 181.

_____ (2001). The ageism survey. *The Gerontologist,* 41(5), 572-575.

_____ (2002). Ageism in Canada and the United States. *The Center Report,* 22(3), 2.

Polisar, D. (1982). Figurative aging. Paper presented at the Southern Sociological Meeting, April. Unpublished.

Richmond, J. and Tallmer, M. (1977). The foolishness and wisdom of age: Attitudes toward the elderly as reflected in jokes. *The Gerontologist,* 17, 210.

Smith, M. (1979). The portrayal of elders in magazine cartoons. *The Gerontologist,* 19, 408.

HYPERTENSION

Hayden B. Bosworth

Hypertension is associated with increased cardiovascular morbidity (e.g., stroke, congestive heart failure) and mortality in older persons. Physicians' behavior affects rates of blood pressure (BP) control and health care costs. After decades of improvement in BP control, this trend has declined since the early 1990s (Joint National Committee on Detection, 1997); only one-quarter of those individuals aware of having hypertension have controlled BP (<140/90 mm/hg) (Burt et al., 1995).

Physicians do not treat hypertension aggressively enough despite the clear benefits of pharmacological and nonpharmacological treatments (Berlowitz et al., 1998). This is particularly problematic for older adults because rates of hypertension and poor BP control increases with age. Hypertension prevalence ($\geq$140/90 mm/hg or under a physician's care for hypertension) in persons aged sixty-five and seventy-five years in the United States is 60 percent and is 70 percent among those seventy-five years and older (Wolz et al., 2000).

Despite the increase incidence of hypertension with age and the inadequacy of BP control, a significant proportion of physicians do not seek BP treatment goals as recommended. More troubling is that physicians tolerate higher BP in older patients (Hyman and Pavlik, 2000) despite evidence of the advantage of treatment is greater in older than in younger patients (Psaty et al., 1997). A misperception persists that because BP increases with age, it is normal for older adults to have higher BPs than younger adults. In fact, 35 percent of members of the American Geriatrics Society who responded to a survey reported that increase in BP with age is a normal process of aging (Hajjar, Millar, and Hirth, 2002). This misperception contributes to the lack of appropriate treatment among older adults (Gifford, 1987). High BP is abnormal at any age and reflects a pathological process associated with increased risk of morbidity.

The providers' role in outcomes of hypertension treatment may be overt, as in their medication prescription patterns. Physicians may confound BP control by inadvertently abetting patient nonadherence with overly complicated medication regimens or by not addressing side effects. Physicians also may be unable to teach and monitor lifestyle changes because of an excessive number of patients, infrequent follow-up appointments, and assume that elevated office BP values do not reflect the true levels at home (DiMatteo et al., 1993). Physicians also may provide less time for consultation to older as compared to younger adults (Clark, Porter, and McKinlay, 1990).

The causes of inadequate BP control are unclear, but age is not one of them. Although patient nonadherence may partially explain poor BP control rates (Bosworth and Oddone, 2002), age is not a reliable factor for predicting treatment adherence (Lorenc and Branthwaite, 1993). Age also should not affect treatment. Clinical trials have demonstrated the benefit of treating hypertension in the elderly (Staessen et al., 1997), and that all classes of antihypertensive drugs are effective in lowering BP in older individuals.

Because of the high prevalence of hypertension in older persons, recognition and treatment of this disease should be a priority for physicians. Although hypertension treatment in the elderly has been less examined than other age groups, the benefits of treating older adults are clear. A recent meta-analysis, for example, suggests treatment decreased stroke by 34 percent in the oldest-old (Gueyffier et al., 1999).

Multiple explanations exist for the poor BP control rates among older adults. The treatment of chronic diseases such as hypertension requires a team approach. Because of the consistent poor levels of BP control, the promotion and maintenance of BP control requires individuals and their families to assume a leadership role in the treatment of their hypertension and not rely solely on health care providers. Patients and their families be their own case managers and take control of their own BP. Educating and encouraging patients to monitor their hypertension is likely to motivate patients to control their BP.

See also GERIATRICS; HEALTH CARE

REFERENCES

Berlowitz, D., Ash, A.S., Hickey, E.C., Friedman, R.H., Glickman, M., Kader, B., and Moskowitz, M.A. (1998). Inadequate management of blood pressure in a hypertensive population. *New England Journal of Medicine,* 339(27), 1957-1963.

Bosworth, H.B. and Oddone, E.Z. (2002). A model of psychosocial and cultural antecedents of blood pressure control. *Journal of the National Medical Association,* 94, 236-248.

Burt, V., Whelton, P., Roccella, E.J., Brown, C., Cutler, J.A., Higgins, M., Horan, M.J., and Labarthe, D. (1995). Prevalence of hypertension in the U.S. adult population: Results from the third National Health and Nutrition Examination Survey, 1988-1991. *Hypertension,* 25, 305-313.

Clark J.A., Porter, D.A., and McKinlay, J.B. (1990). Bringing social structure back into clinical decision making. *Social Science & Medicine,* 32, 853-866.

DiMatteo, M., Sherbourne, C.D., Hays, R.D., Ordway, L., Kravitz, R.L., McGlynn, E.A., Kaplan, S., and Rogers, W.H. (1993). Physicians' characteristics influence patients' adherence to medical treatment: Results from the Medical Outcomes Study. *Health Psychology,* 12(2), 93-102.

Gifford, R.W. (1987). Myths about hypertension in the elderly. *Medical Clinics of North America,* 71(5), 1003-1011.

Gueyffier, F., Bulpitt, C., Boissel, J.P., Schron, E., Ekbom, T., Fagard, R., Casiglia, E., Kerlikowske, K., and Coope, J. (1999). Antihypertensive drugs in very old people: A subgroup meta-analysis of randomised controlled trials. INDANA Group. *Lancet,* 353(9155), 793-796.

Hajjar, I., Millar, K., and Hirth, V. (2002). Age-related bias in the management of hypertension: A national survey of physicians' opinions on hypertension in elderly adults. *Journal of Gerontology: Medical Sciences, 57*(8), M487-M491.

Hyman, D.J. and Pavlik, V.N. (2000). Self-reported hypertension treatment practices among primary care physicians: Blood pressure thresholds, drug choices, and the role of guidelines and evidence-based medicine. *Archives of Internal Medicine, 160*(15), 2281-2286.

Joint National Committee on Detection, Evaluation, and Treatment of High Blood Pressure (1997). *The sixth report of the Joint National Committee on Detection, Evaluation, and Treatment of High Blood Pressure (JNC VI).* Bethesda, MD: U.S. Department of Health and Human Services, National Institutes of Health.

Lorenc, L. and Branthwaite, A. (1993). Are older adults less compliant with prescribed medication than younger adults? *British Journal of Clinical Psychology, 32*, 485-492.

Psaty, B.M., Smith, M.L., Siscovick, D.S., Koepsell, T.D., Weiss, N.S., Heckbert, S.R., Lemaitre, R.N., Wagner, E.H., and Furberg, C.D. (1997). Health outcomes associated with antihypertensive therapies used as first-line agents: A systematic review and meta-analysis. *Journal of the American Medical Association, 277*(9), 739-745.

Staessen, J.A., Fagard, R., Thijs, L., Celis, H., Arabidze, G.G., and Birkenhager, W.H. (1997). Randomised double-blind comparison of placebo and active treatment for older patients with isolated systolic hypertension. *Lancet, 350*, 757.

Wolz, M., Cutler, J., Roccella, E.J., Rohde, F., Thom, T., and Burt, V. (2000). Statement from the National High Blood Pressure Education Program: Prevalence of hypertension. *American Journal of Hypertension, 13*, 103-104.

INDIVIDUAL SOURCES OF AGEISM

Erdman B. Palmore

There are at least six individual sources of ageism: the authoritarian personality, frustration-aggression theory, ignorance, rationalization, selective perception, and death anxiety (Palmore, 1999).

The Authoritarian Personality

Prejudice against various groups is part of a complicated personality syndrome called *the authoritarian personality* (Adorno et al., 1950). According to this theory, prejudice is often result of insecurity, repressed impulses, a belief that life is capricious and threatening, and an emphasis on competitive power in human relationships. Rigidity of outlook, intolerance of ambiguity, pseudoscientific or antiscientific attitudes, suggestibility, gullibility, and unrealistic perceptions of what will achieve goals also characterize personalities with this syndrome.

Various studies have also found that authoritarian personalities are less intelligent and less educated (Christie and Cook, 1958), and dislike or distrust people in general (Sullivan and Adelson, 1954). Similarly, several studies have found that those with negative attitudes toward elders are often less educated (Palmore, 1998; Thorson, Whatley, and Hancock, 1974).

Kogan (1973) found that among 482 undergraduates tested, "There is a general trend for subjects to be positive or negatively disposed toward a wide variety of groups deviating in some respect from a hypothetical norm of similarity to self" (p. 53).

Although the theory linking authoritarian personalities to ageism has not been thoroughly tested, the existing evidence suggests that the same personality traits that contribute to racism and other prejudices may also contribute to ageism.

Frustration-Aggression Theory

Frustrating events can cause hostile impulses (Simpson and Yinger, 1985). Sometimes this hostility cannot be directed toward the real source of the frustration for various reasons: there may be no human agent, the agent may be unknown, the agent may be too powerful to attack, or the frustration may result from inner conflict.

In such situations, the hostility may be displaced against some innocent minority-group members who are vulnerable to attack. The minority-group members become scapegoats for the hostility generated by the frustration. Such an attack must be justified or rationalized so that the attacker can feel moral and reasonable. Stereotypes rationalize discrimination against the whole group, despite the variation that characterize any human group.

Binstock (1983) described how elders can become scapegoats, "bearing the blame for a variety of economic and political frustrations" (p. 136) such as a depressed economy, high rates of unemployment and inflation, and the budget deficit. He concluded that such scapegoating has three deleterious effects: it diverts our attention from a variety of deficiencies in public leadership and public policy; it engenders intergenerational conflict; and it diverts our attention from issues of reform in government policies.

Ignorance

Various studies have found that those who are more ignorant about the facts on aging are also likely to be more negative toward the aged (Palmore, 1998). The good news is as more information about what aging is really like becomes available, the negative stereotypes based on older assumptions tend to diminish.

Rationalization

Rationalization is the process of attributing one's actions to rational and creditable motives without analysis of the true (and often unconscious) motives. In the area of ageism, forced retirement may be rationalized on the grounds that older workers are no longer competent, or are slowing down, or old-fashioned, or unattractive, when the primary reason is to replace a higher paid (older) worker with a lower-paid (younger) worker. Putting older relatives into a nursing home may be rationalized on the grounds that "it is for their own good," when the real reason is to avoid the burdens of caregiving at home. Doctors may rationalize their neglect of older patients on the grounds that their illness is "due to old age" and will not respond to treatment, when the actual reason is that doctors usually do not get as high a fee from Medicare or Medicaid patients as from younger patients.

Selective Perception

Selective perception is a major explanation for the persistence of stereotypes in the face of contrary evidence. We have a tendency to see what we expect to see. This tendency to perceive confirming evidence and to ignore disconfirming evidence is especially strong in the case of ageism stereotypes, because we do not usually know the actual age of older persons. We usually infer people's age from their characteristics. Thus, when we see people who are gray-haired, wrinkled, stooped, or feeble, we infer that they are old, when in fact they might be younger persons who have had some illness or disability. When we see people who are dark-haired, smooth skinned, erect, and vigorous, we infer that they are young, when actually they may be elders who are in good health, have dyed their hair, and have had a face lift. In either case, our perceptions confirm our stereotypes because we identify as old only those who fit our stereotypes of old people. The fact that most people older than age sixty-five do not fit the negative stereotypes is not perceived, precisely *because* they do not fit the stereotypes.

Death Anxiety

Anxiety about death may be a cause of ageism because aging is associated with death, and many people fear death more than anything else. People fear aging because it is assumed that each year older brings one closer to death. In a sense this is true, but it should be balanced by the equal truth that each year survived extends one's life expectancy (expected age at death) by several months. For example, each year survived beyond age sixty-five increases one's life expectancy by about five months (National Center for Health Statistics, 2000).

See also AGE DENIAL; BLAMING THE AGED; CULTURAL SOURCES OF AGEISM

REFERENCES

Adorno, T., Frenel-Brunswick, E., Levinson, D., and Sanford, R. (1950). *The authoritarian personality.* New York: Harper & Row.

Binstock, R. (1983). The aged as scapegoat. *The Gerontologist, 23,* 136.

Christie, R., and Cook, P. (1958). A guide to published literature relating to the authoritarian personality. *Journal of Psychology,* (April), 171.

Kogan, N. (1973). Attitudes toward old people. *Journal of Abnormal and Social Psychology,* 62, 44.

National Center for Health Statistics (2000). *Vital statistics of the United States: Life tables.* Washington, DC: U.S. Government Printing Office.

Palmore, E. (1998). *The facts on aging quiz.* New York: Springer.

_____ (1999). *Ageism.* New York: Springer.

Simpson, G. and Yinger, J. (1985). *Racial and cultural minorities.* New York: Plenum.

Sullivan, P. and Adelson, J. (1954). Ethnocentrism and misanthropy. *Journal of Abnormal and Social Psychology,* (April), 246.

Thorson, J., Whatley, L., and Hancock, K. (1974). Attitudes toward the aged as a function of age and education. *The Gerontologist,* 14, 316.

INTERGENERATIONAL PROJECTS

Erdman B. Palmore

One of the most effective ways to reduce prejudice is equal-status personal contact in a cooperative activity (Simpson and Yinger, 1985). All three aspects of this kind of activity must be present for it to be effective. It must be equal-status because unequal-status activity may only reinforce the prejudices against the lower-status participants (e.g., slavery). It must be personal contact, not some abstract theorizing. Third, it must be cooperative activity, because competitive activity may increase hostility and prejudice.

Intergenerational projects usually fit all three criteria: the older and younger participants have more or less equal status; there is personal contact; and the participants work together cooperatively. Aday and colleagues (1996) found that an intergenerational project involving several activities shared by fourth-grade students and elderly volunteers resulted in significant attitude improvement toward the elders by the students.

Similarly, an evaluation of a "friendly visitor" program in Ontario, which involved high school students interacting socially with senior citizens in the community, found that general attitudes of the students toward the aged improved. Also the experience of college students working with elders in a laboratory resulted in improved attitudes of the students toward elders (Shoemaker and Rowland, 1993).

Meaningful, equal-status, cooperative, and enjoyable intergenerational projects are time-consuming and difficult to organize; but the resulting improvement in attitudes may be worth it.

See also CHANGE STRATEGIES

REFERENCES

Aday, R. (1996). Changing children's perceptions of the elderly: The effects of intergenerational contact. *Gerontology and Geriatrics Education,* 16, 37.

Shoemaker, A. and Rowland, V. (1993). Do laboratory experiences change college students' attitudes toward the elderly? *Educational Gerontology,* 19, 295.

Simpson, G. and Yinger, J. (1985). *Racial and cultural minorities.* New York: Plenum.

ISOLATION

Erdman B. Palmore

A common stereotype about elders is that they are socially isolated. Nearly 50 percent of respondents to the Facts on Aging Quiz (FAQ) mistakenly thought that "The majority of old people are socially isolated and lonely" and that "The majority of old people live alone" (Palmore, 1998). Two-thirds of persons younger than sixty-five think that loneliness is a very serious problem for most old people (Harris, 1981).

In fact, most elders are not socially isolated. About two-thirds live with their spouse or family (Coward and Netzer, 2001). Only about 4 percent of elders are extremely isolated, and most of these have had lifelong histories of withdrawal (Kahana, 2001). Most elders have close relatives within easy visiting distance, and contacts between them are relatively frequent. A decline does occur in total social activity with age, but the total number of persons in the social network remains steady (Palmore, 1981).

However, some elders react to ageism by attempting to avoid it through isolating themselves from younger persons (Palmore, 1999). They avoid leaving home as much as possible, they order food and supplies by telephone or the Internet to be delivered, they order clothes by mail order catalogs or online. In this way they can avoid facing ageism from younger people.

The costs of such isolation are difficult to estimate, but isolation may contribute to mental and physical illness, unnecessary institutionalization, depression and suicide. The costs to younger people include the loss of the wisdom and guidance that elders have to offer; the loss of personal knowledge of what aging is really like; the development of unrealistic fears and prejudices about aging; and the loss of the emotional support and enjoyment that is provided by normal relations with older people.

See also AGE SEGREGATION; AGE STRATIFICATION; RESPONSES TO AGEISM

REFERENCES

Coward, R. and Netzer, J. (2001). Coresidence. In G. Maddox (Ed.), *The encyclopedia of aging.* New York: Springer.

Harris, L. (1981). *Aging in the eighties.* Washington, DC: The National Council on the Aging.

Kahana, B. (2001). Isolation. In G. Maddox (Ed.), *The encyclopedia of aging.* New York: Springer.

Palmore, E. (1981). *Social patterns in normal aging.* Durham, NC: Duke University Press.

_____ (1998). *The facts on aging quiz.* New York: Springer.

_____ (1999). *Ageism.* New York: Springer.

J

JAPAN

Erdman B. Palmore

Japan provides many examples of *positive ageism* (Palmore, 1999). Most older people are respected and honored *because* of their age. This respect is shown in the following traditional customs (Palmore, 1985):

- The oldest male in the household is usually given the seat of honor (in front of the *tokonoma,* the alcove in which scrolls, flowers, or art objects are displayed). The oldest female is seated in the next highest seat of honor.
- The same order of prestige is followed in serving food: the oldest male first and the oldest female second.
- The same order of prestige is followed in going through doorways.
- The same order of prestige is followed in bathing: the older persons get to use the family *ofuro* (hot tub) before younger persons.
- Older persons walk in front of younger persons on the street.
- There is a special national holiday called Respect for Aged Day *(Keiro no hi).*
- On buses and trains, special seats are reserved for the elderly.
- Younger people show their deference to older people by bowing lower and longer than do the older people.
- Japanese also show deference to elders by using a different set of words and grammar when a younger person is talking to an older person.

In fact, some have said that Japan has a *gerontocracy* in which the elders rule by virtue of their age. This is an exaggeration, but the leaders in business, education, religion, and other institutions do tend to be older.

On the other hand, resentment appears to be growing against the power of older people, and against the onerous duties of caring for infirm parents. As the Japanese culture becomes more Westernized, the traditional respect and honor for older persons appears to be waning.

See also CROSS-CULTURAL AGEISM; TYPOLOGIES

REFERENCES

Palmore, E. (1985). *The honorable elders revisited.* Durham, NC: Duke University Press.

_____ (1999). *Ageism.* NY: Springer.

JOURNALISM

Erdman B. Palmore

Until the 1970s, journalists tended to ignore the aged (Kleyman, 2001; Palmore, 1999). When they did write about older people they wrote about one of two extremes: either the severely disadvantaged (human sympathy stories) or the "exotics," those elders who were interesting because they accomplished feats not considered in keeping with their age (e.g., hang gliding or skydiving). Sometimes elders were praised for their accomplishments *despite* their age—as if it is unusual for older people to accomplish anything. These approaches reinforced stereotypes and ageism.

Journalists now have begun to respond more sensitively to older people, both as subjects and as readers (Vesperi, 1994). Four formats have been used to accomplish this:

- An age page that targets older readers
- Monthly or occasional special sections devoted to aging
- The "aging beat," which uses age-related stories as news

- Integrated coverage that tries to integrate political, medical, and social information about aging by reporting on such issues for a general readership

Another format that developed toward the end of the twentieth century is the newsmagazine for the "mature audience." In 2004 three such magazines existed: the AARP's *Modern Maturity,* the *Readers Digest New Choices,* and *Mature Outlook.* Numerous locally distributed free newsmagazines are available such as *Fifty Plus,* which is distributed in North Carolina. These magazines try to avoid ageist images and treatments of elders.

In 1995 the North American Mature Publisher's Association (NAMPA) was founded, which brought together the owners of more than 200 local and regional senior newspapers and magazines. One goal of the group is to improve the uneven quality of journalism devoted to elders, which would include the avoidance of stereotypes and other biased reporting about issues in aging.

In 1993 the Journalists Exchange on Aging (JEoA) was formed and now has more than 600 members who exchange information about aging (Kleyman, 2001). Such exchanges reduce the neglect and the misinformation about aging that was typical of journalism in the past.

However, widespread opinion recognizes that most mainstream media outlets continue to neglect the information and entertainment needs and interests of older persons because of the owner's desire to reach people age eighteen to forty-nine (Grossman, 1999).

A problem continues regarding biased reporting on issues in aging, such as Social Security, Medicare, and the need for prescription drugs (Kleyman, 2001). Ekerdt (1998) documented how the *Kansas City Star* formed a partnership with the antientitlement organization, the Concord Coalition, to undermine public confidence in Social Security, Medicare, and related entitlement programs.

Hopefully, the growing interest and exchange of objective information among journalists about aging and the aged will reduce such biased reporting and other forms of ageism in the media.

See also SOCIETAL AGEISM

REFERENCES

Ekerdt, D. (1998). Entitlements, generational equity, and public-opinion manipulation in Kansas City. *The Gerontologist,* 38, 525.

Grossman, L. (1999). Journalism. In R. Butler, L. Grossman, and M. Oberlink (Eds.), *Life in an older America.* Washington, DC: Twentieth Century Fund.

Kleyman, P. (2001). Journalism and aging. In G. Maddox (Ed.), *The encyclopedia of aging.* New York: Springer.

Palmore, E. (1999). *Ageism.* New York: Springer.

Vesperi, M. (1994). Perspectives on aging in print journalism. In D. Shenk and W. Achenbaum (Eds.), *Changing perceptions of aging and the aged*. New York: Springer.

1

LANGUAGE

Kenneth F. Ferraro
Michael W. Steinhour

Language is one of the primary ways in which ageism is expressed. Every human society has a spoken language that transmits culture and helps interpret reality for its members. Language is used to convey basic information (e.g., facts necessary for survival), but it is also used to communicate the value of objects and expectations of appropriate behavior. In this way, the image of older people can be embedded in the language of everyday life. In some cases, these negative images about older people will be obvious, but more often the usage will be more subtle.

Ageist language is prevalent in everyday contemporary conversation, reflecting norms and images of older people. Phrases such as "she's getting old" and "dirty old man" connect being older with negative personal traits. Even if no negative personal traits are invoked, patronizing speech can be used to control older people, even if done politely (Hummert and Mazloff, 2001) and/or within the family (Morgan and Hummert, 2000).

Speaking of older people in pejorative ways is not new, but Covey's (1988) historical review revealed more terms used to negatively represent older people in modern societies than in traditional societies. Although there is debate about the role of modernization on the use of ageist language, a plethora of negative terms are used for older people. For instance, older men and women have been referred to as animals (e.g., old goat, no spring chicken) or with terms connoting evil (hag), greed (geezer), or grouchiness (old coot).

Ageist language also appears in the mass media of modern societies. In television shows, older adults may be referred to in disparaging terms or used as the punch line of jokes. References to older adults as frail, greedy, or inept abound in television commercials. Ageist language may be observed in newspapers, magazines, greeting cards, and bumper stickers. The intent may be humorous, but the latent effect is often a pejorative view of being old.

Although one might expect ageist language in communication by the popular media, past research shows that even professionals are not immune to using ageist language (Butler, 1994). Terminology learned in many medical schools gives way to medical ageism and prejudicial attitudes, which can potentially affect behavior. The term *crock* is sometimes applied to those people who have no apparent organic basis for their disease. Older people are also more likely to be labeled a *gork* (God only really knows—what the basis of the person's symptoms really are) because of the longer medical history and lifetime of exposure to risk factors.

The use of ageist language by academicians is a problem because the terminology used by researchers has been shown to affect results of studies. A study of undergraduate students found that the use of terms *old* and *elderly* more negatively influenced attitude measurement than with the phrase *seventy to eighty-five years of age* (Polizzi and Millikin, 2002). Within the field of gerontology, two of the major refereed journals, *Journals of Gerontology (Series B)* and *The Gerontologist,* follow the *Publication Manual of the American Psychological Association* regarding the use of terms such as *elderly* or *aged:* "Elderly is not acceptable as a noun and is considered pejorative by some as an adjective" (American Psychological Association, 2001, p. 69). Most gerontologists recommend using any of the following terms: *older people, older adults,* or *older persons.* Parallel to ethnic and racial groupings, the point is to emphasize the humanity of the individuals: *older people.*

See also CULTURAL SOURCES OF AGEISM; EUPHEMISMS; STEREOTYPES

REFERENCES

American Psychological Association (2001). *Publication manual of the American Psychological Association* (Fifth edition). Washington, DC: Author.
Butler, R. N. (1994). Dispelling ageism: The cross-cutting intervention. In D. Schenk and W. A. Achenbaum (Eds.), *Changing perceptions of aging and the aged.* New York: Springer.

Covey, H. C. (1988). Historical terminology used to represent older people. *The Gerontologist,* 28, 291-297.

Hummert, M. L. and Mazloff, D. C. (2001). Older adults' responses to patronizing advice: Balancing politeness and identity in context. *Journal of Language and Social Psychology,* 20, 167-195.

Morgan, M. and Hummert, M. L. (2000). Perceptions of communicative control strategies in mother-daughter dyads across the life span. *Journal of Communication,* 50, 48-64.

Polizzi, K. G. and Millikin, R. J. (2002). Attitudes toward the elderly: Identifying problematic usage of ageist and overextended terminology in research instructions. *Educational Gerontology,* 28, 367-377.

LEGAL REVIEW PROGRAM

Erdman B. Palmore

The AARP Foundation Litigation Volunteer Legal Review Program is available to help members who have been victims of ageism. The program is staffed by volunteer lawyers who do not charge for reviewing cases involving age discrimination in employment, denial of treatment by an HMO (health maintenance organization), nursing home abuse, consumer scam, or predatory-lending schemes.

AARP members wishing this service should send a letter to AARP Legal Review, PO Box 50228-MM, Washington, DC 20091-0028. The lawyers review the letters and let the writers know whether they have a legal claim worth pursuing. The AARP also recommends submitting information online by e-mailing <litigation@aarp.org>.

LEGAL SYSTEM

Erdman B. Palmore

Older people have a much lower crime rate than younger people, regardless of how it is measured. For example, persons over age sixty-five have about one-tenth the arrest rate for all offenses than the arrest rate for younger persons (Cutler, 2001). Several explanations for this include the following:

- Criminals tend to die young or "retire" from crime before reaching old age.
- Elders usually have more assets and financial security than younger people.
- Elders may have learned that "crime doesn't pay."
- When they do commit a crime, it tends to be a minor offense not included in the FBI's Crime Index.
- When arrested, older offenders tend to receive more lenient sentences than their younger counterparts (Steffensmeier and Motivans, 2000).

This latter fact suggests that some of the difference in crime rates between older and younger persons may be due to positive ageism on the part of police, attorneys, juries, and judges. Some evidence suggests that behavior treated as criminal in younger people may be viewed as less serious when committed by older people. Some reports state that police ignore all sorts of strange behavior by the elderly because the police perceive it as harmless and due to senility (Atchley, 1997).

Also positive ageism is shown when attorneys use more plea bargaining for older offenders, juries convict older defendants less often, and judges give more lenient sentences and more parole to older persons, especially when the person has a relatively "clean" record, or appears to have few years left to live.

Such discrimination in favor of older offenders may result from the stereotype that elders are more kind, honest, and trustworthy than younger people are.

A noted criminologist asserts that there is

> a double standard of law enforcement toward older men and women. Except for the most serious crimes, such as murder, police and prosecutors are inclined to overlook offenses by the elderly, especially women. They often don't make arrests, or if they do, the charges are dismissed. (Chaneles, 1987, p. 49)

This positive ageism in the legal system gives older people an advantage, but tends to undermine equality before the law.

See also BENEFITS OF AGING; STEREOTYPES

REFERENCES

Atchley, R. (1997). *Social forces and aging.* Belmont, CA: Wadsworth.

Chaneles, S. (1987). Growing old behind bars. *Psychology Today,* 48(October), 49.

Cutler, S. (2001). Crime (against and by the elderly). In G. Maddox (Ed.), *The encyclopedia of aging.* New York: Springer.

Steffensmeier, D. and Motivans, M. (2000). Older men and older women in the arms of criminal law. *Journal of Gerontology: Social Sciences,* 55B, S141.

LITERATURE

Marla Harris

Traditionally the elders in a community have occupied a respected role as storytellers, passing on familial and communal histories. Yet the stories told about the elderly in Western literature have frequently reduced older people to stereotypes, revering them as "wise and spiritually profound elders" or ridiculing them as "self-indulgent, doddering old fools" (Waxman, 1997, p. 134). By studying the representation of aging in literature, literary gerontologists foster an awareness of how texts perpetuate ageist attitudes toward older people. Despite the historical predominance of negative stereotyping (Falk and Falk, 1997), there is encouraging evidence that since the 1970s the portrayal of the elderly in fiction, poetry, drama, and autobiography has increasingly become more realistic and less ageist.

In addressing ageism in literature, one must begin by recognizing that the elderly are a diverse group, focusing exclusively on how an older character is depicted in a literary text may erase or displace the ways in which that character is also defined by class, gender, race, and ethnicity. Ageism may also be exacerbated by other forms of discrimination, such as gender bias. Waxman (1990), for instance, has found the older woman in Western literature to be a target of negative ageism disproportionately more often than the older man.

Second, literature itself is not a monolithic entity, but is shaped by multiple factors, including generic conventions, literary traditions, and audience. Even the idea of what constitutes literature is subject to change. Hendricks and Leedham (1989) caution readers to "consider statements regarding aging in the context of the works of which they form a part and in light of the literary conventions and the tone in which they are expressed" (p. 12).

Early studies of ageist attitudes in literature often focused on a particular author, single genre, or on a specific time period (Sohngen, 1977; Clark, 1980; Loughman, 1980). More recently, annotated bibliographies of aging in literature have proved useful resources for both gerontologists and literary critics. Yahnke and Eastman (1990, 1995) primarily identify literary texts in which older characters figure prominently, and Waxman and Wyatt-Brown (1999) highlight nonageist depictions of the elderly in literature.

Recognizing the need to examine ageism outside the confines of contemporary English language literature, Porter and Porter (1984) and Bagnell and Soper (1989) have investigated the representation of the elderly in other national literatures. Again Hendricks and Leedham (1989) warn against misreading: "Whether implicitly or explicitly, commentators addressing aging in literature carry with them an orienting model that prompts them to highlight certain dimensions while underplaying others" (p. 7). Much more work remains to be done in the field of cross-cultural comparison of literary representations of the aged.

In conclusion, ageism in literature has not yet received from either literary critics or social scientists the degree of close critical attention accorded to representations of class, race, ethnicity, and gender. Because of the diversity of literary texts, it is difficult to draw wide-ranging conclusions about ageism in literature. It may be, however, that as awareness of ageism is heightened generally, more authors will consciously create works that are not ageist. Thus Waxman (1990) has coined the term *reifungsroman,* or novel of ripening, to describe a late-twentieth-century genre of fiction, pioneered by writers such as May Sarton and Doris Lessing, that "rejects negative cultural stereotypes of the old woman in aging, seeking to change the society that created these stereotypes" (p. 2). In addition, Wyatt-Brown and Rossen (1993) contest the notion that a writer's creativity declines with age, suggesting that old age may instead provoke writers to experiment with new styles and to explore new subject matter. Ultimately, the most effective challenge to ageism in literature may come from older writers themselves, male as well as female, who are incorporating their own multidimensional experiences of aging into their literary works in ways that defy stereotypes of the elderly (Waxman, 1997).

See also CHILDREN'S LITERATURE; JOURNALISM; STEREOTYPES

REFERENCES

Bagnell, P. and Soper, P. (Eds.) (1989). *Perceptions of aging in literature: A cross-cultural study.* New York: Greenwood.

Clark, M. (1980). The poetry of aging: Views of old age in contemporary American poetry. *The Gerontologist, 20,* 188-191.

Falk, U.A. and Falk, G. (1997). *Ageism, the aged and aging in America: On being old in an alienated society.* Springfield, IL: Charles C Thomas.

Hendricks, J. and Leedham, C. (1989). Making sense: Interpreting historical and cross-cultural literature on aging. In P. Bagnell and P. Soper (Eds.), *Perceptions of aging in literature: A cross-cultural study* (pp. 1-16). New York: Greenwood.

Loughman, C. (1980). Eros and the elderly: A literary view. *The Gerontologist, 20,* 182-187.

Porter, L. and Porter, L. (Eds.) (1984). *Aging in literature.* Troy, MI: International Book Publishers.

Sohngen, M. (1977). The experience of old age as depicted in contemporary novels. *The Gerontologist, 17,* 70-78.

Waxman, B. (1990). *From the hearth to the open road: A feminist study of aging in contemporary literature.* New York: Greenwood.

_____(1997). *To live in the center of the moment: Literary autobiographies of aging.* Charlottesville: U. Press of Virginia.

Waxman, B. and Wyatt-Brown, A. (1999). *Aging in literature: A selective annotated bibliography for gerontology instruction.* Washington, DC: Association for Gerontology in Higher Education.

Wyatt-Brown, A. and Rossen, J. (Eds.) (1993). *Aging and gender in literature: Studies in creativity.* Charlottesville: U. Press of Virginia.

Yahnke, R. and Eastman, R. (1990). *Aging in literature: A reader's guide.* Chicago: American Library Association.

_____ (1995). *Literature and gerontology: A research guide.* Westport, CT: Greenwood, 1995.

LIVING WILLS

Ori Ashman
Becca R. Levy

In theory, living wills provide individuals with the means to express a preference for receiving or foregoing life-extending medical procedures in the event they become incompetent when gravely ill. In practice, the option to receive life-extending measures has been increasingly defined out of existence. For instance, it is disregarded in this statement: "Living will instruments provide that, if an individual's views are expressed in a legal document in advance, medical personnel are instructed . . . to withdraw or withhold certain treatments that would prolong life" (Cicirelli, 1998, p. 187). Elders are the age group most likely to fill out living wills, and they do so most often in the direction of foregoing treatment (Gallup, 1992).

Although the original intent behind living wills was to provide patients with a measure of autonomy, elders filling out these documents are subject to a multitude of external pressures. They may find themselves the targets of positive as well as negative ageism, both having the goal of limiting medical treatment—though for entirely different reasons. A manifestation of positive ageism is the belief that elders should be allowed to choose a dignified death without extreme medical intervention when recovery is not expected. Whereas negative ageism is conveyed, as an example, through physicians who are subject to pressures by managed care to contain costs; they tend to view older patients as less entitled than younger patients to these extreme medical interventions (Levinsky, 1996).

Perhaps the most pervasive influence on living-will decisions by elders is societal beliefs about aging, including the perception that they are excessive users of medical resources (Bailly and DePoy, 1995). These views become internalized by elders, as demonstrated by older respondents who indicated in a survey that one reason for rejecting life-prolonging measures is their belief that "Younger people should be afforded more rigorous or extended interventions than elderly people, who had already lived their lives" (Bailly and DePoy, 1995, p. 225).

In addition, an experimental study demonstrated the link between external pressures, namely societally derived age stereotypes, and the willingness of elders to seek life-extending interventions (Levy, Ashman, and Dror, 1999-2000). Participants were presented with circumstances, based on some types of living wills, in which they were asked to imagine that they had been diagnosed with a fatal illness for which they could choose a life-extending intervention. They were also presented with an array of scenarios that varied the types of cost associated with the intervention—both in terms of finances and family-caregiving effort. It was found that regardless of cost, the older participants subliminally exposed to negative age stereotypes were more likely to reject the life-extending procedure, and those subliminally exposed to positive age stereotypes were more likely to choose the life-extending procedure.

This link between negative age stereotypes and foregoing hypothetical life-extending interventions was not found in young participants for whom these stereotypes are not as salient. Furthermore, the young were more willing to seek medical interventions than the old regardless of stereotype exposure. However, elders who were exposed to the positive age stereotypes did not differ significantly from the young participants in their willingness to seek interventions. These findings are made particularly relevant by the prevalence of negative stereotypes of aging in society (Palmore, 1999).

Another aspect of living wills that may be influenced by negative ageism is how closely the wishes expressed in these documents are followed. A researcher, who interviewed emergency room workers and observed 112 resuscitative attempts at two hospitals, found that "Even when the advance directive was present and known, the extent to which the staff followed [it] . . . depended mostly on the assumed social viability of the patient" (Timmermans, 1998, p. 462). Patients who were perceived to have greater social viability were usually younger. In their cases, the possible existence of these documents was not usually discussed among the emergency room staff. In contrast, patients with low social viability had their documents checked, and the staff's frustration was noted when none existed.

Further support for a relationship between ageism and living wills is suggested through cross-cultural research. In Latin American and Asian societies, which hold more positive views of aging than in the United States (e.g., Holmes and Holmes, 1995; Levy and Langer, 1994; Palmore and Maeda, 1985), elders are less likely to fill out living wills (e.g., Matsumura et al., 2002; Perkins et al., 2002). It has also been found that acculturated Japanese-American elders view living wills more positively than nonacculturated Japanese-American elders (Matsumura et al., 2002).

By looking at the issue from various directions, we find justification to conclude that living wills in this country are not so much a means of elders imposing their preferences on society, as they are a means of society imposing its preferences on elders. In a culture that often limits the opportunities of elders to control their lives, ageism may impede their ability to control their deaths.

See also HEALTH CARE

REFERENCES

Bailly, D. J. and DePoy, E. (1995). Older people's responses to education about advance directives. *Health and Social Work,* 20, 223-228.

Cicirelli, V. G. (1998). Views of elderly people concerning end-of-life decisions. *Journal of Applied Gerontology,* 17, 186-203.

Gallup, J. (1992). *That Gallup Poll: Public opinion 1991.* Wilmington, DE: Scholarly Resources Inc.

Holmes, E. R. and Holmes, L. D. (1995). *Other cultures, elder years.* Thousand Oaks, CA: Sage.

Levinsky, N. G. (1996). The purpose of advance medical planning—Autonomy for patients or limitation of care? *The New England Journal of Medicine,* 335, 741-743.

Levy, B., Ashman, O., and Dror, I. (1999-2000). To be or not to be: The effects of aging stereotypes on the will to live. *Omega: Journal of Death and Dying,* 40, 409-420.

Levy, B. R. and Langer, E. J. (1994). Aging free from negative stereotypes: Successful memory in China and among the American deaf. *Journal of Personality and Social Psychology,* 66, 989-997.

Matsumura, S., Bito, S., Liu, H., Kahn, K., Fukuhara, S., Kagawa-Singer, M., and Wenger, N. (2002). *Journal of General Internal Medicine,* 17, 531-539.

Palmore, E. B. (1999). *Ageism.* New York: Springer.

Palmore, E. B. and Maeda, D. (1985). *The honorable elders revisited.* Durham, NC: Duke University Press.

Perkins, H. S., Geppert, C. M. A., Gonzales, A., Cortez, J. D., and Hazuda, H. P. (2002). Cross-cultural similarities and differences in attitudes about advance careplanning. *Journal of General Internal Medicine,* 17, 48-57.

Timmermans, S. (1998). Social death as self-fulfilling prophecy: David Sudnow's "Passing On" revisited. *The Sociological Quarterly,* 39, 453-472.

m

MANDATORY RETIREMENT OF JUDGES

Charles F. Blanchard

All United States Supreme Court Justices, all U.S. Circuit Court judges, and all U.S. District Court judges are known as "Article III judges," deriving their names from Section 1 of Article III of the U.S. Constitution and hold their offices during their "good behaviour" or for life. The majority of U.S. Supreme Court Justices are over seventy and two are in their eighties. Likewise, many of the federal lower-court judges are past the age of seventy. Yet not since the days of Franklin D. Roosevelt, when his court-packing proposal failed, have any serious objections been raised to the advanced ages of many of the federal judges.

The main reason that almost no efforts have been made to require mandatory retirements of federal judges is the existance of very liberal retirement benefits offered to these judges that permit them to use a judicial program whereby when the age of the judge plus his or her length of service equals eighty the judge may retire on full salary plus cost of living adjustments for the life of the judge as well as for his or her spouse, as long as the spouse remains unmarried after the judge's death. Despite this bountiful provision, many federal judges continue to serve long after they reach the age of seventy-two because they simply like what they do.

For many years there were no age provisions for State judges, but in the past few decades the majority of states have passed statutes or changes to their constitutions requiring that State judges retire at a certain age, generally between the ages of sixty-eight and seventy-two. There have been many challenges to the legality of these mandatory retirement provisions, most of which have concentrated on the application of the Federal Age Discrimination in Employment Act (ADEA). Other attacks against such provisions focus on the constitutional guarantee of equal protection.

With only a few exceptions, these attacks have failed primarily because the retirement plans were deemed to be a legitimate way to maintain a vigorous and efficient judiciary and to eliminate the unpleasant need to remove unfit, elderly judges *(Keefe v. Eyrich)*.

In *Malmed v. Thornburg,* upholding a compulsory retirement statute, the court observed that individual removal proceedings were exceptional. Moreover, even if they were regularly and efficiently used to remove judges disabled by senility or other causes, concern for the harmful effects on the judicial system of even one senile judge and the desire to avoid the unpleasantness and public humiliation associated with an individual removal support the preference for employing mandatory retirement to address the problems of the senility of even a few older judges.

In the landmark case of *Gregory v. Ashcroft,* the U.S. Supreme Court affirmed a Missouri statute requiring compulsory retirement of judges reaching the age of seventy. The court held that the statute did not violate the Equal Protection Clause of the Fifth Amendment and that the appointed Missouri judges were not protected by the provisions of ADEA. As justification of mandatory retirement provisions the court decided that the need to draw a line to ensure the high competency required for judicial service, the desire to avoid difficult decisions and determining when judges are not physically and mentally qualified to continue service, increasing the opportunity for other persons to serve in the judiciary, and providing predictability in ease establishing and administering retirement plans for judges.

"The People of Missouri rationally can conclude that the threat of deterioration at age 70 is sufficiently great, and the alternatives for removal sufficiently inadequate, that they will require all judges to step aside at age 70" *(Gregory v. Ashcroft,* p. 452).

On the state level there are two categories of judges: *elected* and *appointed*. Most state court decisions have held that both elected and appointed judges may be compelled to retire at a specified age and do not have protection under ADEA. Since both groups fall within the appointees on the policymaking level exception to the ADEA, the rational that the decision making engaged in by common law judges such as petitioners, places them on the policymaking level. A minority of the states considering the question has concluded that appointed state judges are protected by ADEA because they are not elected state officials and are not on the policy making level under the provisions of ADEA.

The problem with most of the cases concerning this subject is that the mandatory retirement treats all judges who have reached the age of seventy (or seventy-two) as if they were incompetent. As Severson has noted, "that to assume that these older judges are unfit to perform their judicial duties, simply because some persons of like age have certain characteristics, is to condemn by statistical stereotype" (p. 858). By upholding mandatory retirement at a specific age is to adhere to "an obsolete scheme of retirement reflected in ancient, illogical, and now repudiated policy substituting chronological age for individualized physical/mental evaluation" (Severson, 1994, p. 882). ADEA has eliminated age discrimination for some judges (except federal) but seem to remain a suspect group when reaching age seventy or seventy-two. Generally, they are entitled to no relief because of this arbitrary disability forced down upon them.

Most states have provided for liberal pay for judges who involuntarily retire after long service or when reaching the age of seventy or seventy-two. Their retirement pay is generally on a much less generous basis than is available to federal judges. These provisions, however, are not nearly so helpful to judges who serve in the latter parts of their careers, in which case the amount of compensation after retirement can be somewhat meager compared to that of their federal counterparts.

See also EMPLOYMENT DISCRIMINATION

REFERENCES

Gregory v. Ashcroft 501U.S.452 (1991).
Keefe v. Eyrich, 22 Ohio St. 3d 164, 489 NE 2d 259 (1986).
Malmed v. Thornburg, 621F 2d 565, CA3Pa (1980).
Severson, Darlene M. (1994). 17 Mitchell Law Review, 858, 882.

MEASURING AGEISM IN CHILDREN

Sheree T. Kwong See
Robert B. Heller

Children's ageist attitudes are comprised of their feelings about older people and their beliefs and expectations (stereotypes) about what older people are like. These attitudes are manifested in differential treatment or behavior directed at older people compared to younger people. Charting the development of ageist attitudes in children is useful for isolating mechanisms that contribute to ageism and provides the groundwork for the design and evaluation of early interventions aimed at promoting positive attitudes toward aging (Montepare and Zebrowitz, 2002).

The study of ageism among young adults has had a long history and has been a key focus in the social gerontological literature (Kite and Wagner, 2002). Ageism in children, however, has received relatively less attention. The latter partly reflects methodological challenges inherent in measuring ageism in children. Here we briefly summarize common methods that have been used to examine ageism in children, what these techniques have revealed about children's attitudes, and limitations associated with methods we call direct assessments (see Kwong See and Ryan, 1999). Direct assessments measure ageism by first prompting children to think about older people, for example by using verbal instructions or pictures as cues, and then asking for conscious (direct) judgments on attitude measures. Indirect techniques, in contrast, do not ask children to make conscious decisions about older people themselves but rather, allow one to infer children's beliefs and feelings about older people by observing children's behavior toward older persons, usually in the context of performing tasks that in no way appear to be measures of ageism. We conclude that indirect assessments offer a new direction for measuring ageism in children.

Direct Assessments

Direct assessments measure attitudes using self-report on open-ended questions (e.g., What will it be like to be old?), closed-ended questions (e.g., Which person is the oldest?), semantic differential scales (e.g., making judgments on a scale bound by bipolar adjectives such as good-bad, rich-poor), Likert statements (e.g., indicating degree of agreement to statements such as "Old people are nice"), and by having children rank their preferences (e.g., rank pictures of persons differing in age in terms of with whom one would most like to interact). Combinations of these measures are found in published instruments that have been specially developed to measure attitudes in children and include the "Children's Attitude Toward the Elderly" (Jantz et al., 1977), "Children's Views on Aging" (Marks, Newman, and Onawola, 1985), social attitude scale of ageist prejudice (Isaacs and Bearison, 1986), and children's perception of aging and the elderly (Rich, Myrick, and Campbell, 1983).

In a recent review of the children's attitude literature, Montepare and Zebrowitz (2002), concluded that children as young as four years of age (1) possess negative feelings toward older adults, (2) have beliefs (stereotypes) that are similar to the beliefs of younger adults in that children expect losses in physical and cognitive attributes but gains in social characteristics in aging, and (3) indicate a preference for behavioral activities that discriminate against older adults. (See Kite and Johnson, 1988, for a review of the young-adult literature.)

Montepare and Zebrowitz (2002) also identify an important methodological issue unique to the developmental literature. The use of visual stimuli significantly increases the likelihood of finding negative attitudes toward the elderly in children. One explanation for this finding may be in how images are selected. For example, the drawings on the widely used children's attitudes toward the elderly instrument (Jantz et al., 1977) were constructed to control for gender (male) and facial expression (neutral). However, the neutral expressions of older adults are often perceived to be sadder than neutral expressions in younger adults (Malatesta, Fiore, and Messina, 1987). This bias in the stimulus materials may lead to further negative effects that generalize to other attitude measures on the instrument.

Another possibility is based on the work of Hummert, Garstka, and Shaner (1997), who showed that photographs can easily be classified into negative and positive age-related stereotypes by college students and that older adults and adults with neutral expressions were more likely to be categorized into a negative age stereotype.

In the developmental literature, photographs and drawings of older adults, especially those with neutral expressions, may have led to the prompting of negative stereotypes associated with aging as opposed to positive stereotypes, and ultimately an overly negative depiction of children's beliefs and feelings about aging.

Finally, it is generally known in the developmental literature that children are heavily influenced by visual information and may respond more strongly to the negative features often associated with facial ageing. Consistent with this statement, children almost universally express a negative attitude toward physical aspects of aging (Montepare and Zebrowitz, 2002). Using images as prompts may be a useful point of reference for preliterate populations, however, more work needs to be done on identifying the key variables that influence measures of attitudes that are derived from images.

Another methodological issue involves the widespread use of semantic differential scales to investigate attitudes in children (e.g., Caspi, 1984; Chapman and Neal, 1990; Couper, Sheehan, and Thomas, 1991; Fillmer, 1984; Jantz et al., 1977; Krause and Chapin, 1987; Marks, Newman, and Onawola, 1985; Thomas and Yamamota, 1975). The semantic differential task is based on the classic work of Osgood, Suci, and Tannenbaum (1957), who found that attitudes toward many objects could be characterized along universal dimensions labeled *evaluative, potency,* and *activity.* They determined this by having many respondents rate a number of stimulus objects using a large set of bipolar adjectives and used statistical techniques to reduce the large set of adjectives into this smaller set of dimensions or factors.

Despite the widespread use of the semantic differential in the children's literature with young persons and old persons as attitudinal objects, there is no consensus on which set of bipolar adjectives items should be included or how the attitudinal object (older person) should be presented (visually using pictures or a verbal description). Moreover, there has been little research on the validity and reliability of a semantic differential in children.

It is interesting to note that Rosencrantz and McNevin (1969) developed the aging semantic differential instrument for use with adults as a means of measuring attitudes. Their instrument was developed by piloting a large set of adjective pairs on a large number of participants to produce a thirty-two-item scale that was further validated on an additional sample of participants to reveal three unique attitudinal dimensions toward the elderly (instrumental-ineffective, autonomous-dependent, and personal acceptability-unacceptability). Unfortunately, there has been no comparable instrument developed for use with children.

From a developmental perspective, many of the direct assessments found on instruments for children place heavy demands on their cognitive and language capabilities. Children are often asked to consider multiple visual stimuli (pictures) at once in rank-order tasks, and both Likert statements and semantic differential measures require children to either compare abstract concepts (e.g., good-bad, rich-poor) simultaneously in order to render judgments or to entertain multiple possibilities. Given the significant developments in children's memory and attention capacity between five and twelve years of age (Shaffer, Wood, and Willoughby, 2002), any more than general conclusions based on very young children's responses on such measures are suspect.

Perhaps the biggest drawback of direct assessments is that the methodology is transparent and subject to demand awareness (Dobrosky and Bishop, 1986; Kwong See and Ryan, 1999). That is, children may give responses they believe the researcher is looking for and as a result, it may appear that children are ageist. Arguably, the results from direct assessments indicate that children *know* cultural stereotypes about aging and older adults but it is unclear from direct assessments that children *believe* the stereotypes and would subsequently behave in a prejudicial way toward older people. The evidence from direct assessments would be strengthened if it could be shown that children behave differently toward older adults in situations in which the goal of measuring ageism is not transparent. Moreover, behavioral evidence would provide support for the interpretation from direct assessments that children actually do believe what they report on attitude measures.

Indirect Assessments

Indirect measures of attitudes infer children's feelings about older adults and their beliefs about aging based on differential behavior with older as opposed to younger persons. Very few studies have used this approach. In one study, four-, six-, and eight-year-old children were asked to work with either a younger (thirty-five-year-old) or older (seventy-five-year-old) adult on a puzzle (Isaacs and Bearison,

1986). Ageism was measured indirectly using several behavioral measures. Showing ageism, children sat farther from the older person, initiated eye contact less often, spoke fewer words, initiated conversation less frequently, and made fewer appeals for assistance or verification with the older person compared to the younger person. Nicely, this study also used an attitude measure (a direct measure) and found that scores on the attitude scale and the behavioral measures correlated such that children who indicated more negative attitudes on the direct measure sat farther from the older person and initiated eye contact less (indirect measures).

An indirect approach to assessing children's ageism was also taken by Kwong See and Rasmussen (2002). These researchers used a modified Piagetian number conservation task to assess young children's attitudes. In a Piagetian number conservation task a preoperational-age child (spanning ages four to seven years approximately) is asked if two aligned rows of objects have the same number or if one of the rows has more. After the child agrees that the lines are the same, the experimenter transforms one of the lines so that it is longer and the child is asked the question a second time. Five-year-old children typically indicate that the longer row has more after the transformation. Rather than reflecting failure to conserve number, it has been shown that children's responses reflect beliefs about the experimenter's reason for asking the same question twice in short succession (e.g., McGarrigle and Donaldson, 1975).

To indirectly probe children's beliefs about aging, five-year-old children were tested according to the standard procedure but either a young experimenter (female in her twenties) or older experimenter (female in her seventies) asked the second question after the transformation. Kwong See and Rasmussen (2002) reasoned that if children believe the young experimenter is competent, they think she is not likely duped by the transformation and must be asking about length. If children associate older age with incompetence, however, they may believe the older experimenter is asking the question because she is confused by the transformation and is legitimately asking for information about number. The expectation that a focus on length or number should differ across the experimenter conditions was supported. In the young experimenter condition 62 percent of children said the longer line had more. Only 20 percent of the children in the old experimenter condition gave this response, with 80 percent of the children providing answers focused on number.

Together the few studies assessing children's attitudes indirectly indicate an early start to ageism in children (seen as early as four and five years of age). The Kwong See and Rasmussen (2002) study suggests that as has been found in the young adult literature, children associate older age with incompetence (Kwong See, Hoffman, and Wood, 2001). The Isaacs and Bearison (1986) study suggests that negativity toward aging and older persons can be shown not only on attitude scale measures but also in prejudicial behavior of children toward older people.

Conclusions and Future Direction

Studies that have assessed children's attitudes directly and indirectly provide converging evidence for ageism in children and that ageism has an early start. Studies taking an indirect approach are few in number but the examples highlighted in this article demonstrate the potential of such approaches for revealing ageism in very young children because the key measures are behavioral and do not place heavy cognitive and language demands on children as the attitude measures typically used in direct assessments. Direct approaches are also fraught with a number of methodological limitations that make the development of direct assessments challenging.

Fruitful avenues for future research on ageism in children include more focused examination of the characteristics of older adults that cue ageist behaviors well as cross-cultural comparisons to ascertain the universality amongst children. Indirect assessments will likely feature prominently in these emerging research directions.

(*Note:* Preparation of this article was supported by grant G124130227 from the Social Sciences and Humanities Research Council of Canada. Correspondence concerning this article can be addressed to Sheree T. Kwong See, Department of Psychology, P220 Biological Sciences Building, University of Alberta, Edmonton, Alberta, Canada, T6G 2E9. Email: <kwongsee@ualberta.ca> or to Robert Heller, Centre for Psychology, Athabasca University, Athabasca, Alberta, Canada, T9S 3A3. Email: <bobh@athabascau.ca>.)

See also CHILDREN'S ATTITUDES; STEREOTYPES; UNCONSCIOUS AGEISM

REFERENCES

Caspi, A. (1984). Contact hypothesis and inter-age attitudes: A field study of cross-age. *Social Psychology Quarterly,* 47, 74-80.

Chapman, N. and Neal, M. (1990). The effects of intergenerational experiences on adolescents and older adults. *The Gerontologist,* 30, 825-832.

Couper, D., Sheehan, N., and Thomas, E. (1991). Attitude toward old people: The impact of an intergenerational program. *Educational Gerontology,* 17, 41-53.

Dobrosky, B. and Bishop, J. (1986). Children's perception of old people. *Educational Gerontology,* 12, 429-439.

Fillmer, H. (1984). Children's descriptions of and attitudes toward the elderly. *Educational Gerontology,* 10, 99-107.

Hummert, M., Garstka, T., and Shaner, J. (1997). Stereotyping of older adults: The role of target facial cues and perceiver characteristics. *Psychology and Aging,* 12, 107-114.

Isaacs, L. W. and Bearison, D. J. (1986). The development of children's prejudice against the aged. *International Journal of Aging and Human Development,* 23, 175-194.

Jantz, R., Seefeldt, C., Galper, A., and Serock (1977). Children's attitudes toward the elderly. *Social Education,* 41, 518-523.

Kite, M. E. and Johnson, B. T. (1988). Attitudes toward older and younger adults: A meta-analysis. *Psychology and Aging,* 3, 233-244.

Kite, M. E. and Wagner, L. S. (2002). Attitudes toward older adults. In T. D. Nelson (Ed.), *Ageism: Stereotyping and prejudice against older persons* (pp. 129-161). Cambridge, MA: MIT Press.

Krause, D. and Chapin, R. (1987). An examination of attitudes about old age in a sample of elementary school children. *Gerontology and Geriatrics Education,* 7, 81-91.

Kwong See, S. T., Hoffman, H. G., and Wood, T. L. (2001). Perceptions of an old female eyewitness: Is the older eyewitness believable? *Psychology and Aging,* 16, 346-350.

Kwong See, S. T. and Rasmussen, C. (2002). An early start to age stereotyping: Children's beliefs about an older experimenter. Paper presented at the annual meeting of the Gerontological Society of America. Boston, MA. November.

Kwong See, S. T. and Ryan, E. B. (1999). Intergenerational communication: The survey interview as a social exchange. In N. Schwarz, D. Park, B. Knauper, and S. Sudman (Eds.), *Cognition, aging, and self-reports* (pp. 245-262). Philadelphia: Psychology Press.

Malatesta, C., Fiore, M., and Messina, J. (1987). Affect, personality and expressive characteristics of older people. *Psychology and Aging,* 2, 64-69.

Marks, R., Newman, S., and Onawola, R. (1985). Latency-aged children's views of aging. *Educational Gerontology,* 11, 89-99.

McGarrigle, J. and Donaldson, M. (1975). Conservation accidents. *Cognition,* 3, 341-350.

Montepare, J. M. and Zebrowitz, L. A. (2002). A social-developmental view of ageism. In T. D. Nelson (Ed.), *Ageism: Stereotyping and prejudice against older persons* (pp. 77-125). Cambridge, MA: MIT Press.

Osgood, C., Suci, G., and Tannenbaum, P. (1957). *The measurement of meaning.* Urbana: University of Illinois Press.

Rich, P., Myrick, R., and Campbell, C. (1983). Changing children's perception of the elderly. *Educational Gerontology,* 9, 483-491.

Rosencrantz, H. and McNevin, T. (1969). A factor analysis of attitudes toward the aged. *The Gerontologist,* 9, 55-59.

Shaffer, D. R., Wood, E., and Willoughby, T. (2002). *Developmental psychology: Childhood and adolescence* (First Canadian edition). Scarborough, Ontario: Nelson.

Thomas, E. and Yamamoto, K. (1975). Attitudes toward age: An exploration in school-age children. *International Journal of Aging and Human Development,* 6, 117-129.

MEDICAL STUDENTS

Kathryn R. Remmes
Becca R. Levy

Acquiring negative views of older patients seems be an unofficial component of the learning experience at medical schools. Accordingly, Robert Butler (Congress, 2002) writes that it is "important to address the ageism that is rooted in medical schools and pervades the medical system. In fact, it is there that a medical student may first become conscious of the medical profession's prejudice toward age" (p. 5). As an example, in medical school, students are exposed to code words for older patients that may help to shape their views of them, including "COP" (crotchety old patient), "LOL in NAD" (little old lady in no apparent distress) and "toad," which is defined as a patient who is "old, debilitated, and sometimes incontinent" (Coombs et al., 1993, p. 991).

Even though entering medical students may have spent more than twenty years being exposed to the negative ageism that is prevalent in society, they are initially resistant to its appearance in medical school. The pejorative terms are at first considered demeaning to older patients, but this resistance gives way to accommodation: one student described the jargon as a means to becoming "indoctrinated into the language and culture" of the medical community (Parsons et al., 2001, p. 547).

As products of this acculturation, medical students hold myriad misconceptions, mostly negative, regarding their older patients. For example, more than 90 percent of 517 medical students interviewed labeled the typical seventy-year-old person as ineffective, dependent, and unacceptable (Rueben et al., 1995). In addition, medical students have described older patients as disagreeable, inactive, socially undesirable, socially withdrawn, more emotionally ill, and economically burdensome by acting as a drain on public resources and by abusing the health care system (Spence et al., 1968; Tarbox, Connors, and Faillace, 1987). It therefore follows that medical students often prefer younger patients to older patients (Perrotta et al., 1981).

These perceptions may influence interactions with older patients. One study found that medical students tend to lack empathy toward older patients (Pendergast et al., 1984). Moreover, medical students are less likely to aggressively treat life-threatening illnesses of older patients, as compared to younger patients (e.g., Madan, Aliabadi-Wahle, and Beech, 2001).

Formal training in geriatrics in medical school is quite limited. Pediatric training is required at all 145 medical schools in the nation, but less than 10 percent of them require geriatric courses, and only three have geriatric departments (Butler et al., 2002; Kovner, Mezey, and Harrington, 2002). Although individuals sixty-five years and older account for 23 percent of all ambulatory visits and for 45 percent of all days of care spent in hospitals (Reuben et al., 1995), the older patient is rarely a focus of study in medical schools; instead the focus is most often on the young, healthy male (Mendelsohn et al., 1994). In the two years of coursework, one of the few exposures that a medical student may have to elders is during the dissection of a cadaver.

Medical students participate in clinical training during their third and fourth years, which usually consist of one-month rotations through different types of medical settings. Geriatric clinical rotations have had limited success in generating more positive views of older patients or in encouraging the students to pursue a career in geriatric medicine (Griffith and Wilson, 2001; Powers et al., 2002). This may be due to the difficulty in reversing the preceding two years of negative attitude formation in medical school. Also, many of the geriatric rotations involve only seriously ill patients, including those in hospices, rather than a mixture of inpatients and outpatients (Griffith and Wilson, 2001).

However, an intervention study showed that second-year medical students who attended a course on the health of elders in their first year had increased positive attitudes toward the older patient, as compared to their peers who did not take the course (Wilson and Hafferty, 1980). Furthermore, this cohort was reassessed after its fourth year of medical school, and it was found that positive views of the older patient had been maintained (Wilson and Hafferty, 1983).

It appears, then, that even a modicum of institutional change is effective in helping to mitigate the culture of negative ageism that has characterized medical school training. If this approach becomes the rule, rather than the exception, medical schools will be in a better position to help future physicians cope with an aging population.

See also GERIATRICS; HEALTH CARE

REFERENCES

Butler, R. N., Estrine, J., Honig, M., Lifsey, D., Muller, C., and O'Brien, N. (2002). *A national crisis: The need for geriatric faculty training and development.* New York: International Longevity Center.

Congress (2002).The image of aging in media and marketing: Hearing before Special Committee on Aging, Senate, 107th Congress, 2nd Session.

Coombs, R. H., Chopra, S., Schenk, D. R., and Yutan, E. (1993). Medical slang and its function. *Social Science and Medicine,* 36, 987-998.

Griffith, C. H. and Wilson, J. F. (2001). The loss of idealism in the 3rd-year clinical clerkships. *Evaluation and the Health Professions,* 24, 61-71.

Kovner, C. T., Mezey, M., and Harrington, C., (2002). Who cares for older adults? Workforce implications of an aging Society: Geriatrics needs to join pediatrics as a required element of training the next generation of health care professionals. *Health Affairs,* 21, 78-89.

Madan, A. K., Aliabadi-Wahle, S., and Beech, D. J. (2001). Ageism in medical students' treatment recommendations: The example of breast-conserving procedures. *Academic Medicine,* 76, 282-284.

Mendelsohn, K. D., Nieman, L. Z., Isaacs, K., Lee, S., and Levison, S. P. (1994). Sex and gender bias in anatomy and physical diagnosis text illustrations. *Journal of the American Medical Association,* 272, 1267-1270.

Parsons, G. P., Kinsman, S.B., Bosk, C. L., Sankar, P., and Ubel, P. A. (2001). Between two worlds: Medical student perceptions of humor and slang in the hospital setting. *Journal of General Internal Medicine,* 16, 544-549.

Pendergast, C., Coe, R. M., Eschner, C., and Galofré, A. (1984). Analysis of practice interviews of medical students with elderly persons. *Journal of Medical Education*, 59, 600-602.

Perrotta, P., Perkins, D., Schimpfhauser, F., and Calkins, E. (1981). Medical student attitudes toward geriatric medicine and patients. *Journal of Medical Education*, 56, 478-483.

Powers, C. S., Savidge, M. A., Allen, R. M., and Cooper-Witt, C. M. (2002). Implementing a mandatory geriatrics clerkship. *Journal of the American Geriatrics Society*, 50, 369-373.

Reuben, D. B., Fullerton, J. T., Tschann, J. M., and Croughan-Minihane, M. (1995). Attitudes of beginning medical students toward older persons: A five-campus study. *Journal of the American Geriatrics Society*, 43, 1430-1436.

Spence, D. L., Feigenbaum, E. M., Fitzgerald, F., and Roth, J. (1968). Medical student attitudes toward the geriatric patient. *Journal of the American Geriatrics Society*, 16, 976-983.

Tarbox, A. R., Connors, G. J., and Faillace, L. A. (1987). Freshman and senior medical students' attitudes toward the elderly. *Journal of Medical Education*, 62, 582-591.

Wilson, J. F. and Hafferty, F. W. (1980). Changes in attitudes toward the elderly one year after a seminar on aging and health. *Journal of Medical Education*, 55, 993- 999.

_____ (1983). Long-term effects of a seminar on aging and health for first-year medical students. *The Gerontologist*, 23, 319-324.

MEMORY AND COGNITIVE FUNCTION

Katherine J. Follett

Memory is the retention of information over time. One of the common fears of growing old is loss of memory and so the loss of the essential self. Unfortunately, a myth of growing old is that an inverse relationship occurs between gray hair and memory; and that the decline in memory interferes with everyday functioning. This ageist myth pictures the older adult as senile, foolish, and confused. What we believe about aging can become our truth (Cavanaugh, 2000), even when the extant literature does not coincide with ageist beliefs. Although evidence supports that general cognitive ability slows in old age (Salthouse, 2000), this slowing is often measured in extra milliseconds needed for processing and does not impinge on the everyday functioning of older adults.

Common Beliefs About Aging and Memory

CRS Syndrome

This "syndrome" (Can't Remember S * * *) may actually peak in middle age when the stresses and hassles of life are often at their greatest. Nevertheless, it is claimed to be a common ailment of old age. It is said that when we lose our car keys at twenty, it is only an ir- ritation; but at forty-five, we think it is a sign of aging. By seventy, we fear it is a sign of dementia. Many older adults claim to be suffering from CRS syndrome. Memory decline is accepted as a natural fact. Cognitive decline, the "mother of memory," is also known to decline. Both of these beliefs are somewhat false and somewhat true; it de- pends on the type of memory. Some memory becomes better with age, some stays the same, and some declines.

Senior Moment

This is also known as a "refrigerator moment," as it occurs all across the life span as soon as one is old enough to stand in front of the open refrigerator and wonder why.

Senility

In their book on successful aging, Rowe and Kahn (1998) categori- cally state, "There is no such thing as senility" (p. 91). Furthermore, they explain that the majority of people maintain their full cognitive functioning with modest, age-related changes in memory. Dementia is not a part of normal aging and afflicts only about 10 percent of peo- ple who are over sixty-five (Rowe and Kahn, 1998). Healthy adults of any age do not show signs of dementia.

Use It or Lose It

Unlike some other sayings related to memory in old age, this has some basis in fact. Keeping mentally active—stretching one's mem- ory while also keeping physically active—appears to be related to mental acuity in middle and old age.

The Nuts and Bolts of Memory

Before further tackling the misconceptions of aging and memory, we must understand a bit more about memory. Memory involves both cognitive mechanics—the hardware of the mind, and cognitive pragmatics—the software of the mind (Baltes, 1993, 1996). Cognitive mechanics, which is biological, involving speed and accuracy of processing as well as other processes such as the abilities related to the senses, tends to decline over time. On the other hand, cognitive pragmatics, including knowledge about life, skills, our self, reading, and writing, and language comprehension, may improve or at least not decline over time (Santrock, 2000).

The information-processing approach to memory presents memory as being comprised of multiple processes. Atkinson and Schiffrin (1968) suggest that memory is structured in three stages: sensory memory, short-term memory, and long-term memory. The processes of memory are sensing, encoding, and retrieval. *Sensing* is effortless and automatic. *Encoding* is either automatic or effortful. Automatic processing happens without our thought or control, whereas effortful processing requires rehearsal (repetition), mnemonics (memory devices, imagery, and cues), and organization (chunking and hierarchies) (Meyers, 2000). *Retrieval* is crucial to memory. An important aspect of retrieval is processing speed. What good is it if a memory is stored but cannot be accessed? Retrieval appears to be where older adults feel they are most challenged.

Long-term memory, the workbench of memory (Baddeley, 1992), is of at least two types: explicit memory (also known as declarative memory), and implicit memory (also know as nondeclarative or procedural memory). *Explicit memory,* memory we are aware of, can be broken down into two substructures, episodic memory and semantic memory. Episodic memory, the where and when of life's happenings (Tulving, 2000), a sort of personal diary (Kausler, 1994; Smith, 1996), is the type of memory that helps us retain our past. Two types of episodic memory are recall and recognition. Semantic memory is our encyclopedia, our store of academic knowledge, expert knowledge, and everyday knowledge. Unlike episodic memory, semantic memory is not directly involved in our sense of self.

The second type of long-term memory, *implicit memory,* is our memory for motor skills, such as riding a bicycle or driving a car, and things we have been conditioned to respond to. This explains why someone who has lost all memory of self might retain the ability to play the piano, swim, or treat a kitten with the utmost gentleness.

Some types of memory, such as prospective memory, which involves remembering to do something in the future, seem to improve with age (Moscovitch, 1982; Patton and Meit, 1993; Zacks, Hasher, and Li, 2000). In addition, older adults were found to have better prospective memory than middle-aged adults (Park et al., 1999). Thus, older adults were found to be more reliable in taking medications than middle-aged adults, presumably because of middle-aged adults' hectic lifestyles.

Other memory, such as autobiographical memory, an aspect of episodic memory, seems to show little decline over time (Bahrick, Bahrick, and Wittlinger, 1975). Implicit memory also appears to be relatively unaffected by age but there are contradictory findings and the verdict is still not in on whether conceptually based implicit memory or perceptually based implicit memory are impacted differentially by age or at all. When written material is well organized, clearly structured, and focuses on main ideas, younger and older adults are similar in remembering the gist of the information (Cavanaugh and Blanchard-Fields, 2002).

Although some decline has been found in working memory (Light, 2000), Schimamura and colleagues (1995) found that professors show very little decline in working memory. Thus, working memory decline is not universal but is perhaps, in part, dependent upon the "use it or lose it" rule.

The assumption that memory declines with age is not without foundation. Salthouse (2000) has demonstrated that perceptual speed and working memory show declines in late adulthood. This is one of those actual facts of aging and thought by some to underlie much of any measurable decline seen in other areas of memory and cognitive functioning in healthy older adults (Earls and Salthouse, 1995; Salthouse, 2000).

In the realm of episodic memory, when challenged with fast-paced and disorganized information, older adults are disadvantaged relative to younger adults (Cavanaugh and Blanchard-Fields, 2002). How often does this happen to older adults in the real world? Older adults also have more tip-of-the tongue experiences when they are searching for a word and they just cannot seem to get hold of it (MacKay and Abrams, 1996; Smith and Earles, 1996).

Relative to older adults, younger adults appear to be better at processing and retaining knowledge relating to the temporal and spatial contexts in which information was acquired (Light, 1992). Source memory (Spencer and Raz, 1995) and false memories (Jacoby, 1999) are problems in old age. Source memory deals with how you came to know something and whether it was real or imagined. False memory is the memory of things that did not happen. These decrements in old age can be dangerous when scam artists turn them to their advantage. Activity memory declines with age and can be predicted by processing speed (Earles and Coon, 1994; Salthouse, 1992). Therefore, older adults are more apt to have difficulty remembering what activities they have actually done.

Keeping Memory at Its Peak

Training

Rowe and Kahn (1998) explain that even people who have already experienced cognitive decline "can, with appropriate training, improve enough to offset approximately two decades of memory loss" (p. 137).

Education

Numerous researchers have demonstrated that memory and cognition in aging adults is better in those who have higher levels of education (Stern and Carstensen, 2000). In addition, Schaie (1996) found that even the most dramatic age-related decline that may occur in seventy-year-olds is less noticeable in people with higher education.

Lifestyle Choices

In a study of nearly 6,000 women who were all sixty-five or older, Kristine Yaffe found there was a 13 percent reduced chance of cognitive decline for each extra mile walked per week (Underwood and Watson, 2001). Exercise is also known to decrease depression, which is a known factor in poor memory. Rowe and Kahn (1998) emphasize the importance of lung function, physical fitness, attitude, training, social support, and diet in maintaining and improving overall cognitive functioning and memory.

The Bottom Line

Some cognitive decline and loss of memory occurs in old age. However, this decline is little more than an irritation and can, in part, be prevented by lifestyle choices. The belief that all memory seriously declines with age is just an ageist stereotype that is contrary to the facts.

See also MEMORY STEREOTYPES; MENTAL ILLNESS

REFERENCES

Atkinson, R. and Schiffrin, R. (1968). Human memory: A control system and its control processes. In K. Spence (Ed.), *The psychology of learning and motivation,* Volume 2. New York: Academic Press.

Baddeley, A. (1992). Working memory. *Science,* 255, 556-569.

Bahrick, H., Bahrick, P., and Wittlinger, R. (1975). Fifty years of memory for names and faces: A cross-sectional approach. *Journal of Experimental Psychology,* 104, 54-75.

Baltes, P. B. (1993). The aging mind: Potentials and limits. *The Gerontologist,* 33, 580-594.

_____ (1996). On the incomplete architecture of human ontogeny: Selection, optimization, and compensation as foundations of developmental theory. Invited award address presented at the meeting of the American Psychological Association, Toronto, November.

Cavanaugh, J. (2000). Commentary. *American Psychologist,* 31(January), 25.

Cavanaugh, J. and Blanchard-Fields, F. (2002). *Adult development and aging,* (Fourth edition). Belmont, CA: Wadsworth/Thomson Learning.

Earls, J. L. and Coon, V. E. (1994). Adult age differences in long-term memory for performed activities. *Journal of Gerontology: Psychological Sciences,* 49, P32-P34.

Earls, J. and Salthouse, T. (1995). Interrelations of age, health, and speed. *Journal of Gerontology: Psychological Sciences,* 50B, P33-P41.

Jacoby, L. L. (1999). Ironic effects of repetition: Measuring age-related differences in memory. *Journal of Experimental Psychology: Learning, Memory, and Cognition,* 25, 3-22.

Kausler, D. H. (1994). *Learning and memory in normal aging.* San Diego: Academic Press.

Light, L. (1992). The organization of memory in old age. In F. I. M. Craik and T. A. Salthouse (Eds.), *Handbook of aging and cognition.* Mahwah, NJ: Erlbaum.

_____(2000). Memory changes in adulthood. In S. H. Qualls and N. Abeles (Eds.), *Psychology and the aging revolution*. Washington, DC: American Psychological Association.

MacKay, D. and Abrams, L. (1996). Language, memory, and aging: Distributed deficiencies and the structure of new-vs-old connect. In J. E. Birren and K. W. Schaie (Eds.), *Handbook of the psychology of aging* (Fourth edition) (pp. 251-265). San Diego: Academic Press.

Meyers, D. (2000). *Psychology*. New York: Worth Publishers.

Moscovitch, M. C. (1982). A neuropsychological approach to perception and memory in normal and pathological aging. In F. I. M. Craik and S. Trehub (Eds.), *Aging and cognitive processes*. New York: Plenum.

Park, D., Hertzog, C., Leventhal, H., Morrell, R., Leventhal, E., Birchmore, D., Martin, M., and Bennett, J. (1999). Medication adherence in rheumatoid arthritis patients: Older is wiser. *Journal of the American Geriatric Society*, 47, 172-183.

Patton, G. and Meit, M. (1993). Effect of aging on prospective and incidental memory. *Experimental Aging Research*, 19, 165-176.

Rowe, J. and Kahn, R. (1998). *Successful aging*. New York: Pantheon Books.

Salthouse, T. A. (1992). Influences of processing speed on adult age differences in working memory. *Acta Psychologica*, 79, 155-170.

_____(2000). Adulthood and aging: Cognitive processes and development. In A. Kazdin (Ed.), *Encyclopedia of psychology*. Washington, DC, and New York: American Psychological Association and Oxford University Press.

Santrock, J. (2000). *Life-span development*. New York: McGraw Hill.

Schaie, K. (1996). *Intellectual development in adulthood: The Seattle longitudinal study*. New York: Cambridge University Press.

Schimamura, A., Berry, J., Mangels, J., Rusting, C., and Jurica, P. (1995). Memory and cognitive abilities in university professors: Evidence for successful aging. *Psychological Science*, 6, 271-277.

Smith, A. D. (1996). Memory. In J. E. Birren (Ed.), *Encyclopedia of gerontology*, Volume 2. San Diego: Academic Press.

Spencer, W. D. and Raz, N. (1995). Differential effects of aging on memory for content and context: A meta-analysis. *Psychology and Aging*, 10, 527-539.

Stern, P. and Carstensen, L. (2000). *The aging mind: Opportunities in cognitive research*. Washington, DC: National Academy Press.

Tulving, E. (2000). Concepts of memory. In E. Tulving and F. I. M. Craik (Eds.), *The Oxford handbook of memory*. New York: Oxford University Press.

Underwood, A. and Watson, R. (2001). Thanks for the memories. In H. Cox (Ed.), *Annual Editions: Aging* (Fifteenth edition). Guilford CT: McGraw-Hill/ Dushkin.

Zacks, R. T., Hasher, L., and Li, K. (2000). Human memory. In F.I.M. Craik and T. A. Salthouse (Eds.), *Handbook of aging and cognition* (Second edition). Mahwah, NJ: Erlbaum.

MEMORY STEREOTYPES

Becca R. Levy

The stereotype about inevitable memory loss in old age is so prevalent that it has been found to influence the thinking of children. Five-year-olds were more likely to assume an elderly researcher has an unreliable memory than does a young researcher (Kwong See, 2002). Once the initial stereotype is encoded in memory, it forms a structure that continues to influence perceptions about the memory of older adults. For example, young adults were more likely to remember the word old after it was briefly flashed on a computer screen, compared to right after seeing the word young (Perdue and Gurtman, 1990).

It has been shown that an "age-based double standard" exits in interpretations of forgetfulness experienced by younger and older adults (Erber and Prager, 1999). Both age groups were more likely to judge a memory problem in younger individuals as a temporary lapse, due to lack of effort, whereas the same problem in older individuals was more likely to be considered a chronic state of incompetence (Erber, Szuchman, and Rothberg, 1990).

Studies of memory performance in elders fall into two main camps. One group of research suggests that memory inevitably declines in old age, due to hardwired changes in the aging mind. However, the age decrements in memory that these studies report may be due, at least in part, to the researchers selecting methodologies that favor younger adults. For example, memory studies rely on computers, although younger adults tend to have greater competence with them. In addition, memory studies are often in the form of tests, which college students are more oriented toward, giving them an advantage when compared to the performance of elders. In support of this, a study found that age differences in memory were eliminated when a memory task was no longer presented as a memory test (Rahhal, Hasher, and Colcombe, 2001).

The other camp provides research that rejects generalizations about the inevitability of memory decline in old age. These studies include quite specific ones, such as the finding that when older and younger adults were matched on chess skill levels, the older adults, apparently building on their experience, took less time to select an equally good chess move (Charness, 1981).

Research of a more generalized nature points to variations in memory processes among elders. For example, it has been shown that whereas memory that is based on the "hardware" of the human brain (e.g., visual memory) tends to consistently decline in old age, this is not the case with memory that is based on the culturally acquired "software" of the mind (e.g., procedural memory) (see Baltes, 1997). Yet even the first type of cognition can be improved with sufficient training (Willis and Nesselroade, 1990).

Furthermore, evidence suggests that memory decline may be associated with societal beliefs about aging. This was found by comparing two cultures that have a relatively positive perception of elders, the Mainland Chinese and the American deaf, to hearing Americans (Levy and Langer, 1994). Younger participants from the three cultures performed similarly, but the older Chinese and older deaf Americans outperformed the older hearing Americans. Moreover, the older Chinese (who had the most positive stereotypes of aging among the elderly groups) did not score significantly lower than the younger Chinese participants.

The influence of age stereotypes on elders' memory performance has also been established by experimental studies. When older adults were subliminally exposed to either positive or negative age stereotypes, those in the positive-age-stereotype group performed significantly better on memory tasks than those in the negative-age-stereotype group (Levy, 1996). Another study demonstrated that older adults who read an article about memory decline in old age performed significantly worse on a memory task than those who read an article about older adults performing as well as younger adults (Hess et al., 2003).

The damaging effects of negative stereotypes about memory extend to those who have not yet reached old age. In a recent study, middle-aged participants were either asked to compare themselves to older adults, compare themselves to younger adults, or were not asked to make a comparison (Hummert and O'Brien, 2002). The memory performance of those who compared themselves to older adults was worse than those in the other two groups. The effect was strongest for participants who had the most pronounced old age identity, suggesting that the old-age comparison intervention activated an age stereotype that led to worse memory performance.

There is reason to question the inevitability of memory loss in old age. To the extent that stereotypes about aging prevent this questioning, the cognitive well-being of every age level may be at risk.

See also FACTS ON AGING AND MENTAL HEALTH; MEASURING AGEISM IN CHILDREN; MENTAL ILLNESS; STEREOTYPES; UNCONSCIOUS AGEISM

REFERENCES

Baltes, P. B. (1997). On the incomplete architecture of human ontogeny: Selection, optimization, and compensation as foundation of developmental theory. *American Psychologist,* 52, 366-380.

Charness, N. (1981). Aging and skilled problem solving. *Journal of Experimental Psychology: General,* 110, 21-38.

Erber, J. T. and Prager, I. G. (1999). Age and memory: Perceptions of forgetful young and older adults. In T. M. Hess and F. Blanchard-Fields (Eds.), *Social cognition and aging.* Boston: Academic Press.

Erber, J. T., Szuchman, L. T., and Rothberg, S. T. (1990). Everyday memory in failure: Age differences in appraisal and attribution. *Psychology and Aging,* 5, 236-241.

Hess, T. M., Auman, C., Colcombe, S. J., and Rahhal, T. A. (2003). The impact of stereotype threat on age differences in memory performance. *Journal of Gerontology: Psychological Science.*

Hummert, M. L. and O'Brien, L. T. (2002). Age self-stereotyping, stereotype threat, and memory performance in middle-aged adults. Annual meeting of the Gerontological Society of America. Boston, MA, November.

Kwong See, S. T. and Rasmussen, C. (2002). An early start to age stereotyping: Children's beliefs about an older experimenter. Annual meeting of the Gerontological Society of America. Boston, MA, November.

Levy, B. (1996). Improving memory in old age by implicit self-stereotyping. *Journal of Personality and Social Psychology,* 71, 1092-1107.

Levy, B. and Langer, E. (1994). Aging free from negative stereotypes: Successful memory among the American Deaf and in China. *Journal of Personality and Social Psychology,* 66, 935-943.

Perdue, C. W. and Gurtman, M. B. (1990). Evidence for the automaticity of ageism. *Journal of Experimental Social Psychology,* 26, 199-216.

Rahhal, T. A., Hasher, L., and Colcombe, S. (2001). Instructional manipulations and age differences in memory: Now you see them, now you don't. *Psychology and Aging,* 16, 697-706.

Willis, S. L. and Nesselroade, C. S. (1990). Long-term effects of fluid ability training in old-old age. *Developmental Psychology,* 26, 905-910.

MENTAL ILLNESS

Erdman B. Palmore

Two of the frequent misconceptions about aging is that mental abilities tend to decline from middle age onward and that most elderly suffer from some form of senility or mental illness (Palmore, 1998). It is often believed that older people are unable to learn new things ("You can't teach an old dog new tricks"). Another belief is that memory loss is typical, if not inevitable, in old age. There are many jokes about memory loss in old age (Palmore, 1999). Another aspect of such stereotypes is the belief that mental illness among the aged is untreatable.

Such beliefs can become self-fulfilling prophecies in which the belief that mental illness is inevitable and untreatable leads to lack of prevention and treatment, which, in turn, tends to confirm the original belief. This helps to explain why elders use mental health facilities at only one half the rate of the general population (Lebowitz, 2001). Elders themselves and many health professionals think that most mental illness in old age is untreatable.

All these beliefs are false and simply manifestations of ageism. In fact, most elders are not senile, and mental illness is neither common, inevitable, nor untreatable in old age. Only about 3 percent of persons age sixty-five or older are institutionalized with mental disorders (Kahana, 2001). Community studies agree that less than 10 percent of elders have significant or severe mental illness, and another 10 percent have moderate mental impairment (Gurland, 2001).

In fact, community surveys find that when all mental illnesses are counted, fewer elders have mental impairments than do younger persons. It is true that rates of dementia climb steeply with advancing age; but this is counterbalanced by decreases in major depressions, schizophrenia, paranoid disorders, alcoholism and other substance abuse, and anxiety disorders.

So, contrary to the stereotype about senility and mental illness, elders actually have *less* mental illness than younger people do. If this fact were more widely known, it would reduce this common form of ageism.

See also MEMORY STEREOTYPES; SELF-FULFILLING PROPHECY; STEREOTYPES

REFERENCES

Gurland, B. (2001). Psychopathology. In G. Maddox (Ed.), *The encyclopedia of aging*. New York: Springer.

Kahana, E. (2001). Institutionalization. In G. Maddox (Ed.), *The encyclopedia of aging*. New York: Springer.

Lebowitz, B. (2001). Mental health services. In G. Maddox (Ed.), *The encyclopedia of aging*. New York: Springer.

Palmore, E. (1998). *Facts on aging quiz.* New York: Springer.

_____ (1999). *Ageism.* New York: Springer.

MODERNIZATION THEORY

Erdman B. Palmore

Modernization theory claims that the changes involved in the development of industrial societies also cause declines in the status of elders and the development of ageism (Cowgill, 1974). These changes include the following:

- Falling birth and death rates cause a rapid increase in the proportion of aged in the society. In a sense, the supply of old people exceeds the demand for them. There are more old people than the society can support.
- Technology and automation decreases the demand for older workers, leading to unemployment and competition between the generations for jobs.
- New technology and changing occupational structure make the job skills of older workers obsolete.
- These trends cause more retirement, which in turn lowers the income and status of elders.
- Public education and rapid social change may make obsolete much of the knowledge that formerly was a basis for prestige of elders.
- Urbanization and suburbanization leave old people behind in rural areas and deteriorating parts of the city, leading to their isolation and loss of status.

Some historians argue that these changes occurred after the general decline in status of the aged and so were not the cause of ageism

(Achenbaum, 2001; Fischer, 1978). They contributed to the decline in status of the aged, which is related to the rise of ageism.

Two modifications were proposed to this basic theory (Palmore, 1999). First, there are some societies, such as Japan, in which the culture (filial piety and respect for elders) and the social structure (vertical rather than horizontal) counteract the effects of modernization so that the respect and prestige of elders remain relatively high (Palmore, 1985). Second, in postindustrial societies, such as the United States, the prestige and status of elders increased in recent years because of increased income, education, and health (Palmore, 1998). Also the increasing research and knowledge about aging in postindustrial societies diminishes the old negative stereotypes.

Thus, the effects of modernization on the status of the aged probably form a U-shaped curve, in which the early effects caused a decline, but after industrialization was complete, there was an increase in the status of elders and a decline in ageism.

See also AGE CONFLICT; CULTURAL SOURCES OF AGEISM; HISTORY

REFERENCES

Achenbaum, W. (2001). Modernization theory. In G. Maddox (Ed.), *The encyclopedia of aging.* New York: Springer.

Cowgill, D. (1974). Aging and modernization. In J. Gubrium (Ed.) *Late life, communities, and environmental policy.* Springfield, IL: Charles C Thomas.

Fischer, D. (1978). *Growing old in America.* New York: Oxford University Press.

Palmore, E. (1985). *The honorable elders revisited.* Durham, NC: Duke University Press.

_____ (1998). *The facts on aging quiz.* New York: Springer.

_____ (1999). *Ageism.* New York: Springer.

NURSING

Charlene Harrington
Eric Collier
Anna Burdin

Substantial amount of literature suggests that ageism is prevalent in the nursing field (Courtney, Tong, and Walsh, 2000). This phenomenon contributes to perceptions of low status for nurses working in long-term care settings and reduces the desire by nurses to specialize in geriatric nursing. Factors related to a high prevalence of ageism include

1. nurses who lack previous associations or contact with older adults,
2. nursing school curricula that lack content in gerontology,
3. professional and industry stereotypes about aging,
4. institutional factors, such as low pay and difficult work, and
5. other factors.

This entry reviews some of these key issues.

The demand for nursing care of older persons is growing as the population is rapidly aging. In the United States, almost half of the hospital days and most of the home health services and nursing facility care are provided to the elderly (Kovner, Mezey, and Harrington, 2002). Yet evidence suggests a critical shortage of nurses trained in geriatrics and gerontology, exacerbated by a general shortage of nurses. Only 1 percent of the nation's 2.2 million practicing registered nurses (RNs) are certified in geriatrics and most baccalaureate nursing programs do not have a geriatrics course or specialty programs in gerontology (Kovner, Mezey, and Harrington, 2002).

The lack of interest in geriatric nursing (Burnside, 1981) and the lack of geriatric nursing education (Kovner, Mezey, and Harrington, 2002), in part, reflect the ageism within nursing and the broader society. Until nursing schools are required to design and incorporate curriculum requirements for basic education in gerontology and specialized geriatric training, the needs of older people will not be adequately met and the quality of care for older people may suffer. This current situation raises serious questions about the availability and training of nurses who can provide services to older people in the future.

Within nursing, ageism is a common phenomenon that is fueled by negative stereotypes. Nurses have been shown to stereotype older people by labeling them as complainers who are inflexible, and unwilling to compromise. These misconceptions can negatively influence the type and quality of care that elderly individuals receive from providers (Courtney, Tong, and Walsh, 2000). Such negative attitudes can be spread within nursing if education and work experiences are not directed to the problem. These problems are compounded by the long-term care industry, which has contributed to ageism and stereotypes by describing older people as the least capable, least healthy, and least alert (Cohen, 1988).

Institutional barriers often cause nurses to dislike working with older adults. The heavy workloads, difficult work environment, and low wages and benefits that are endemic to nursing homes and other long-term care settings can also contribute to a negative attitude toward working in long-term care (Wunderlich and Kohler, 2001). Pursey and Luker (1995) found that the high dependency levels of older people and the structure of nursing work in hospitals meant that some nurses did not have favorable impressions about work with older patients.

Previous associations with older adults are seen as an important marker for how nurses or nursing students will feel about older adults. Haight, Christ, and Dias (1994) found through surveying student nurses in a graduate program, that a positive influence in the students' attitudes toward the elderly was their interaction with older adults, especially their grandparents. Furthermore, the students who were exposed to well-adjusted and healthy elderly persons tended to have a more favorable impression of the elderly and aging. Hope

(1994) found that positive attitudes toward older people were associated with: post–basic gerontological education, age of respondents, and knowledge of older people.

A number of recommendations to combat ageism have been described in the literature. Formalized geriatric nursing as a specialty throughout nursing schools and educational requirements in gerontology for all basic registered nursing programs would improve the preparation of nurses to work with older people (Kovner, Mezey, and Harrington, 2002; Wade, 1999). Training experiences that refute the idea that old age must involve disability and illness also can be valuable in helping nurses understand the individual needs of older people (Reed and Clarke, 1999). Changes in the long-term care settings are also needed to improve wages and benefits and working conditions (Wunderlich and Kohler, 2001). If these few recommendations were adopted, it would enhance the quality of care for elderly patients, and improve relations between nurses and patients in the long-term care settings that so many elderly patients frequent.

See also ABUSE IN NURSING HOMES; GERIATRICS; HEALTH CARE; MEDICAL STUDENTS; NURSING HOMES

REFERENCES

Burnside, I. (1981) Gerontological Nursing. In I. Burnside (Ed.), *Nursing and the aged.* Second edition. New York: McGraw Hill.

Cohen, E., S. (1988) The elderly mystique: Constraints on the autonomy of the elderly with disabilities. *The Gerontologist,* 28(Suppl), 24-31.

Courtney, M., Tong, S., and Walsh, A. (2000) Acute-care nurses' attitudes toward older patients. *International Journal of Nursing Practice,* 6, 62-69.

Haight, B., Christ, M., and Dias, J. (1994). Does nursing education promote ageism? *Journal of Advanced Nursing,* 20, 382-390.

Hope, K. (1994). Nurses' attitudes toward older people: A comparison between nurses working in acute medical and acute care of elderly patient settings. *Journal of Advanced Nursing,* 20, 605-612.

Kovner, C., Mezey, M., and Harrington, C. (2002). Who cares for older adults? Workforce implications of an aging society. *Health Affairs,* 21(5), 78-89.

Pursey, A. and Luker, K. (1995). Attitudes and stereotypes: Nurses' work with older people. *Journal of Advanced Nursing,* 22, 547-555.

Reed, J. and Clarke, C. (1999). Nursing older people: Constructing need and care. *Nursing Inquiry,* 6, 208-215.

Wade, S. (1999). Promoting quality of care for older people: Developing positive attitudes to working with older people. *Journal of Nursing Management, 7*, 339-347.

Wunderlich, G.S. and Kohler, P. (Eds.) (2001). *Improving the quality of long term care.* Washington, DC: National Academy Press.

NURSING HOMES

Diana K. Harris

Ageism is manifested in nursing homes in a number of ways. A common one is infantilizing patients and treating them like children instead of mature adults. It is not unusual for nursing aides to act as if female patients were little girls. For example, some aides fix their patients' hair in pigtails tied with ribbons and give them dolls to which the aides refer to as the patients' "babies" (Kimsey, Tarbox, and Bragg, 1981). Nursing aides often speak to their patients in baby talk. Such speech patterns have a detrimental effect on the self-esteem of the patients, convey less respect, and support dependent behavior. Nursing staff who view patients as dependent are also more likely to use baby talk than those who do not (Pasupathi and Lockenhoff, 2002).

Infantilization of nursing home patients includes patting patients on the head and addressing them by their first names whether they request it or not. Researchers have found that those staff who treated the patients like children were at greatest risk of engaging in psychologically abusive behavior (Pillemer and Moore, 1989).

Ageism is also manifested in nursing homes by depersonalization. It is not unusual for patients to be treated as if they were nonpersons without an identity. This is done by failing to communicate and ignoring them. For instance, a patient sitting in the lounge repeatedly said, "Good morning" to the aides as they walked by and none of them replied to her greeting; they acted as if she weren't there (Kayser-Jones, 1981).

Finally, many of the nursing staff reflect the societal view that the patients belong to a socially stigmatized category and are devalued as a result of their physical and mental impairments. These views create an environment in the nursing home in which ageist attitudes toward patients are seen as justifiable.

See also ABUSE IN NURSING HOMES; ABUSE BY ELDERS IN NURSING HOMES

REFERENCES

Kayser-Jones, J. (1981). *Old, alone, and neglected.* Berkeley: University of California Press.

Kimsey, L.,Tarbox, A., and Bragg, D. (1981). Abuse of the elderly: The hidden agenda. *Journal of the American Geriatrics Society,* 29, 465-472.

Pasupathi, M. and Lockenhoff, C. (2002). Ageist behavior. In T. Nelson (Ed.), *Ageism: Stereotyping and prejudice against older people* (pp. 201-246). Cambridge, MA: MIT Press.

Pillemer, K. and Moore, D. (1989). Abuse of patients in nursing homes: Findings from a survey of staff. *The Gerontologist,* 29, 314-320.

O

ORGANIZATIONS OPPOSING AGEISM

Erdman B. Palmore

The following is a list of the major national organizations working to reduce negative ageism.

Administration on Aging (AoA)
Washington, DC 20201
phone: (202) 619-0724
www.aoa.gov

American Association of Retired Persons (AARP)
601 E. Street, NW
Washington, DC 20049
phone: (888) 687-2277
www.aarp.org

American Federation for Aging Research (AFAR)
70 West 40th Street, 11th Floor
New York, NY 10018
phone: (888) 582-2327
www.afar.org

American Society on Aging (ASA)
833 Market Street
Suite 511
San Francisco, CA 94103
phone: (800) 537-9728
www.asaging.org

Americans Discuss Social Security (ADSS)
2001 Pennsylvania Avenue, NW
Suite 825
Washington, DC 20006
phone: (202) 955-9000
www.americansdiscuss.org

Association for Gerontology in Higher Education (AGHE)
1030 15th Street, N
Suite 240
Washington, DC 20005-1503
phone: (202) 289-9806
www.aghe.org

Gerontological Society of America
1030 15th St., NW
Suite 250
Washington, DC 20005-1503
phone: (202) 842-2088
www.geron.org

Gray Panthers
733 15th Street, NW
Suite 437
Washington, DC 20005
phone: (800) 280-5362
www.graypanthers.org

National Association for Hispanic Elderly
234 East Colorado Boulevard
Suite 300
Pasadena, CA 91101
phone: (626) 564-1988
www.nia.nih.gov

National Caucus on Black Aged (NCBA)
1220 L Street, NW
Suite 800
Washington, DC 20005

phone: (202) 637-8400
www.ncba-aged.org

National Council on the Aging (NCOA)
300 D Street, SW
Suite 801
Washington, DC 20024
phone: (202) 479-1200
www.ncoa.org

National Council of Senior Citizens (NCSC)
8403 Colesville Road
Suite 1200
Silver Spring, MD 0910-3314
phone: (301) 578-8800
www.ncscinc.org

National Institute on Aging (NIA)
Building 31, Room 5C27
31 Center Drive, MSC 2292
Bethesda, MD 20892
phone: (301) 496-1752
www.nia.nih.gov

National Senior Citizen's Law Center (NSCLC)
1101 14th St., NW
Suite 400
Washington, DC 20005
phone: (202) 289-6976
www.nsclc.org

Older Women's League (OWL)
1750 New York Ave., NW
Suite 350
Washington, DC 20006
phone: (202) 783-6686
www.owl-national.org

See also CHANGE STRATEGIES

P

PATRONIZING

Erdman B. Palmore

Patronizing is adopting an air of condescension toward others. This common form of ageism is practiced by younger people toward the elderly, especially if the elder is frail or infirm in some way. Since nursing home staff and other medical personnel routinely deal with such infirm elders, they are especially prone to patronizing elders. Such patronizing may take several forms as in the following:

- Calling elders by their first names when they prefer the dignity of surnames prefaced by Mr., Mrs., or Ms.
- Calling elders "darling," "dearie," "honey," or even "baby," when elders do not wish such implied intimacy.
- Elders are "talked down to" by oversimplified sentences and words.
- The use of "we" or "our" when the speaker really means "you" or "your;" as in "It's time for our bath."
- Speaking loudly on the assumption that elders cannot hear well, when that assumption is not warranted.
- Repeating the same thing over and over on the assumption that elders do not understand the first time.
- Insincere flattery, as in "You're doing wonderfully!"
- Offering to help the elders when they do not need or want any help.

Such patronizing destroys elders' sense of dignity and self-esteem, as well as encouraging learned helplessness.

See also AGEISM SURVEY; EXAMPLES; NURSING HOMES

PENSION BIAS

Erdman B. Palmore

In 1992, Ron Arnett, a Freemont, California, patrol officer injured his back, which forced him to retire. However, when he applied for a disability retirement pension, he found out that he would be awarded only 32 percent of his former pay from the California Public Employees' Retirement System (CalPERS), because he had joined the force at a relatively late age, when he was forty-three. In contrast, others with a similar history, who joined the force when they were twenty-nine, were awarded 50 percent of their former pay (Harris, 2003).

Arnett filed an age-discrimination complaint with the Equal Employment Opportunity Commission (EEOC). The EEOC used Arnett's case to file a class-action suit for 1,700 others who had suffered similar pension discrimination based on their age. The case went through several federal courts, and in January 2003, a settlement was made in which CalPERS agreed to pay $50 million in retroactive benefits, or about $30,000 to each of the 1,700 affected officers—half of what they would have gotten had the discriminatory policy not been in place.

The pension fund is to pay another $200 million in future benefits. This $250 million settlement is by far the largest in the EEOC's history.

See also EMPLOYMENT DISCRIMINATION; MANDATORY RETIREMENT OF JUDGES

REFERENCE

Harris, D. (2003). Simple justice: The inside story of the biggest age bias win in U.S. history. *AARP,* July/August, 58-66.

PERPETUAL YOUTH

Robert Kastenbaum

The most intimate form of ageism is the rejection of one's own future self. This attitude has been on display from the earliest historical documents to the present time. For example, an Egyptian papyrus promised to show how a man of eighty could become a youth of twenty. It was, in fact, a cosmetic enhancement formula.

Ancient Greeks recoiled at the prospect of growing old. No god of aging was included in their crowded pantheon: the mighty deities were spared age as well as death. Surveying the tales of Homer, poetry, and plays, Falkner and de Luce (1992) find aging described in relentlessly negative terms such as accursed, hateful, sorrowful, dishonored, and pitiless. The idea of dying young became relatively popular because no joy was anticipated in becoming a futile caricature of one's vigorous youthful self. Not everybody was enthusiastic about an early death, however. How to stay alive and not grow old—that became a prime subject for reflection, but also a goad for efforts to defeat aging through magic, religion, or diabolically clever experiments.

The quest for perpetual youth has often been accompanied by efforts to roll back the clock after one has already aged. Rejuvenation (becoming a juvenile version of one's aging adult self) becomes a priority when age has already taken its toll. History most frequently offers masculine examples with more than a dollop of sexual ambition (e.g., Solomon sending for virgins to lie beside him, or nineteenth-century gentlemen investigating the possibility of monkey gland transplants). The pioneering alchemists in Asian as well as Western traditions were keen on transforming base metals into gold, but even more urgently seeking a way to prevent or reverse aging (Gruman, 1966). From the most ancient spells and incantations to the latest antiaging elixers, few causes have been as enduring as the desire to achieve perpetual youth. Some lessons have been learned along the way, as we shall see.

"Be Careful What You Wish For"

This well-known phrase applies well to the quest to vanquish both aging and death. Consider, for example, Tithon, the Struldbrugs, Dr. Faustus, Dorian Gray, Emilia Marty, and Axel Bernstein.

Aurora, the dawn goddess, was enamoured of Tithon. She pleaded with her father to grant this handsome mortal immunity from death. Zeus agreed, but played a horrible trick. Nothing had been in the contract about keeping her lover young. Tithon soon became the most miserable of creatures.

> The woods decay, the woods decay and fall,
> The vapors weep their burden to the ground,
> Man comes and tills the field and lies beneath,
> And after many a summer dies the swan
> Me only cruel immortality consumes (Tennyson, 1895)

Here is a lesson drawn repeatedly from attempts to alter *The Journey of Life* (Cole, 1992). Not to accept aging and death is to remove ourselves from both nature and society.

Captain Gulliver was at first delighted to meet a Struldbrug. How marvelous it must be for such a rare and fortunate person who was born immortal, and for the society that would benefit from the endless wisdom acquired through time. Other Luggnaggians, however, quickly disabused him of this misconception. The Struldbrugs were "not only opinionative, peevish, covetous, morose, vain, and talkative, but uncapable of friendship, and dead to all natural affection . . . despised and hated by all sorts of people" (Swift, 1963 [1726], p. 233).

The Struldbrugs were much more an affront to human pride than the unfortunate Tithon. Swift was suggesting that a longer life, like a longer rope, is something we would only use to hang ourselves out to dry. We would just continue to perfect our faults and quirks. Dr. Faustus, though, was portrayed as a visionary alchemist who had grown old in the quest for perpetual youth (as imagined by Marlowe, 1994 [1604], and Goethe, 1962 [1808]). Having fallen in love with a beautiful and virtuous maiden, Faust barters his soul to the devil in exchange for another chance at youth. He has his moments of bliss, but anguish and dishonor soon follow and, literally, all hell breaks loose. The Tithon/Struldbrug warning now sounds another note: the desire for returned or extended youth is not only ill advised, but violates God's plan.

Alchemy also figures in the tale of Emilia Marty (first portrayed in a play by Karel Capek, now better known through Leo Janacek's opera, *The Makropolus Affair* (Janacek, 1978). As a sixteen-year-old she is forced to imbibe a concoction to see whether it was safe to give the emperor and provide him with three hundred years of youthful life. Emilia nearly dies—but 300 years later she is the one who is still a "young" beauty. Her emotions have eroded, however, and she abandons lovers and children along a trail of sorrow until she chooses death to a meaningless continuation as a person who has almost everything—youth, beauty, talent, wealth—but no longer her humanity. A person who does not age along with her generation may be doomed to alienation.

Other compelling examples of the folly of seeking perpetual use include the friends who participate in "Dr. Heidegger's experiment" (Hawthorne, 1991), and Axel Bernstein (Weisman, 2002), the only outsider truly accepted and respected by the Highland tribes of Papua New Guinea. In Nathaniel Hawthorne's story, the friends of an aged physician assure him they would live their lives more wisely if given a second chance at youth. Immediately upon feeling young again, they—well, just as you would expect—gleefully set off on the same course of foolishness and dysfunction that had already ruined their lives once. An aging but vigorous man, Bernstein is saved from a nearly fatal illness by native medicine, but then continues beyond his recovery into renewed youth. Unfortunately, having shed his age, he also shed his maturity and regressed into an impulsive and thought-less youth until his loss of wisdom led to death. The author's message is clear. There is a reason that people advance beyond youth: *perpet-ual immaturity* is not entirely a blessing.

Dorian Gray and the Perpetual Youth Theme Today

The poster boy for perpetual youth for more than a century has been Oscar Wilde's (1982 [1890]) memorable creation Dorian Gray. A handsome fellow idling through life, he came under the influence of a cynical friend who feared his own aging. Dorian let himself be persuaded to devote himself entirely to pleasure. His opportunities ex-panded immensely when his own aging and misdeeds were inflicted upon his portrait while others aged but he enjoyed perpetual youth. Dorian's character became increasingly ugly despite his charming ap-pearance. It need hardly be added that eventually fate dealt with him harshly, like all those before him who had attempted to escape from the natural journey of life.

Dorian was shaped by the specific social forces and fantasies of the late-Victorian period as well as the persistent general fascination with perpetual youth. A comparison of Dorian and his times with societal conditions a century later has produced the following observations (Kastenbaum, 1995):

- Anxiety about leaving one's youth behind has decreased because middle age is now associated with continued health and vigor. More people now desire to stay middle-aged.
- The later adult years have become more familiar and less threatening because there are more elderly men and women about who are strongly engaged with life. The older person is becoming less marginal, less a victim, and more a political force.
- There is more recognition that youth is not all fun and games: risks, conflicts, frustrations, and vulnerabilities sometimes make this phase of life highly stressful. The comparison of an idyllic version of youth and a catastrophic version of age is less persuasive than ever.
- The "youth" that Dorian wanted to keep is artificial: a split-off zone of suspended time, a stalled vehicle with its motor running but no destination. The natural, continuous flow of life is threatened by both the idealization of youth and the marginalization of age.
- Dorian in retrospect looks less like an elite dandy than a slacker who fears commitment and responsibility: not ready even to become an adult, let alone a senior member of society.
- Research and experience have indicated that age is better suited than youth for the integration of experiences and the evaluation of meanings. There is also more awareness of the total life course (as, for example, in Erikson's influential theory, 1963, 1979), so thoughtful people are more likely to grow up with the prospect of their elder selves waiting to welcome them further on down the road.

Persistence of the Perpetual Youth Theme

Despite the changes previously noted, the perpetual youth and rejuvenation theme continues to flourish. One of the more curious forms is the widespread use of human growth hormone (HGH) derivatives by athletes, some still in their teens. In this endeavor, being young is not enough: one must also have that competitive edge. Unfortunately, this potion exacts its price, as did most of the others that have been favored through the centuries. The same HGH stream that carries children to physical maturity has a toxic effect after nature's date of recommended use has been exceeded. The details are different, but the basic story similar: the quest for unlimited youth has its way of turning around and biting us.

Extended childbearing is another emerging example of holding back or reversing time. There is not yet sufficient information to understand the corollaries and consequences of this endeavor. Much more active and lucrative is the invitation to lift that face, landscape that nose, tuck that tummy, and enhance that breast. Many people, though, ease their way through life transitions, making early discoveries of elder wisdom, and bringing elements of youth with them all the way through life's journey. One's past-, present-, and future-self can find themselves as boon companions rather than distrustful strangers.

See also ANTIAGING MEDICINE; LITERATURE

REFERENCES

Cole, T. R. (1992). *The journey of life.* Cambridge and New York: Cambridge University Press.

Erikson, E. H. (1963). *Childhood and society* (Second edition). New York: W. W. Norton.

_____ (1979). Reflections on Dr. Borg's life cycle. In D. D. Van Tassel (Ed.), *Aging, death, and the completion of being* (pp. 29-68). Philadelphia: University of Pennsylvania Press.

Falkner, T. M. and de Luce, J. (1992). A view from antiquity: Greece, Rome, and Elders. In T. R. Cole, D. D. Van Tassel, and R. Kastenbaum (Eds.), *Handbook of the humanities and aging* (pp. 3-39). New York: Springer.

Goethe, J. W. V. (1962 [1808]). *Goethe's Faust.* New York: Anchor.

Gruman, G. J. (1966). *A history of ideas about the prolongation of life: The evolution of prolongevity hypotheses to 1800.* Philadelphia: The American Philosophical Society.

Hawthorne, N. (1991). *The celestial railroad and other stories.* San Antonio: Buccaneer Books.

Janacek, L. (1978). *Vec Makropulos* (The Makropulos affair). London (2CDs) 430-372-2.

Kastenbaum, R. (1995). *Dorian, graying: Is youth the only thing worth having?* Amityville, NY: Baywood.

Marlowe, C. (1994 [1604]). *Dr. Faustus.* New York: Dover.

Swift, J. (1963 [1726]). *Gulliver's travels.* Boston: Beacon Press.

Tennyson, A. (1895). *The works of Alfred, Lord Tennyson,* Volume 2. Boston: Estes and Lauriat.

Weisman, A. D. (2002). *The next taboo: Curing cancer through cannibalism.* First Books Library. <www.1stbooks.com>.

Wilde, O. (1982 [1890]). *The picture of Dorian Gray.* New York: Penguin.

PHYSICAL THERAPY

Kathy M. Shipp

In the absence of age bias, older patients who need rehabilitation services would receive these services in frequency, duration, and intensity equivalent to younger patients who have similar medical problems and levels of disability. This is not the current reality, but evidence that would allow either confirmation or denial regarding equal access to and provision of rehabilitation services for older patients is sparse.

Age bias in rehabilitation for older people exists on at least two levels: the societal and the individual. Ageist attitudes can be manifest in terms of health care policy and procedural regulations. For example, Centers for Medicare and Medicaid Services (CMS) limits Medicare reimbursement for rehabilitation services for physical and speech therapy to an amount of approximately $1,600 per calendar year regardless of medical diagnoses or extent of disability (Centers for Medicare and Medicaid Services, 2003). This limitation has the effect that older Americans often do not receive as much rehabilitation services as younger people with the same diagnoses. Furthermore, treating patients covered by Medicare takes more administrative time for physical therapists because of the increased complexity and amount of documentation required to meet Medicare compliance standards compared to compliance standards of private medical insurers. As a result, some physical therapists do not treat patients insured by Medicare, thus limiting access for older patients.

Ageist attitudes held by individual health care providers are another potential source of differential rehabilitation opportunity and outcomes for older people. Studies show that health professionals in general describe working with older patients as less desirable than working with younger patients (Kosberg and Harris, 1978; Glasspoole and Aman, 1990; Wilderom et al., 1990); agree that the goals of care for older people should be limited to palliative concerns (Coe, 1967); or anticipate poorer therapeutic outcomes for older patients (James and Haley, 1995). However, only a few studies have focused on rehabilitation providers or physical therapists.

Age bias among rehabilitation professionals takes several forms: lower expectations of rehabilitation potential, less-intensive treatment, and negative attitudes. Two studies demonstrated that therapists view older patients as having less potential for return to high-level functioning. A study of 127 physical therapists presented two case vignettes of a patient following traumatic amputation that varied only by the age of the patient, either twenty-eight or seventy-eight years old (Kvitek et al., 1986). The results were that the therapists rated lower-level goals as being appropriate for the older patient. Another study using case vignettes, which varied only by age of the patient, found that rehabilitation professionals rated the younger patient to be 12.5 percent more likely to meet treatment goals (Kee et al., 1998).

Regarding treatment intensity, Osberg and colleagues (1990) found that younger stroke patients had higher costs associated with rehabilitation than older stroke patients. The authors interpreted this finding as evidence that the older patients' treatment was less aggressive.

Finally, negative attitudes toward older patients have been reported. One study of 1,063 rehabilitation professionals found that the subjects viewed older people as less motivated and more psychologically needy (Nicholas et al., 1998). Rybarczyk and colleagues (2001) used a professional-bias questionnaire in a sample of 974 rehabilitation professionals (176 were physical therapists). They found that the respondents had more negative attitudes of depressed and noncompliant older patients in comparison to depressed and noncompliant younger patients.

Fortunately, some evidence supports that specific aspects of professional training can reduce age bias. An educational program designed to increase understanding of older people improved medical students' attitudes about rehabilitation potential of this population (Holtzman, Beck, and Coggan, 1978). A study of physical therapy students found that adding geriatric mock clinics to the curriculum improved negative attitudes toward older people (Brown et al., 1992). Professional training programs should train future practitioners to provide equal rehabilitation care to older adults.

See also GERIATRICS; HEALTH CARE; NURSING

REFERENCES

Brown, D. S., Gardner, D. L., Merritt, L., and Kelly, D. G. (1992). Improvement in attitudes toward the elderly following traditional and geriatric mock clinics for physical therapy students. *Physical Therapy, 72,* 251-260.

Centers for Medicare and Medicaid Services (2003). Program memorandum intermediaries/carriers. Transmittal AB-03-085, CMS-Pub AB. *United States Department of Health and Human Services.* June 10.

Coe, R. M. (1967). Professional perspectives on the aged. *The Gerontologist, 7,* 114-119.

Glasspoole, L. S. and Aman, M. G. (1990). Knowledge, attitudes, and happiness of nurses working with gerontological patients. *Journal of Gerontological Nursing,* 16, 11-14.

Holtzman, J. M., Beck, J. D., and Coggan, P. G. (1978). Geriatric program for medical students. II. Impact of two educational experiences on student attitudes. *Journal of the American Geriatric Society,* 26, 355-359.

James, J. W. and Haley, W. E. (1995). Age and health bias in practicing clinical psychologists. *Psychology of Aging,* 10, 610-616.

Kee, W. G., Middaugh, S. J., Redpath, S., and Hargadon, R. (1998). Age as a factor in admission to chronic pain rehabilitation. *Clinical Journal of Pain,* 14, 121-128.

Kosberg, J. and Harris, A. (1978). Attitudes toward elderly clients. *Health and Social Work,* 3, 66-90.

Kvitek, S. D. B., Shaver, B. J., Blood, H., and Shepard, K. F. (1986). Age bias: Physical therapists and older patients. *Journal of Gerontology,* 41, 706-709.

Nicholas, J. J., Rybarczyk, B., Meyer, P. M., Lacey, R. F., Haut, A., and Kemp, P. J. (1998). Rehabilitation staff perceptions of characteristics of geriatric rehabilitation patients. *Archives of Physical Medicine Rehabilitation,* 79, 1277-1284.

Osberg, J. S., Haley, S. M., McGinnis, G. E., and DeJong, G. (1990). Characteristics of cost outliers who did not benefit from stroke rehabilitation. *American Journal of Physical Medicine Rehabilitation,* 69, 117-125.

Rybarczyk, B., Haut, A., Lacey, R. F., Fogg, L. F., and Nicholas, J. J. (2001). A multifactorial study of age bias among rehabilitation professionals. *Archives of Physical Medicine Rehabilitation,* 82, 625-632.

Wilderom, C. P. M., Press, E. G., Perkins, D. V., Tebes, J. A., Nichols, L. Calkins, E., et al. (1990) Correlates of entering medical students' attitudes toward geriatrics. *Educational Gerontology,* 16, 429-446.

POLITICS

Robert H. Binstock

For the past several decades a "senior power" model of politics has been widely used by journalists, politicians, political advisors, political observers and some academicians to describe the political behavior and impact of older people and old-age-based organizations (Binstock, 1995; Peterson and Somit, 1994). This model is a manifestation of ageism in two respects. First, it inaccurately stereotypes older people as being homogeneous politically. Second, when applied as an interpretive framework, it can be and has been used to suggest that older people are an undesirable and destructive political force (Preston, 1994; Thurow, 1996) that should be countered by changing electoral rules (Stewart, 1970; Carballo, 1981; Peterson, 1999).

The senior power model builds on the fact that older people constitute a numerically significant portion of the electorate and then assumes that their political behavior is guided by their self-interests, and that most of them perceive their interests to be the same. Applying these assumptions, one expects older people to be homogeneous in political attitudes, cohesive in their voting behavior and, consequently, through sheer numbers, to be a powerful, perhaps dominating, electoral force. Moreover, the model also assumes that interest groups representing older people can swing the votes of older persons and thereby intimidate politicians. Based on all these assumptions one can believe that older voters and old-age interest groups function effectively as a powerful gray lobby (Pratt, 1976), able to exert substantial control over policies on aging and indirectly affect other policy decisions.

Some of the key assumptions in the senior power model, however, are wrong. First, contrary to this ageist model, older people *do not* vote cohesively. They are as diverse in their voting decisions as any other age group; their votes divide along the same partisan, economic, social, gender, racial, ethnic, and other lines as those of the electorate at large. Accordingly, the various cohorts of older Americans during the past fifty years have tended to distribute their votes among presidential candidates, for instance, in roughly the same proportions as other age groups do; exit polls show sharp divisions within each age group, and very small differences between age groups (see Campbell and Strate, 1981; Connelly, 2000). The empirical evidence from European nations is similar (Naegele and Walker, 1999).

The senior power model also mistakenly assumes that old-age policy issues play a major role in affecting the electoral choices of older voters because all elderly people have a common self-interested stake in government policies that provide old-age benefits. In fact, the self-interests of older people in relation to old-age policy issues, as well as the intensity of their interests, vary substantially. Consider, for example, that Social Security benefits are extremely important as a source of income for poor and near-poor older persons, but of relatively negligible importance to wealthy older persons. Some older individuals have much more at stake than others do in policy proposals that would reduce, maintain, or enhance Social Security benefit payments.

No evidence from exit polls indicates that old-age policy issues critically influence older persons' votes for candidates, and there are many reasons to expect that they would not be so influenced. Old age is only one of many personal characteristics of aged people with which they may identify themselves and their self-interests. Even if some older voters primarily identify themselves in terms of their age status, this does not mean that their self-interests in old-age policies are the most important factors in their electoral decisions. Other policy issues, strong and long-standing partisan attachments, underlying political attitudes, and many other electoral stimuli can be of equal or greater importance. Overall, the weight of the evidence indicates that older people's voting choices have rarely, if ever, been based on age-group interests.

An element of the senior power model that does have some empirical validity is the assumption that old-age-based interest groups, casting themselves as "representatives" of a large constituency of older voters, have some forms of political influence (Binstock, 1997; Day, 1998). Although they have not demonstrated a capacity to swing the votes of older persons, they do play a role in the policy process. Public officials find it both useful and incumbent upon them to invite an organization such as AARP that has more than 30 million members—or some of the more than forty other old-age interest groups—to participate in policy activities. This provides public officials with a ready means of "being in touch" symbolically with tens of millions of older persons, thereby legitimizing subsequent old-age policy actions and inactions. It also affords old-age interest groups an opportunity to put forward their views.

Perhaps the most important form of power available to the old-age interest groups might be termed *the electoral bluff*. Although these organizations have not demonstrated a capacity to swing a decisive bloc of older voters, members of Congress are hardly inclined to risk upsetting the existing distribution of votes that puts them and keeps them in office. Few politicians, of course, want to call the bluff of the aged or any other latent mass constituency if it is possible to avoid doing so.

Nonetheless, these forms of power have been quite limited in their impact. The old-age interest groups have had little to do with the enactment and amendment of major old-age policies such as Social Security and Medicare. Rather, such actions have been largely attributable to the initiatives of public officials in the White House, Congress, and the bureaucracy who were focused on their own agendas for social and economic policy (Binstock, 1995). Moreover, the old-age organizations have not been able to prevent significant policy reforms that have been perceived to be adverse to the interests of an artificially homogenized constituency of "the elderly" (Binstock, 1994; Day, 1998).

Despite these facts, the notion of so-called senior power persists because it serves certain purposes. It is marketed by the leaders of old-age-based organizations who have many incentives to inflate the political importance of the constituency for which they speak, even if they need to homogenize it artificially in order to do so. It is used as a straw man by those who would like to see greater resources allocated to their causes and who depict the power of elderly people as the root of many of society's problems (e.g., Preston, 1994; Peterson, 1999). And journalists purvey it as a tabloid symbol that simplifies the complexities of politics.

Perhaps the most influential perpetuators of the ageism embodied in the senior power model are politicians. They are always hopeful that they can capitalize on a potential cohesiveness of older voters, and are worried that older voters might turn against them en masse. So candidates for office actively woo the "senior vote" by positioning themselves on old-age policy issues in a fashion that they think will appeal to the self-interests of older voters, and they also take care that their opponents do not gain an advantage in this respect. Thus, during election campaigns, journalists inevitably write stories emphasizing the critical importance of elderly voters, which tend to perpetuate the ageist myth of "senior power."

See also AGE CONFLICT; GENERATIONAL EQUITY; JOURNALISM; ORGANIZATIONS OPPOSING AGEISM; PUBLIC POLICY; STEREOTYPES; SUBCULTURES

REFERENCES

Binstock, R. H. (1994). Changing criteria in old-age programs: The introduction of economic status and need for services. *The Gerontologist,* 34, 726-730.

_____ (1995). Policies on aging in the post–cold war era. In W. Crotty (Ed.), *Post-cold war policy: The social and domestic context* (pp. 55-90). Chicago: Nelson-Hall Publishers.

_____ (1997). The old-age lobby in a new political era. In R. B. Hudson (Ed.), *The future of age-based public policy* (pp. 56-74). Baltimore, MD: Johns Hopkins University Press.

Campbell, J. C. and Strate, J. (1981). Are older people conservative? *The Gerontologist,* 21, 580-591.

Carballo, M. (1981). Extra votes for parents? *The Boston Globe,* December 17, 35.

Connelly, M. (2000). Who voted: A portrait of American politics, 1976-2000. *The New York Times,* November 12, wk4.

Day, C. L. (1998). Old-age interest groups in the 1990s: Coalition, competition, strategy. In J. S. Steckenrider and T. M. Parrott (Eds.), *New directions in old-age policies* (pp. 131-150). Albany: State University of New York Press.

Naegele, G. and Walker, A. (1999). Conclusion. In A. Walker and G. Naegele (Eds.), *The politics of old age in Europe* (pp. 197-209). Buckingham, PA: Open University Press.

Peterson, P. G. (1999). *Gray dawn: How the coming age wave will transform America—and the world.* New York: Times Books.

Peterson, S. A. and Somit, A. (1994). *Political behavior of older Americans.* New York: Garland.

Pratt, H. J. (1976). *The gray lobby.* Chicago: University of Chicago Press.

Preston, S. H. (1994). Children and the elderly in the U.S. *Scientific American,* 251(6), 44-49.

Stewart, D. J. (1970). Disenfranchise the old: The lesson of California. *The New Republic,* 163(8-9), 20-22.

Thurow, L. C. (1996). The birth of a revolutionary class. *New York Times Magazine,* May 19, 46-47.

POSITIVE AGING NEWSLETTER

Erdman B. Palmore

Positive Aging Newsletter published by Kenneth and Mary Gergen on the internet (www.healthandage.com), is "Dedicated to productive dialogue between research and practice." In fact, it emphasizes positive aspects of aging and thus attempts to counteract negative ageism. A typical issue contains the following sections:

Commentary
Research
Book Alert
In The News
Readers Respond
Announcements and Upcoming Events

The newsletter is sponsored by the Novartis Foundation for Gerontology and the Taos Institute.

See also JOURNALISM

PUBLIC POLICY

Robert H. Binstock

From the New Deal of the 1930s through the late 1970s, U.S. public policy issues concerning older people were framed by an underlying ageism—the attribution of the same characteristics, status, and just deserts to a heterogeneous group that was artificially homogenized and labeled *the aged*. The lowest levels of economic status, health, and functional capacities that could be found among older persons became familiar as common denominators in public discourse (Neugarten, 1974). Elderly persons were seen as poor, frail, dependent, objects of discrimination, and above all *deserving* (Kalish, 1979).

The stereotypes expressed through this ageism were compassionate—unlike those of racism or sexism—and have not been wholly prejudicial to the well-being of its objects, older people. Indeed, throughout more than five decades the American polity implemented this construct of compassionate ageism by creating many old-age government benefit programs, as well as by enacting laws against age discrimination. During the 1960s and 1970s, just about every issue or problem affecting some older persons that could be identified by advocates for the elderly became a governmental responsibility. Programs were enacted to provide older Americans with health insurance; nutritional, legal, supportive, and leisure services; housing; home repair; energy assistance; transportation; help in getting jobs; protection against being fired from jobs; public insurance for employer-sponsored pensions, special mental health programs; and on, and on. By the late 1970s, if not earlier, American society had learned the catechism of compassionate ageism very well and had expressed it through a great many policies. A committee of the U.S. House of Representatives (1977), using loose criteria, identified 134 programs benefitting the aging, overseen by forty-nine committees and subcommittees of Congress. Today, more than one-third of the federal budget is spent on benefits to older persons (Binstock, 2002).

Although many of the old-age policies enacted during that period made distinctions among older person in determining their eligibility for assistance (e.g., through low-income and asset tests for participation in the Medicaid health insurance program, public housing, and energy assistance), a number of them treated all older persons exactly the same regardless of their personal circumstances. All persons age sixty-five and older were entitled to an extra personal deduction in filing their federal income tax. The nearly 100 percent of persons in this age category who were eligible for Medicare, a national health insurance program, received precisely the same benefits and paid precisely the same premiums in order to participate in the supplemental portion of the program, regardless of economic status. All persons age sixty and older were eligible for the supportive services and nutrition programs funded through the Older Americans Act (OAA).

Beginning in the late 1970s, however, the use of compassionate ageism in public policy was criticized. A leading gerontologist, Bernice Neugarten, sharply challenged the use of old age as a marker for determining a person's need for governmental assistance. At a major policy conference in Washington she argued against the implicit ageism in public policy:

> In a society in which age is becoming increasingly irrelevant as a predictor of lifestyle or as a predictor of need, policies and programs formulated on the basis of age are falling increasingly wide of the mark. Income and health care and housing and other goods and services should be provided, not according to age, but according to relative need. (Neugarten, 1979, pp. 50-51)

Neugarten recognized the political complexities of transforming the many old-age-based programs—many of them massive, such as Social Security and Medicare—into need-based programs, so she assembled a number of policy analysts and scholars to thoughtfully address these complexities in a compendium titled *Age or Need: Public Policies for Older People* (Neugarten, 1982).

Shortly thereafter, in the early 1980s, Congress revised some of the ageist features of policies on aging. Through a new legislative trend that has continued through today, policies on aging have been reformed incrementally to reflect the diverse economic and social characteristics of older persons.

The impetus for the first step in this trend was a financial problem in maintaining the Old-Age and Survivors Insurance (OASI) benefits of the Social Security program in the early 1980s. Sustained high rates of inflation and unemployment had brought about a short-term crisis in financing benefit payments (see Light, 1985). As part of a package of 1983 Social Security reforms to deal with that problem and anticipated future problems, the OASI benefits received by wealthier older persons were made subject to taxation, but those of other OASI recipients were not.

Once this 1983 taxation provision broke the traditional barrier against treating older persons differently in nonwelfare policies, further reforms in old-age policies began to distribute benefits according to economic status. The Tax Reform Act of 1986 eliminated the extra personal exemption that had been available to all persons age sixty-five and older when filing their federal income tax returns, and replaced it with new income tax credits for low-income older persons on a sliding scale. OAA programs and services have gradually been targeted to low-income older persons through a series of congressional amendments. In addition, policy changes have permitted OAA programs to charge for supportive services (through *cost sharing*) based on the income level of clients, and to accept *donations* from participants in congregate meal programs. Various amendments to the OAA have also targeted programs and services to minority older persons and those in the greatest *social need.*

Sensitivity to the economic status of older persons was also applied to the health policy arena beginning in 1988 with a change affecting Medicare. A provision of the Medicare Catastrophic Coverage Act established a Qualified Medicare Beneficiary program that requires the federal/state Medicaid program to pay premiums, deductibles, and coinsurance payments for Medicare enrollees who have incomes and assets that are below specific levels of federal guidelines for classifying individuals as poor. Medicaid assistance with health care expenses has subsequently been extended to additional older persons (with somewhat higher income levels) through the Omnibus Budget Reconciliation Act of 1990 and the Balanced Budget Act of 1997.

These various policy reforms firmly established the principle that it is politically feasible for nonwelfare policies on aging to treat older people differently based upon their economic status. Today, proposals for new polices on aging almost invariably make distinctions among elderly persons with respect to their economic and other characteristics. The compassionate ageism that historically characterized many policies on aging continues to erode.

See also BENEFITS OF AGING; COSTS OF AGEISM; SOCIAL SECURITY; TAX BREAKS

REFERENCES

Binstock, R. H. (2002). The politics of enacting reform. In S. H. Altman and D. I. Shactman (Eds.), *Policies for an aging society* (pp. 346-377). Baltimore, MD: Johns Hopkins University Press.

Kalish, R. A. (1979). The new ageism and the failure models: A polemic. *The Gerontologist,* 19, 398-407.

Light, P. C. (1985). *The politics of Social Security reform.* New York: Random House.

Neugarten, B. L. (1974). Age groups in American society and the rise of the young-old. *Annals of the American Academy of Political and Social Science,* 415, 187-198.

_____ (1979). Policy for the 1980s: Age or need entitlement? In J. P. Hubbard (Ed.), *Aging: Agenda for the eighties, a national journal issues book* (pp. 48-52). Washington, DC: Government Research Corporation.

_____ (Ed.) (1982). *Age or need? Public policies for older people.* Beverly Hills, CA: Sage.

U.S. House of Representatives, Select Committee on Aging (1977). *Federal responsibility to the elderly: Executive programs and legislative jurisdiction.* Washington, DC: U. S. Government Printing Office.

REDUCING AGEISM

Erdman B. Palmore

Strategies for reducing ageism can be divided into those focused on changing individuals and those focused on changing the social structure. Strategies for reducing ageism in individuals include the following (Palmore, 1999):

- *Testing ageism.* This is useful to determine what prejudices and misconceptions about aging the individual holds and need to be corrected. The Facts on Aging Quiz (FAQ) has been widely used for this purpose (Palmore, 1998).
- *Education, propaganda, and exhortation.* These are three related methods of trying to change the individual's attitudes and misconceptions.
- *Slogans.* These may be used to counteract the prejudices and misconceptions that many people have. Their advantage is that they are usually catchy and easy to remember.
- *Benefits of aging.* A listing of these benefits may be used to counteract the negative aspects of aging of which most people are aware, and which are usually exaggerated into stereotypes. Most people are usually not aware of the many benefits of aging.
- *Religion.* Religious organizations are uniquely able to use exhortation to reduce ageism. They can influence more people than any other type of institution; they can call on the authority of the Bible and other teachings of their religion, as well as the authority of the church and synagogue leaders.

- *The media.* Print and electronic media (including television) influence more people for more hours of the day than any other one mass influence. It can be used to correct misconceptions, change images, and reduce stereotypes and discrimination by individuals.
- *Personal contact.* When personal contact is equal and cooperative, it is the most effective strategy for reducing prejudice and discrimination in the areas of racism and sexism. It would be equally effective in reducing ageism.
- *Models of successful aging.* When elders themselves model successful aging by being healthy, active, involved, and productive, they set examples that challenge the old negative stereotypes about aging.
- *Therapy.* If ageism is caused by some emotional personality problem (as in the authoritarian personality), individual or group therapy may be needed to reduce the ageism.

Social structures that need to be changed in order to reduce ageism include the following:

- *The economy.* Ageism in the economy that needs to be reduced includes employment discrimination, Social Security, Supplemental Security Income (SSI), and taxation.
- *The government.* Ageism in the government includes negative and positive ageism in various government agencies and programs; and the legal system.
- *The family.* Ageism in the family is found in marriage (older men marrying only younger women); the norms against remarriage for widowed or divorced elders; and elder abuse by family members.
- *Housing.* Ageism in housing includes residential segregation, subsidized housing for elders only, and "architecture" for the elderly.
- *Health care.* Ageism needs to be reduced in the exclusion of younger people from Medicare; in the discrimination against handicapped elders by rehabilitation programs; in the forcing of elders into nursing homes against their will; and the prejudice and misconceptions about aging among health professionals.

See also AGE-SPECIFIC PUBLIC PROGRAMS; BENEFITS OF AGING; CHANGE STRATEGIES; CHURCHES; EDUCATION; EMPLOYMENT DIS-

CRIMINATION; HEALTH CARE; HOUSING; JOURNALISM; SLOGANS; TELEVISION

REFERENCES

Palmore, E. (1998) *Facts on aging quiz.* New York: Springer.
_____ (1999). *Ageism.* New York: Springer.

RESPONSES TO AGEISM

Erdman B. Palmore

In the face of the prejudice and discrimination of ageism, elders respond with acceptance, denial, avoidance, or reform.

Acceptance

This response may range from reluctant submission to complete endorsement. Some elders voluntarily disengage from social and other activity, but remain satisfied with their lives (Havighurst, 1968). They are contented to "retire to the rocking chair."

Another type of acceptance is called the *apathetic.* This type disengages reluctantly and are not happy with their role. They feel they are imprisoned in a "roleless role"; but think they can do nothing about it (Burgess, 1960).

Both of these acceptance types have internalized role expectations and stereotypes in the same way as they were socialized to accept other role expectations related to earlier roles. Throughout life there are subtle and sometimes overt sanctions to "act your age." In old age, these age norms are more flexible and the sanctions may be more informal, but they are nonetheless real and potent (Back, 2001).

This type of elder may not even be aware of ageism and may simply accept the role restrictions of old age as normal and natural. Many responders to the Ageism Survey denied that they had ever experienced any ageism. This is a denial, or unawareness, of *ageism,* in contrast to the second type who deny their *age.*

Denial

The response of denial is similar to the minority group response of *passing*. In this case, elders try to deny their membership in the devalued group (the aged) and "pass" for younger persons. This may take the form of lying about their true age, dyeing their gray hair, getting face lifts and tummy tucks, attempting to minimize wrinkles with Botox, etc.

Some of this denial is a result of confusing aging with deterioration—these elders try to deny their age because they are denying that they have deteriorated. They equate healthiness with youth and therefore try to claim they are still young. Age denial should not be confused with attempts to stay healthy and vigorous.

Avoidance

Elders may try to avoid ageism through age segregation, isolation, alcoholism, substance abuse, mental illness, or even suicide (Palmore, 1999).

Age-segregated retirement communities separate elders from the prejudice and discrimination of younger people. Fear of victimization and violence is often given as a reason for moving to a retirement community (Jacobs, 1974). The slights and indignities experienced by elders in their dealings with younger people can be minimized in segregated communities.

Elders may also isolate themselves from contact with younger people even though living in an age-integrated community. They avoid leaving their home as much as possible. In this way they can avoid face-to-face contact with younger people as effectively as if they lived in an age-segregated community.

Alcoholism and other substance abuse are other ways to avoid ageism. When a person is drunk or high on drugs he or she may not notice the ageism of younger people.

Mental illness may be another kind of escape from ageism. If the problems of old age become unbearable, one can escape into a fantasy world of psychosis. This has been called *avoidance psychosis* (Payne, Gibson, and Pittard, 1969). The symptoms of avoidance psychosis may be indistinguishable from those of organic dementia.

Suicide is the ultimate escape from ageism. Suicide rates increase sharply with age among males in the United States and other industrialized countries, but not among older women (Kastenbaum, 2001). The typical profile of the older suicide victim is a man who is depressed, socially isolated, not married, downwardly mobile, residing in an urban area, and suffering from illness or disability. It is probable that much of this isolation and depression is caused, at least in part, by ageism.

Reform

Reform recognizes the prejudice and discrimination of ageism and seeks to eliminate it, or at least to reduce it. This response has not been as prevalent as the other three, but signs indicate that more elders are becoming aware of ageism and working to reduce it. Many organizations are now devoted to combating ageism. Neugarten (1970) suggests that attempts to reduce ageism may grow as elders become increasingly educated, healthier, and affluent:

> As they become accustomed to the politics of confrontation they see around them, they may also become a more demanding group. There are signs that this is already so, with, for example, appeals to "senior power" . . . and with more older people picketing and protesting over such local issues as reduced fares or better housing projects. (p. 17)

Many elders quietly challenge the ageist stereotypes by engaging in activities that do not conform to these stereotypes. They continue to be athletic, healthy, romantic, clever, involved, and active. They usually are proud of their age, rather than trying to deny it. Such challenge of ageism by personal example may be more effective than all the activities of organizations attempting to reduce ageism.

See also AGE DENIAL; AGE NORMS; ALCOHOLISM; ORGANIZATIONS OPPOSING AGEISM; ROLE EXPECTATIONS; RETIREMENT; SUICIDE

REFERENCES

Back, K. (2001). Age norms. In G. Maddox (Ed.), *The encyclopedia of aging.* New York: Springer.

Burgess, E. (Ed.) (1960). *Aging in western societies.* Chicago: University of Chicago Press.

Havighurst, R. (1968). Personality and patterns of aging. *The Gerontologist, 8, 20.*

Jacobs, J. (1974). *Fun city.* New York: Holt, Rinehart, and Winston.

Kastenbaum, R. (2001). Suicide. In G. Maddox (Ed.), *The encyclopedia of aging.* New York: Springer.

Neugarten, B. (1970). The old and young in modern societies. *American Behavioral Scientist,* 14, 13.

Palmore, E. (1999). *Ageism.* New York: Springer.

Payne, R. Gibson, F., and Pittard, B. (1969). Social influences in senile psychosis. *Sociological Symposium,* 1, 137.

RETIREMENT COMMUNITIES

James T. Sykes

Do retirement communities reflect another form of ageism in society? Some older persons, with the financial resources to do so, have chosen to live in retirement communities usually open only to retired persons. Critics have called retirement communities age-segregated housing and assert that those who live there are, somehow, victims of discrimination, or at least misguided for having chosen such an environment. To address the question of whether a form of ageism underlies the concept and development of retirement communities requires that one understand the motivations of both those who develop retirement communities and the retired persons who decide to move into one.

Note should be taken that although retirement communities have been developed to appeal to persons looking for a special place to live for their retirement years, over time other communities become—when more than 50 percent of the households are headed by persons of retirement age—what have been called "naturally occurring retirement communities" (Hunt and Gunter-Hunt, 1996, p. 3). In addition, given the various ages at which people retire, a retirement community might be home to persons as young as fifty or as old as 100. Even the term *retirement community* needs to be understood as including a wide variety of living environments including planned communities, retirement communities near to college campuses, large complexes developed privately to appeal to upper income retirees eager for an active lifestyle, and continuing-care retirement communities that serve active older persons as well as those who need support and health care services. A subsidized housing project for older residents is also a retirement community. With such diversity among residents and living arrangements, from intentional retirement communities to naturally occurring retirement communities, one cannot easily discern forms of ageism in the communities themselves or in the decisions retirees make when they choose to live in a retirement community.

The term *age-segregated* has often been applied to developments designed for retirees with little regard to the negative connotations the term implies. Those who have decided—for whatever reason—to live in such a facility or community have been subject to criticism for choosing to live among people, generally, of their own age, as though by so doing they have rejected the benefits of living in age-integrated communities. Astute observers have noted that retirees living in the midst of diverse communities may have little or no contact with their neighbors. Those familiar with retirement communities acknowledge that often two or three generations of retirees live side by side in retirement complexes. With special efforts, people from the surrounding neighborhoods are drawn to the retirement community, thus providing residents with more opportunities for engagement with people of all ages than may be true for those living in the midst of so-called age-integrated neighborhoods or communities.

Applying a definition such as "ageism is the systematic stereotyping and discrimination against people because they are old" (Butler, 1969, p. 243), one must push this definition to find ageism implicit in the concept of retirement communities or in the motivations of those living in retirement communities, whether purpose-built or naturally occurring. Of course, one may argue that retirement communities discriminate against people who are young. However, if one allows that people who live in gated communities are not discriminating against other people, but simply exercising their freedom to live where they choose, and can afford to live, then one must allow that retirees who choose and can afford to live in communities and facilities designed especially for older persons are not discriminating against younger people—an obvious form of ageism—but simply choosing a living arrangement they have a right to choose without being labeled victims of ageism or judged to be discriminating against younger people.

However, one form of ageism, *gerontophobia,* can be found in retirement communities: when some residents become quite frail and need services, other residents may resent living among persons with disabilities, fearing the consequences of their own aging (Palmore, 1972). To resolve this problem, both within a retirement community and in society generally, requires a major effort to educate people to the realities associated with long life and for older persons to learn not only to cope, but also to understand and accept their own aging as well as the fact that some of their neighbors may be frail.

Those who apply the term ageism to retirement communities or seek to establish a connection between the perverse effects of age discrimination and stereotyping to retirement communities will find it difficult to provide evidence to support that claim. As a concept and as an alternative living arrangement—among many—retirement communities provide the environment and amenities that some retirees have chosen. Unfortunately, the fact is that to live in most retirement communities, a retiree must have a fairly high income. Unfortunately, that means many who would like to consider moving into a retirement community will face discrimination based not on age, but on being unable to afford a retirement community.

See also AGE SEGREGATION; AGE STRATIFICATION; SUBCULTURES

REFERENCES

Butler, R. N. (1969). Ageism: Another form of bigotry. *The Gerontologist,* 9, 243-246.
Hunt, M. E. and Gunter-Hunt, G. (1986). Naturally occurring retirement communities. *Journal of Housing for the Elderly,* 3(3), 3-21.
Palmore, E. (1972). Gerontophobia versus ageism. *The Gerontologist,* 12, 213.

ROLE EXPECTATIONS

Diana K. Harris

A role may be defined as a pattern of behavior built around certain specific rights and obligations associated with the position one holds in a group (e.g., spouse or grandparent). A role refers to a set of expectations for behavior held by the person occupying the role as well as the expectations of others. For example, the role of grandparent carries with it certain expectations. These include staying in regular contact with one's grandchildren, giving them affection, serving as role models for them, and telling them about their family history.

Role expectations may vary along a wide range of behavior but if persons deviate too much from what is considered culturally acceptable behavior by others, they will be negatively sanctioned. In the case of grandparents, deviations would include ignoring their grandchildren's birthdays, seldom seeing them, and not helping their grandchildren when they are in financial need even though they can afford to do so.

Role expectations may be a form of ageism when they are contrary to what the older person can do and wants to do. For example, the expectation that older workers are obligated to retire at a certain age regardless of their ability or their desire to continue working would be an ageist role expectation. Another example of an ageist role expectation would be that older persons should have *no* role that has been referred to as the *roleless role* of persons at retirement (Burgess, 1960). This expectation would deprive older people of *all* activity.

Role expectations consist of rights and obligations. For instance, the rights of retirees include having economic support without working and the freedom to manage their own time. The obligations of retirees include taking care of their health and remaining independent as long as possible. In addition, they should manage their financial resources wisely and not need assistance from their families or the community. Retirees are expected to engage in activities that indicate effort toward worthwhile goals of their own choosing. Such activities may include home maintenance and gardening, going back to school, doing volunteer work, or taking a part-time job.

See also AGE NORMS; SUBCULTURES

REFERENCE

Burgess, E. (1960). *Aging in Western societies.* Chicago: University of Chicago Press.

S

SCAPEGOATING

Robert H. Binstock

Prior to the early 1980s, the predominant stereotypes of older people in American public discourse were sympathetic (Kalish, 1979). But then, rather suddenly, these compassionate stereotypes underwent an extraordinary reversal. Older Americans were depicted by negative stereotypes and, as a group, became a scapegoat for a variety of societal problems. This scapegoating of older people is a form of ageism in which elders are both depicted unfavorably and falsely blamed for various problems in our society.

A key precipitating factor in the development of older people as a scapegoat was that in the late 1970s journalists (e.g., Samuelson, 1978) and academicians (e.g., Hudson, 1978) discovered "the graying of the budget," a tremendous increase in the proportion of federal dollars expended on public benefits to older citizens. The funds spent on older people had grown to be more than one-quarter of the annual federal budget and comparable in size to spending for national defense.

Whereas elderly persons had previously been stereotyped as poor and deserving, they now began to be portrayed as flourishing and a burden to society. As *Forbes* magazine succinctly and patronizingly expressed the new wisdom concerning "old folks": "The myth is that they're sunk in poverty. The reality is that they're living well. The trouble is there are too many of them—God bless 'em" (Flint, 1980, p. 51).

Throughout the 1980s and well into the 1990s, the new stereotypes, readily observed in popular culture, presented older people as prosperous, hedonistic, politically powerful, and selfish. For example, "Grays on the Go," a 1988 cover story in *Time,* described older persons as America's new elite—healthy, wealthy, powerful, and "staging history's biggest retirement party" (Gibbs, 1988, p. 66).

A dominant theme in such accounts of older people was that their selfishness was ruining the nation. The *New Republic* highlighted this motif in 1988 with a drawing on the cover caricaturing older persons, and captioned "greedy geezers" (Fairlie, 1988). The theme was widely echoed, and the epithet "greedy geezers" became a familiar adjective in journalistic accounts of federal budget politics (e.g., Salholz, 1990). *Fortune* magazine went so far as to declaim that the "Tyranny of America's Old" was "one of the most crucial issues facing U.S. society" (Smith, 1992, p. 68).

In this unsympathetic climate of opinion, "the aged" emerged as a scapegoat for an impressive list of American problems. Demographer Samuel Preston (1984) and various advocates for children blamed the political power of elderly Americans for the plight of youngsters who had inadequate nutrition, health care, and education, and insufficiently supportive family environments. One children's advocate even proposed that parents receive an "extra vote" for each of their children in order to combat the pernicious impact of older voters (Carballo, 1981). A former secretary of commerce (Peterson, 1987) suggested that a prerequisite for the United States to regain its stature as a first-class power in the world economy was a sharp reduction in programs benefitting older Americans.

The blame for spiraling U.S. health care costs was redirected, in part, from the health care providers, suppliers, administrators, and insurers—the parties responsible for setting the prices of care—to elderly people. For instance, a prominent biomedical ethicist, Daniel Callahan (1987), depicted health care costs for older persons as a "great fiscal black hole" (p. 17) that would absorb an unlimited amount of national resources. Accordingly, he scapegoated the elderly population as a "new social threat" and a "demographic, economic, and medical avalanche . . . that could ultimately . . . do great harm" (p. 20). He and a number of other academicians and public figures, including politicians, urged vigorously that American society set limits to health care for older people (see Binstock and Post, 1991).

In 1989 a distinguished "executive panel" of American leaders convened by the Ford Foundation designated older persons as the only group of citizens responsible for financing a broad range of social programs for persons of all ages. In its report the panel recommended a series of policies costing $29 billion, to be financed solely by taxing the Social Security benefits of older individuals (Ford Foundation, 1989). In fact, every financing alternative considered in the report assumed that elderly people should be the exclusive financiers of the $29 billion in costs. Apparently, the Ford panel felt that the reasons for this assumption were self-evident; it did not even bother to justify its consideration of just these financing options as opposed to other sources.

The various problems for which the elderly had become a scapegoat were thematically unified as issues of so-called "intergenerational equity"—really, intergenerational *inequity*—through the efforts of Americans for Generational Equity (AGE). Formed in 1985, AGE was led by several congressman and scapegoaters such as Preston and Callahan who were board members. Most of its funding came from insurance companies, health care corporations, banks, and other private-sector businesses and organizations that were in competition with Medicare and Social Security (Quadagno, 1989) and therefore would benefit financially from their curtailment or elimination.

Central to AGE's credo was the proposition that older people were locked in an intergenerational conflict with younger-age cohorts regarding the distribution of public resources. The organization disseminated this viewpoint effectively from its Washington office through press releases, media interviews, and a quarterly publication, *The Generational Journal,* as well as through conferences with such titles as "Children At Risk: Who Will Support an Aging Society?" Although AGE faded from the scene in the early 1990s, its themes of intergenerational equity and conflict were carried forward by a new organization, the Concord Coalition, which favored scaling back Social Security benefits (Concord Coalition, 1993).

The theme of a war between the generations was adopted by the media, academics, and a variety of commentators on public affairs as a routine perspective for describing many social-policy issues (Cook et al., 1994). It also gained currency in elite sectors of American society. The president of the prestigious American Association of Universities, for instance, asserted that the shape of the domestic federal budget pits programs for the retired against every other social purpose dependent on federal funds (Rosenzweig, 1990, p. 6).

During the two terms of William Clinton's presidency in the 1990s, when the U.S. economy was prosperous and the federal budget began to develop annual surpluses, scapegoating of older people diminished somewhat. Politicians, academicians, and the media began to turn their attention to issues of how to finance Social Security and Medicare for baby boomers when they join the ranks of old age in the first half of the twenty-first century (see Altman and Shactman, 2002).

Even then, however, some prominent public figures hastened to portray future cohorts of older people as a danger to society. Economist Lester Thurow (1996) envisioned elderly baby boomers and their self-interested pursuit of government benefits as a fundamental threat to democratic political systems, and warned, "In the years ahead, class warfare is apt to be redefined as the young against the old, rather than the poor against the rich" (p. 47). And at the turn of the century, former presidential cabinet member Peter Peterson (1999) warned that population aging in developed countries could "enthrone organized elders as an invincible political titan," and that " 'intergenerational war' . . . should not be ruled out anywhere in the developed world" (p. 209). Such scapegoating perpetuates a series of false stereotypes that make it an especially pernicious form of ageism.

See also: GENERATIONAL EQUITY; GERONTOCRACY; POLITICS; PUBLIC POLICY

REFERENCES

Altman, S. H. and Shactman, D. I. (Eds.) (2002). *Policies for an aging society*. Baltimore, MD: Johns Hopkins University Press.

Binstock, R. H. and Post, S. G. (Eds.) (1991). *Too old for health care?: Controversies in medicine, law, economics, and ethics*. Baltimore, MD: The Johns Hopkins University Press.

Callahan, D. (1987). *Setting limits: Medical goals in an aging society*. New York: Simon & Schuster.

Carballo, M. (1981). Extra votes for parents? *The Boston Globe,* December 17, p. 35.

Concord Coalition (1993). *The zero deficit plan: A plan for eliminating the federal budget deficit by the year 2000*. Washington, DC: The Concord Coalition.

Cook, F. L, Marshall, V. M., Marshall, J. E., and Kaufman, J. E. (1994). The salience of intergenerational equity in Canada and the United States. In T. R. Marmor, T. M. Smeeding, and V. L. Greene (Eds.), *Economic security and international justice: A look at North America* (pp. 91-129). Washington, DC: Urban Institute Press.

Fairlie, H. (1988). Talkin' 'bout my generation. *New Republic,* 198(13), 19-22.

Flint, J. (1980). The old folks. *Forbes,* February 18, 51-56.

Ford Foundation (1989). *The common good: Social welfare and the American future.* New York: The Ford Foundation.

Gibbs, N. R. (1988). Grays on the go. *Time,* 131(8), 66-77.

Hudson, R. B. (1978). The "graying" of the federal budget and its consequences for old age policy. *The Gerontologist,* 18, 428-440.

Kalish, R. A. (1979). The new ageism and the failure models: A polemic. *The Gerontologist,* 19, 398-407.

Peterson, P. G. (1987). The morning after. *Atlantic,* 260(4), 43-69.

_____ (1999). *Gray dawn: How the coming age wave will transform America—and the world.* New York: Times Books.

Preston, S. H. (1984). Children and the elderly in the U.S. *Scientific American,* 251(6), 44-49.

Quadagno, J. (1989). Generational equity and the politics of the welfare state. *Politics and Society,* 17(3), 353-376.

Rozensweig, R. M. (1990). Address to the President's Opening Session, 43rd Annual Scientific Meeting, Gerontological Society of America, Boston, MA, November 16.

Salholz, E. (1990). Blaming the voters: Hapless budgeteers single out "greedy geezers." *Newsweek,* October 29, 36.

Samuelson, R. J. (1978). Aging America: Who will shoulder the growing burden? *National Journal,* 10, 1712-1717.

Smith, L. (1992). The tyranny of America's old. *Fortune,* 125(1), 68-72.

Thurow, L. C. (1996). The birth of a revolutionary class. *New York Times Magazine,* May 19, 46-47.

SELF-FULFILLING PROPHECY

Diana K. Harris

Proposed by Robert K. Merton (1957), the self-fulfilling prophecy is based on the theorem attributed to W. I. Thomas: "If men define situations as real, they are real in their consequences." A false definition of a situation, or belief which one acts upon, actually manifests itself as truth and further strengthens the belief. Definitions of a situation become a part of the situation and thus have an effect on the actual consequences. The self-fulfilling prophecy is a false definition of the situation that results in a new behavior in which the originally false conception become true. The self-fulfilling prophecy goes a long way in explaining the plight of many of the elderly in our society today.

For example, because of ageism, people frequently label the elderly as incompetent, obsolete, sexless, and so on. As a result, they treat them as if they were. In time the elderly begin to accept such negative labeling and then they begin to think of themselves in this way and begin to act as if these labels were true. This sets the stage for the vicious cycle of increasing incompetence, etc. In other words, the label then proves to be a self-fulfilling prophecy.

Related to the self-fulfilling prophecy is the *social breakdown syndrome* proposed by Kuypers and Bengtson (1973). This syndrome explains how ageism reinforces itself. It consists of a four-stage cycle. The first stage is based on the premise that the elderly are highly susceptible to social labeling because they are deprived of positive feedback and support from others. This susceptibility is due to ambiguous norms, their loss of roles, and their lack of reference groups. Second, because of this lack of positive feedback and support from family, friends, and significant others, the elderly become dependent for self-labeling on the larger society that often stereotypes and characterizes them as incompetent, obsolete, sexless, etc. Third, those older persons who accept such negative labeling learn to act as if the labels are true and they begin to think of themselves in this way. This sets the stage for the vicious cycle of increasing social and psychological incompetence.

Kuypers and Bengtson (1973) note that the breakdown of competence in elderly persons can be reversed by *social reconstruction syndrome.* This syndrome is accomplished by giving older persons improved and supportive environment along with helping them to develop a sense of personal strength.

See also ROLE EXPECTATIONS; STEREOTYPES

REFERENCES

Kuypers, J. and Bengtson, V. (1973). Social breakdown and competence: A model of normal aging. *Human Development,* 16, 181-201.

Merton, R. (1957). *Social theory and social structure.* Glencoe, IL: Free Press.

SEMANTIC DIFFERENTIAL SCALE

Erdman B. Palmore

This scale is one of the best ways to measure ageism or attitudes toward elders (Rosencranz and McNevin, 1969). It consists of a series of polar adjectives such as "weak—strong" and "sad—happy," which are arranged at the ends of a continuum, and responders are asked to place a mark along the line to represent where they think older people are on that continuum. Thus, it is clearly a measure of attitudes and feeling toward older people, rather than a measure of knowledge or facts about aging. Palmore concludes that this scale is a clearer and more direct measure of attitudes than his Facts on Aging Quiz (FAQ) (Palmore, 1998).

The FAQ was designed to be primarily a measure of knowledge about aging and older persons, but it can be used as an indirect measure of attitudes if one assumes that incorrect answers on some items show negative or positive bias toward the aged. For example, if one responds with "True" to the statement, "The majority of old people are senile (have defective memory, are disoriented, or demented)," this probably indicates a negative bias toward old people.

The Semantic Differential Scale is also a clearer measure of attitudes than the Kogan "Attitudes Toward Old People" Scale (1961), because the Kogan scale confuses factual statements with attitudinal statements, all of which are arbitrarily scored as being "favorable" or "unfavorable." For example the statement, "Most old people would prefer to continue working just as long as they can, rather than be dependent on anybody," is probably false, depending on what is meant by "working" and "dependent." In fact, most old people are content to be retired and dependent on their Social Security and other retirement income. Yet a "disagree" response is scored as showing an "unfavorable" attitude toward the aged. Unfortunately, some negative stereotypes about the aged are generally true, and some of the positive statements are generally false.

Numerous studies have used and validated the Semantic Differential Scale as a measure of attitudes toward elders.

See also DEFINITIONS; FACTS ON AGING QUIZ; STEREOTYPES

REFERENCES

Kogan, N. (1961). Attitudes toward old people. *Journal of Abnormal Psychology,* 62, 44-54.

Palmore, E. (1998). *The facts on aging quiz* (Second edition). New York: Springer.

Rosencranz, H. and McNevin, T. (1969). A factor analysis of attitudes toward the aged. *The Gerontologist,* 9, 55-59.

SENIOR CENTERS

Erdman B. Palmore

Age-segregated facilities, such as senior centers, discriminate against younger people and therefore are a form of ageism. It is a kind of *positive ageism* in that it discriminates in favor of older people. From the standpoint of younger people who are not admitted and who pay most of the taxes that support the centers, senior centers are a negative kind of ageism, or *reverse ageism.*

Unquestionably, senior centers perform many good services from information and referral, through congregate meal services, to fitness and social activities. In fact, the average number of activities and services offered is more than 30 percent (Krout, 2001).

Nevertheless, several problems exist with the policy of restricting senior centers to seniors:

- They discriminate against younger people. This is by definition a kind of ageism and is as ethically wrong as a policy of restricting community centers to younger persons.
- They waste community resources by providing duplicate facilities for different age groups, which could be served by one facility: a community center for all ages.
- They are based largely on the old stereotype that most seniors are frail or disabled, senile, poor, or otherwise in need of special programs. This stereotype is in fact true of only a small minority of persons over sixty-five—probably about 20 percent. The other 80 percent are able to engage in their normal activities, are mentally competent, and have incomes well above the poverty line.

- Activities or programs that require older persons to define themselves as "old" or in any way incapable or inferior, are unattractive to most seniors. This may be the main reason that about 85 percent of persons over sixty-five do not participate in any senior centers.

The solution to these problems is to open up the senior centers to all ages, making them *community centers,* and thus eliminating the ageism involved in restricting the centers to seniors.

See also AGE SEGREGATION; AGE-SPECIFIC PUBLIC PROGRAMS; TYPOLOGIES

REFERENCE

Krout, J. (2001). Senior centers. In G. Maddox (Ed.), *The encyclopedia of aging.* New York: Springer.

SEXISM

Marla Harris

Although all elderly are potentially subject to prejudice because of ageism, elderly women must combat the *double standard* of aging, in which the discriminatory effects of ageism are compounded with those of sexism (Sontag, 1972). This double standard is not uniquely modern but has been found in preindustrial societies, as well as in industrialized ones (Markson, 1997; Haber, 1997). In colonial America, for instance, elderly widows independent by virtue of wealth, property, or business were frequently viewed with suspicion, and sometimes accused of witchcraft; more often elderly women found themselves dependents in the homes of relatives, with relatively little freedom (Haber, 1997).

In modern times the persistent antipathy toward older women has had wide-ranging implications, including low self-esteem. It is evident even in the realm of humor, where old women are the target of negative jokes, disproportionately more often than older men (Palmore, 1971). Internalizing this cultural bias, younger women may discriminate against older women by ignoring, avoiding, or otherwise marginalizing them (Macdonald and Rich, 2001). Matthews (1979) reports on older women's reluctance to self-identify themselves as old women, which they perceive to be a stigmatized group, and their strategies to differentiate themselves from other old women.

According to Sontag, the problem arises from the way that femininity has been equated with youthful attractiveness. Historically women have been valued according to their fertility; the older woman, no longer (re)productive, is deemed no longer feminine (Markson, 1997). Unlike the older man, whose financial or social status may enhance or redefine his sex appeal, the older woman is rarely considered sexually eligible or desirable. Moreover, the increasing medicalization of the female reproductive cycle has encouraged the pathologization of the postmenopausal female body (Gannon, 1999).

Quite apart from cultural prejudices that devalue the older woman, socioeconomic inequities contribute to the older woman's being, on the whole, more disadvantaged than the older man. Lesnoff-Caravaglia (1984) asserts that "The problems of old age in the industrialized world are largely the problems of older women" (p. 17). Indeed older women in the industrialized world in general, and in the United States in particular, significantly outnumber older men and will continue to do so (Administration on Aging, 2000). Furthermore, "most women will, under present conditions, become poor if they live long enough" (Lesnoff-Caravaglia, 1984, p. 17). Older women are almost twice as likely to face poverty as older men (Administration on Aging, 2000). One reason for the higher poverty rate is that women have historically worked for no pay or for lower pay than men. Another reason is that women live longer than men, typically marry men slightly older than themselves, and so are more likely to be widowed. Palmore (1997) stresses, however, the need to determine "whether the inferior status of older women is due to present sexism against older women or to a lifetime of past sexism" (p. 4).

Although older women are the most obvious sufferers of inequities between the sexes, Thompson (1994) charges that older men are also victims of sexism, for "Ironically, as older women's lives and their profound needs gained visibility, older men became more marginal and invisible. In fact, being elderly appears in some quarters to have become synonymous with being female" (p. 14). Feminizing aged men belies the extent to which "men's personal experiences of age are challenged by cultural double binds and structurally induced conflicts about masculinities" (p. 14). It has been suggested, however, that old age brings with it not so much a loss of gender identity as a convergence of gender roles that affects women as well as men; just as men adopt some traits culturally associated with femininity, so women take on some traits identified as masculine (Palmore, 1997).

As is evident from even a brief review of the literature, sexism joined to ageism is demoralizing whether it affects men or women. With increasing numbers of younger and middle-aged women balancing motherhood and careers outside the home, it seems likely that social biases and economic inequities between the sexes will diminish over time, which should in turn reduce the negative stereotyping of elderly women. The challenge will be meeting the different needs of older men and older women instead of placing them in competition with one another.

See also AGE INEQUALITY; FACE-LIFTS; SEXUALITY

REFERENCES

Administration on Aging (2000). Older women. Washington, DC: Administration on Aging. <http://www.aoa.gov/NAIC/Notes/olderwomen.html>.

Coyle, J. M. (Ed.) (1997). *Handbook on women and aging.* Westport, CT: Greenwood.

Gannon, L. (1999). *Women and aging: Transcending the myths.* London: Routledge.

Haber, C. (1997). Witches, widow, wives, and workers: The historiography of elderly women in America. In J. M. Coyle (Ed.), *Handbook on women and aging* (pp. 29-40). Westport, CT: Greenwood.

Lesnoff-Caravaglia, G. (1984). Double stigmata: Female and old. In G. Lesnoff-Caravaglia (Ed.), *The world of the older woman: Conflicts and resolutions* (pp. 11-20). New York: Human Sciences Press.

Macdonald, B. and Rich, C. (2001). *Look me in the eye: Old women, aging, and ageism.* Denver: Spinsters Ink.

Markson, E. (1997). Sagacious, sinful, or superfluous? The social construction of older women. In J. M. Coyle (Ed.), *Handbook on women and aging* (pp. 53-71). Westport, CT: Greenwood.

Matthews, S. (1979). *The social world of old women: Management of self-identity.* Beverly Hills, CA: Sage.

Palmore, E. (1971). Attitudes toward aging as shown by humor. *The Gerontologist,* 11, 181.

_____ (1997). Sexism and ageism. In J. M. Coyle (Ed.), *Handbook on women and aging* (pp. 3-13). Westport, CT: Greenwood.

Sontag, S. (1972). The double standard of aging. *Saturday Review,* 55, 29-38.

Thompson, E. H. Jr. (1994). Older men as invisible men in contemporary society. In E. H. Thompson Jr. (Ed.), *Older men's lives* (pp. 1-21). Thousand Oaks, CA: Sage.

SEXUALITY

Diana K. Harris

One of the least-understood aspects of life in the later years has been sexuality. As a result, many erroneous beliefs and stereotypes exist concerning the sexual behavior of older people, which in turn has contributed to ageist attitudes about the topic.

One of the more common beliefs is that older persons are not interested in sex and do not think about it. Old age is often thought of as a period devoid of sexuality in which elderly persons are often relegated to a neuter status. Contributing to this view is the fact that many older people are embarrassed to talk about their sexuality for fear of disapproval.

Another belief that prevails in our society is that sexuality of any kind in the later years is disgusting and contemptible. It is felt that sex is only for the young. For example, an older man who shows interest in sex is quickly censured and given the ageist label of a "dirty old man," and an older female may be labeled a "frustrated, indecent old woman." Sexual activity of any kind on the part of older persons is rarely referred to except in derogatory terms. According to ageist thinking, "what is virility at twenty-five becomes lechery at sixty-five" (Rubin, 1965).

In their study of sex and sexuality among elderly persons, Starr and Weiner (1981) collected questionnaire data from 800 people between the ages of sixty and ninety-one. They found that a substantial majority (75 percent) indicated that sex after sixty was just as satisfying or more satisfying than when they were younger. The respondents believed that sex is important for physical and mental health. Most were satisfied with their lives and saw them remaining much the same as they get even older.

The Duke Longitudinal Studies found that almost half of married women remained sexually active through their sixties, and about half of the married men remained sexually active until their mid-seventies (Palmore, 1981). Furthermore, substantial proportions reported stable or even increasing sexual activity from earlier to later examinations.

However, many older women are forced to give up sexual activity not from the lack of desire but from the lack of a partner. About three-quarters of all married women will be widows at some point in their lives, due to the difference in life expectancy between the sexes and the fact that men usually marry women younger than themselves.

The requirement for sexual expression and the capacity to enjoy it are lifelong. We never outgrow our need to be close to another human being, and to be touched or caressed.

See also FACTS ON AGING QUIZ; SELF-FULFILLING PROPHECY; SEXISM; STEREOTYPES

REFERENCES

Palmore, E. (1981). *Social patterns of normal aging.* Durham, NC: Duke University Press.

Rubin, I. (1965). *Sexual life after sixty.* New York: Basic Books.

Starr, B. and Weiner, M. (1981). *The Starr-Weiner report on sexuality in the mature years.* New York: McGraw-Hill.

SLOGANS

Erdman B. Palmore

Slogans have often been an important part of various movements and attempts to change attitudes. To combat racism, several slogans were popular, such as "Black is beautiful," "Black power," and "We shall overcome." To combat sexism, there is "A man of quality is not threatened by a woman of equality" and "A woman's place is in the House and the Senate."

On the other hand, negative slogans can reinforce prejudice. Several familiar slogans or jokes reinforce negative ageism, such as:

- Five Bs of aging: baldness, bifocals, bridges, bulges, and bunions
- Old age is an incurable disease.
- Old age is when your legs buckle and your belt doesn't.
- There's no fool like an old fool.
- You can't teach an old dog new tricks.
- You're getting old when it takes longer to rest than to get tired.

Recently, many pro-age slogans are appearing on bumper stickers, buttons, birthday napkins, T-shirts, caps, and coffee mugs (Palmore, 1999). These slogans can be used to combat negative ageism.

- Age is a case of mind over matter. If you don't mind, it don't matter.
- Age is important only for wines and cheese.
- Age is just a number.
- Aged for smoothness and taste.
- Aged to perfection.
- Aging is living.
- The best wines come in old bottles.
- Better over the hill than under it.
- Better sixty than pregnant.
- Being young at heart is better than being young.
- Elders have done it longer.
- Fifty is nifty.
- Gray power.
- Grow old with me, the best is yet to be.
- How dare you think I'd rather be younger?
- If aging improves quality, I'm approaching perfection.
- I'm not over the hill. I'm on a roll.
- I'm not a dirty old man; I'm a sexy senior citizen.
- It's never too late to learn.
- It's not how old you are, but how you are old.
- It's no sin to be seventy.
- Old age is better than its alternative.
- Old age is not for sissies.
- Old age is the consummation of life.
- Old wines and violins are the best.
- Older is bolder.
- Over the hill and loving it.

- Over the hill and off the pill.
- People are like cars: their age is less important than how they've been treated.
- Retired: no boss, no worries, no work, no pay.
- Retired: rejuvenated, retreaded, relaxed, and remodeled.
- Senior power.
- Sixty and still sexy.
- The best thing about being a parent is you may get to be a grand-parent.
- The first fifty years are just a rehearsal.
- The older the violin, the sweeter the music.
- There may be snow on the roof, but there's fire in the hearth.
- Things of quality have no fear of time.
- When you're over the hill, you pick up speed.
- You can teach an old dog new tricks.
- Youth is a gift of nature; age is a work of art.

See also REDUCING AGEISM

REFERENCE

Palmore, E. (1999). *Ageism: Negative and positive.* New York: Springer.

SOCIAL PSYCHOLOGY

Linda K. George

Ageism takes two forms: errors of commission and errors of omission. Errors of commission occur when inaccurate, negative stereotypes about aging are applied to older adults. Errors of omission occur when older adults are rendered invisible because of neglect. Both forms of ageism can be observed in the theories and research of social psychology, although this is less common recently than in the past. Both forms of ageism also have serious consequences for understanding aging and the older population. Explicit ageism, or errors of commission, render research flawed from the outset. Implicit ageism, or errors of omission, results in a lack of knowledge about aging and the tendency to assume that knowledge about younger adults applies equally well to older persons.

Social psychology is a broad field, encompassing literally thousands of concepts, resting on a broad range of research goals and methods. It is as inaccurate to discuss social psychology as if it is a homogeneous body of scholarship as it is to assume that older adults represent a homogeneous group. Numerous scholars have tried to develop frameworks that depict the major traditions in social psychology. The best known of these is the *three faces of social psychology* developed by House (1977). It is worth examining these three research traditions separately because they differ in the extent to which they have been and are characterized by explicit and implicit ageism. Thus, the defining characteristics of each tradition will be briefly described, followed by an assessment of the levels and forms of ageism that typify it.

Psychological Social Psychology

The first face of social psychology is what House labeled psychological social psychology. This tradition focuses on intrapsychic states—including mood, motivation, feelings, and perception—as they are affected by the presence and behaviors of other persons. Virtually all psychological social psychology research is experimental, typically, performed under controlled laboratory conditions. The strength of this research tradition is the strong evidence that it generates about causality. Because of the experimental designs used by researchers in this domain of social psychology, the fact that the presence or behaviors of others causally affects the intrapsychic states of research participants is largely irrefutable.

As with all research traditions, psychological social psychology also has weaknesses. The most common criticism of research in this tradition is that the generalizabilty of results to situations outside the laboratory is unknown. Another limitation of all experimental research is that investigators must be able to randomly assign participants to exposure to the independent variable or presumed cause of participants' intrapsychic states. This severely limits the kinds of causal factors that can be investigated. Many of the questions that interest social psychologists cannot be answered by experiments. For example, if we are interested in the effects of age on achievement motivation, we cannot randomly assign study participants to age (or many other characteristics). Another limitation of this research tradition is lack of attention to sampling study participants in a way that assures generalizability to a known population. Finally, despite the fact that the subject matter of psychological social psychology is usually intrapsychic states, investigators typically make inferences about the kinds of mental processing in which participants engage rather than eliciting information about those processes.

Psychological social psychology suffers immensely from implicit ageism or neglect of the older population. Only a very small percentage (far fewer than 10 percent) of studies in this tradition is based on samples of older adults—or even age-heterogeneous samples that include older adults. There also has been a virtual absence of theoretical or conceptual work on the ways in which the aging process might impact on some of the core concepts of psychological social psychology. Numerous examples of unaddressed issues could be provided. The following are offered as illustrations: Are there age-related declines in achievement motivation? Or, alternately, do the domains in which we desire to achieve, change across the life course? Are there age differences in the effects of self-discrepant feedback on mood and task performance?

A very small number of studies in this research tradition are appearing in the gerontological literature. For example, impression formation refers to the ways we develop first impressions when meeting strangers. A broad body of research documents the process of impression formation among younger adults. A recent study compared impression formation among younger and older adults, revealing some distinctive aspects of this phenomenon in late life. For example, older adults rely less on specific traits than their younger peers, focusing instead on more global impressions. Another recent study investigated age differences in the extent to which distraction interferes with impression formation (Mutter, 2000). The results indicated that distraction interfered with memory of specific traits more for older than for younger adults. Nonetheless, no age difference was observed in the overall evaluation of the targets about whom impressions were formed.

The attribution process also is a core concept of psychological social psychology. Attribution is the process by which we decide whether others are responsible for the outcomes that they experience or whether those outcomes are a result of causes external to the individual. Our attributions may or may not be correct, but they strongly affect our behavior toward the persons about whom we make them. Recently, attribution theory has been applied to issues of aging and health, especially dementia. The central issue in this research is whether diagnostic labels have negative or positive effects on assistance provided to ill persons. On the one hand, debilitating illnesses can elicit stigma and lessen the receipt of informal help. On the other hand, illness attributions may elicit sympathy and more help than would occur in the absence of a formal diagnosis. The limited research to date suggests that, in general, diagnostic attributions increase the amount of assistance available to persons diagnosed with dementia, but lessen assistance to depressed persons (Sacco and Dunn, 1990; Wadley and Haley, 2001).

Although small "pockets" of aging research are based on the theories of psychological social psychology, the broader picture is one of neglect. Literally hundreds of concepts central to psychological social psychology have never been replicated on older adults. Ideally, in the future investigators will develop a systematic program of research linking the aging process and older adults with the central tenets of psychological social psychology. Failing that, even less systematic research on selected concepts would help to assuage the implicit ageism that has characterized this field.

Symbolic Interactionism or Interpretive Social Psychology

As described by House (1977), the second face of social psychology is symbolic interactionism. This tradition focuses on the ways in which individuals interpret their social environments and posits that behavior is a direct reflection of those interpretations. From this perspective, the importance of *reality* is not its objective characteristics, but rather its symbolic meanings to individuals.

Because individuals' interpretations of social situations cannot be directly observed, investigators must ask research participants to report their perceptions, using what are commonly referred to as ethnographic or qualitative techniques. These reports are typically elicited in open-ended interviews. Because these kinds of qualitative interviews are used in studies that are not directly linked to symbolic interaction theory, this research tradition is now usually referred to by the broader label of interpretive social psychology.

As with other faces of social psychology, the interpretive approach has both strengths and limitations. Arguably, the greatest advantage of the interpretive approach is its focus on *why* and *how* individuals behave as they do. A related advantage is that knowledge of individuals' interpretations of the situation permits more accurate predictions of behavior than is possible using other methods. Interpretive social psychology also highlights the role of human agency in social life. Both experimental and survey research methods imply a determinism that is not part of interpretive research. A final strength of interpretive social psychology is its focus on processes. Social life is dynamic and interpretive social psychology highlights those dynamics.

Counterbalancing its strengths are the limitations of interpretive social psychology. These limitations are both conceptual and methodological. Conceptually, the scope of this research tradition is very narrow. Although measuring individuals' perceptions and interpretations permits relatively accurate predictions of subsequent behavior, the question of why individuals often interpret the same situation very differently remains unaddressed. In this sense, it is more accurate to view interpretive social psychology as describing rather than explaining individual attitudes and behavior. Methodological concerns fall into two major areas. First, it is difficult to evaluate the validity of research in this tradition. In part this results from the inability to verify respondents' self-reports against any external criterion. In addition, results of interpretive research rest on investigators' interpretations of respondents' self-reports—and different investigators sometimes reach different conclusions when interpreting the same interview data. Second, interpretive studies usually rely on small samples that are not systematically drawn from a defined population. Both of these characteristics make generalization of findings from interpretive studies problematic.

Studies of older adults are well represented in interpretive social psychology. Hochschild's study of *The Unexpected Community* (1978) is not only a classic depiction of late life, but also demonstrates how interpretive research can debunk ageist views of old age. Hochshild studied a low-income senior housing project. When embarking on her research, she expected to find a group of older adults who were bored and lonely, isolated from the work and family roles that defined their earlier lives. Instead, she found a vibrant social structure—a true community—in which members had meaningful roles, developed intimate ties with age peers, and expressed high levels of satisfaction with their lives. Her findings were the exact opposite of what she expected and contradicted common stereotypes about the poor quality of late life.

In *The Social World of Old Women,* Matthews (1979) reports compatible findings. Matthews was surprised to find that when she administered standard scales to a sample of financially strained older widows, most of whom also had chronic health problems, her study participants consistently reported high self-esteem and perceptions of high life quality. Because their reports were at odds with their objective life conditions, Matthews performed an in-depth interpretive study to determine whether the scales had failed to capture the reality of these women's lives or whether in fact they were experiencing high quality of life. Through in-depth interviews, Matthews found that these women were fundamentally satisfied with themselves and their lives. Her book does an admirable job of documenting the creative strategies—some behavioral, but most intrapsychic—that these women used to sustain high quality of life despite objective deprivations in their life conditions.

Interpretive social psychological research also has been used effectively to provide a *voice* for older adults who would otherwise be unlikely to be studied. A classic study in this genre is Gubrium's *Living and Dying at Murray Manor* (1975), a rich ethnographic account of life at a nursing home. Gubrium certainly did not find that conditions were ideal for residents at this facility. But he did find that most residents weren't simply waiting to die. They had personal goals and plans, they had complex relationships with each other and with staff; in short, they had richer and more complex lives than most of us attribute to frail older adults in institutions.

This rich tradition of ethnographic research continues. Charmaz (1991) provides revealing portraits of the strategies that chronically ill people use to sustain a sense of self-worth. Idler, Hudson, and Leventhal (1999) use in-depth interviews to document the ways that severely disabled people use religion and other coping strategies to sustain satisfying lives, although not all of her respondents accomplished this. Kaufman (1998) uses extensive observation and interviews in the intensive care unit (ICU) of a hospital to reveal the complexities and of end-of-life decision making. Her vivid account of the suffering of older patients and their families stands in stark contrast to the premise that advance directives *solve* the issue of end-of-life care and ensure that people die with dignity.

In summary, interpretive social psychology has a long and continuing history of investigating older adults. Interpretive research has played a vital role in helping to debunk myths about aging and to demonstrate the capacity of older adults to lead satisfying lives, even when objective circumstances are less than desirable. It would be helpful, I think, if there were more ethnographic studies of *normal aging.* Reflecting the desire to give the disenfranchised a *voice,* gerontological research in this tradition has focused largely on older adults who are marginal to mainstream society—the sick, the poor, and the dying. As important as those studies are, they need to be balanced by studies of older adults whose experiences are more typical of normal aging.

Social Structure and the Individual

The third, broadest, and most sociological face of social psychology is social structure and the individual (House, 1977). The focus of research in this tradition is the ways that social structures and social processes affect the attitudes and behaviors of individuals. This type of social psychology truly marries the sociological to the psychological. Independent variables of concern are social structures and social processes that are best depicted by sociologists (e.g., social class, family structure, social networks). The dependent variables, however, are individual outcomes, typically either attitudinal or behavioral. Most research in this tradition is based on survey research methods in which large samples, representative of a defined population, are administered questionnaires or standardized interviews. As with experimental research, investigators in the social structure and the individual tradition attempt to make causal inferences. Because they lack the controlled conditions of laboratory research, social psychologists in this tradition use statistical control and sophisticated statistical modeling to buttress their causal inferences.

Social structure and the individual research has both strengths and limitations. The major strengths of research in this tradition are the use of large and representative samples, which facilitates generalizability, and the use of sophisticated statistical models that allow for simultaneous consideration of the wide range of variables that are critical to understanding individual outcomes. Research in this tradition has two major limitations. First, some research topics (e.g., processes of decision making) cannot be addressed by it and some types of research participants (those too ill to complete a questionnaire or interview) cannot be included in survey research. Second, because participants respond to questions with specified categories, survey research can fail to capture the meanings that respondents attach to the questions—that is, the frame of reference is the investigator's rather than the respondent's.

The vast majority of social psychological research on aging and older adults is based on the social structure and the individual perspective. Space limitations prohibit a review of the many topics examined, but examples include the determinants of life satisfaction, the effects of stressors and role loss on physical and mental health, the effects of social networks on health and well-being, and determinants of intergenerational conflict and closeness. These studies consistently report that the older population as a whole experiences high levels of life satisfaction, cope effectively with stress and loss, and are embedded in supportive networks of family and friends. These findings effectively refute early assumptions that older adults would exhibit poorer outcomes than their younger peers.

Especially interesting, perhaps, is the fact that research in this tradition is now the major vehicle by which ageism itself is studied. Some studies of ageism focus on attitudes toward and stereotypes about the elderly. These studies show that large proportions of Americans of all ages endorse negative stereotypes about older people—and older people are as likely to hold these stereotypes as their younger peers (Nelson, 2002). Other studies examine the experience of age discrimination and suggest that institutional ageism (e.g., in the workplace) is relatively rare, but is very common in everyday life in public places. Undoubtedly, the social structure and the individual form of social psychology will continue to be a large and important part of gerontological research. And it will undoubtedly be the face of social psychology that is not only least likely to produce errors of commission and omission, but also that best documents the nature, extent, and consequences of ageism in society.

In summary, evaluating the extent to which social psychology has been characterized by implicit and/or explicit ageism requires separate examination of the major traditions in the discipline. Psychological social psychology has a record of almost virtual neglect of older adults, reflecting implicit ageism. Both interpretive social psychology and the social structure and the individual forms of social psychology began with assumptions or hypotheses that aging poses a crisis and results in lower levels of well-being. Their findings, however, failed to support those assumptions and, since then, these two subfields of social psychology have been critical in helping us to understand the reality, rather than the myths, of aging.

See also ATTRIBUTION THEORY; FACTS ON AGING QUIZ; STEREO-TYPES

REFERENCES

Charmaz, K. C. (1991). *Good days, bad days: The self in chronic illness.* New Brunswick, NJ: Rutgers University Press.

Gubrium, J. F. (1975). *Living and dying at Murray Manor.* New York: St. Martin's.

Hochschild, A. R. (1978). *The unexpected community.* Berkeley: University of California Press.

House, J. S. (1977). The three faces of social psychology. *Sociometry,* 40, 161-177.

Idler, E. L., Hudson, S. V., and Leventhal, H. (1999). The meanings of self-ratings of health: A qualitative and quantitative approach. *Research on Aging,* 21, 458-476.

Kaufman, S. R. (1998). Intensive care, old age, and the problem of death in America. *The Gerontologist,* 38, 715-725.

Matthews, S. H. (1979). *The social world of old women.* Beverly Hills: Sage.

Mutter, S. A. (2000). Illusory correlation and group impression formation in young and older adults. *Journal of Gerontology: Psychological Sciences,* 55B, P224-P237.

Nelson, T. (2002). *Ageism: Stereotyping and prejudice against older persons.* Cambridge, MA: MIT Press.

Sacco, W. P. and Dunn, V. K. (1990). Effect of actor depression on observer attributions: Existence and impact of negative attributions toward the depressed. *Journal of Personality and Social Psychology,* 59, 517-524.

Wadley, V. G. and Haley, W. E. (2001). Diagnostic attributions versus labeling: Impact of Alzheimer's disease and major depression diagnoses on emotions, beliefs, and helping intentions of family members. *Journal of Gerontology: Psychological Sciences,* 56B, P244-P252.

SOCIAL SECURITY

Erdman B. Palmore

The Old Age and Survivors Insurance (OASI) part of our Social Security program is the largest form of ageism in our country today; both in terms of the number of beneficiaries and the money involved. For example, $243.6 billion was paid to retired workers and dependents in 1997 (U.S. Social Security Administration, 1998). The fact that age requirements are needed to become eligible for these benefits makes the program ageist.

Supplement Security Income (SSI) is also partially age-specific. To qualify, one must be over age sixty-five, blind, or disabled, and have a low income. It is a kind of guaranteed income for people who are over sixty-five, blind, or disabled. Of the 6.6 million SSI beneficiaries, 1.4 million qualified on the basis of age, and they were paid $4.5 billion. Thus, SSI is a much smaller program than OASI.

Most people do not realize that OASI and SSI are ageist programs also in the sense that most of the money comes out of the taxes paid by younger people. Many people think of Social Security as an annuity, in which you make *contributions* (FICA taxes) while working and then receive a pension after retirement. In fact, Social Security is basically a *pay-as-you-go* income-transfer program in which the average person receives much more than the value of his or her *investment* plus interest.

The OASI program could be made less ageist by eliminating the age requirement for benefits and using only *years of coverage* (earnings) as the criteria for eligibility. Thus, instead of age sixty-two (for partial benefits) or age sixty-five (for full benefits) qualifying one for retirement benefits, one would need to have worked and earned income for a specified number of years. If forty years were the requirement, one who started working at age twenty could qualify at age sixty; but if one did not start until age twenty-five, one would have to wait until age sixty-five, etc. Thus, the retirement benefits would still go to older people, but the age discrimination would be eliminated.

The ageist aspect of the SSI program could be eliminated by making it a guaranteed minimum income for persons of all ages, as is done in many European countries.

See also AGE-SPECIFIC PUBLIC PROGRAMS; POLITICS; PUBLIC POLICY

REFERENCE

U.S. Social Security Administration (1998). *Annual statistical supplement to the Social Security Bulletin.* Washington, DC: U.S. Government Printing Office.

SOCIETAL AGEISM

Jon Hendricks

Ageism is more than an action or attitude of individuals; it is also a complex tendency woven into the social fabric. Butler (1969), Palmore (1999), and others have drawn fitting attention to behavior and attitudes of individuals as indicators of ageism, but they also note that prejudice and discrimination have roots in shared perceptions not necessarily derived from personal experience. Ageism is pervasive in a wide variety of phenomena, at the institutional as well as at the individual level. To fully understand the epidemiology of ageism, one must look to the social surround and institutionalized patterns that permit ageism to thrive (Butler, 1980, 1987; Palmore, 2001). Societal ageism entails a rescinding of autonomy and opportunities characterizing adulthood and represents a form of domination and control (Braithwaite, 2002).

Individuals immersed in any culture inevitably internalize worldviews, values, and age stereotypes inherent in that culture that shape their perceptions about aging (Levy, 2001). By recognizing linkages between societal conditions and individual expressions of ageism, we can appreciate how categorizations of aged individuals have societal roots and are determined, actualized, and sustained by social practices and social relationships that influence the allocation of social roles, the distribution of benefits, and color the social construction of the life course.

Beyond being expressions by individuals, ageism resides in societal norms, values, public policies, laws, and administrative regulations. A 1977 U.S. Commission on Civil Rights investigation into instances of ageism found the very laws and federal agencies intended to protect against such ageism were infused with instances of age discrimination (Palmore, 1999). Ageism is apparent in roles gained, changed, or lost and in the nature of social interactions, relationships, and labels assigned. These ageist predilections occur in the world of work, family life, and in access to one or another form of social resource. Ageism, thus, exists in the institutionalized foundations and taken-for-granted assumptions that undergird ordered worldviews and individual manifestations of either positive or negative ageism (Butler, 1987; Levin and Levin, 1980).

The conventional understanding about what is fair and equitable plays out in social interaction, reflecting collective notions of moral economy (Thompson, 1964). The latter furnishes the underlying principles behind social organization, resource allocation, and the distribution of opportunities. Looking beyond utilitarian explanations justifying age-based decision making in terms of the greater good, there is a concentration of advantage revolving around current or prospective economic potential (Callahan, 1987; Daniels, 1985; Lamm, 2000). So for example, one formula showing up in calculations used by the White House Office of Management and Budget (Borenstein, 2002) places a value on an older person's life at roughly 63 percent of the value assigned to younger persons.

A further indicator of how a market-based logic pervades public policy can be seen in the gradual evolution of *covered occupations* within the purview of Social Security, wherein coverage came slowly or not at all to marginal workers in economically peripheral occupations and excludes those, primarily women, who provide essential services yet are not employed in the realm of paid labor. Another illustration may be seen in patterns for midlife unemployment among persons age fifty-five to sixty-four in countries in the European Union, and in the numbers of older workers classified as discouraged and out of the labor market for more than one year (Callasanti, 2002; Kinsella and Velkoff, 2001). Despite the fact that the United States passed an Age Discrimination in Employment Act in 1967, more than 20 percent of the complaints filed with the Equal Employment Opportunity Commission (EEOC) for the period 1995 to 1998 addressed age discrimination in employment (McCann and Giles, 2002).

The spread of such market-based logics is far-reaching, coloring our view of people, their worth, and their potential (Palmore, 1999). Moving into the twenty-first century, all manner of decisions are seemingly couched in terms of cost-benefit ratios and bottom-line outcomes. Such an ideology and its role in the valuation of people have become ascendant in diverse cultures not by coercion but by virtue of the active consent of all participants. As a consequence, age-based entitlements, accommodations, or benefits are designed in terms of organizing principles reflecting presumed worth, work histories, and related social priorities. People and things not embodying these values are denigrated, saddled with pejorative adjectives labeling them as irrelevant by those able to wield definitional power to create a prescriptive thesis that absolves those who manifest ageism from personal responsibility (Armon-Jones, 1986; Greene, 1989).

Public policies, as with all social practices, are important social constructions insofar as they help frame perceptions of those who fall within their purview. The definitional power of public policy is enveloping and in the case of age-based policies, serves to underpin both perceptions and self-perceptions of age-related changes. The same holds true for both public insurance and public assistance. The residualist focus of needs-based public assistance, aimed at ameliorating the situations of the least well off, provide poverty-level sustenance, at best, thereby sending an unmistakable message even while intending to provide aid. Sense of worth, for self and others, reflects worth defined by public pronouncements, including policies. With more than 100 state and federal policies affecting older persons in the United States alone, it is not surprising that they promote a bureaucratic rationality on the definitions of what it means to be old. As with boundaries of any sort, age-based policies are emblematic, imparting credence to perceived commonalities among those on one side and to ostensible differences from those on the other (Braithwaite, 2002; Hendricks, 1994, 1995; Johnson and Michaelsen, 1997). With eligibility for age-based benefits, people enter a legally recognized category and, as Estes (2001) notes, doing so delineates rights of those who fall within their purview and are determinative of life changes and social relationships.

Having knowledge of the connection between social forces and individual expressions of any attitude or belief is helpful in recognizing that personal predilections and public pronouncements are interrelated sets. Referring to age as the cause of whatever ills older people encounter is to risk making assumptions not subjected to critical examination. In fact, some portion of the typical experience of older persons is a result of the way societies organize themselves and accoutrements of that organization, including the allocation of roles and opportunities, rather than reflecting personal or physiological declines (Estes, 1979; Levin and Levin, 1980). We need to recognize that societal practices are in part the reason why older persons have lower incomes, greater rates of unemployment when they want to work, fewer medical benefits, less tractable medical conditions, and less power to control their own fates.

No doubt age provides useful categorizations and facilitates administrative management of well-intentioned policies. However, once age becomes stigmatizing for either biological or social reasons, ageism may result. Also, when age results in undifferentiated categorization, the process verges on a composition fallacy—the assumption that all members of a category are identical when they may be comparable on certain criteria only. It is likely that lifelong differentiations do not dissipate but are actually exacerbated or even masked by the assignment of age as incontestable evidence.

When age is stigmatizing or becomes a primary determinant of an individual's master status, supplanting previous categorical components, then all manner of outcomes are explained by age and reified by a kind of circular logic. One consequence is once a person is categorized as elderly, the nonelderly are likely to apply a host of negative stereotypes (Greenberg, Schimel, and Mertens, 2002). As sociologists have long maintained, having an assemblage of outsiders is an important dynamic for insiders, it helps distinguish their own commonalities (Falk, 2001; Levy and Banaji, 2002). It may be that ageism serves a comparable end, by stigmatizing older persons, a condition the elderly are hard-pressed to counter, resources can justifiably be directed to in-group members as old age is depicted as a place across a chasm.

If ageism is to be ameliorated, we must also look to societal conditions and the institutionalized foundations that create the context of ageism. Individualized expressions of ageism are symptomatic of underlying factors, not their causes (Levy and Banaji, 2002; Vincent, 1999).

See also AGE SEGREGATION; AGE STRATIFICATION; CULTURAL SOURCES OF AGEISM; MODERNIZATION THEORY; SCAPEGOATING; STEREOTYPES; SUBCULTURES; TYPOLOGIES

REFERENCES

Armon-Jones, C. (1986). The thesis of constructionism. In R. Harre (Ed.), *The social construction of emotions* (pp. 32-56). Oxford, UK: Basil Blackwell.
Borenstein, S. (2002). Elderly less valuable in cost-benefit analysis. *The Miami Herald,* December 19.

Braithwaite, V. (2002). Reducing ageism. In T. D. Nelson (Ed.), *Ageism: Stereotypes and prejudice against older persons* (pp. 311-337). Cambridge, MA: MIT Press.

Butler, R. (1969). Age-ism: Another form of bigotry. *The Gerontologist,* 9, 243-246.

_____ (1980). Ageism: A forward. *Journal of Social Issues,* 36, 8-11.

_____ (1987). Ageism. In G. L. Maddox (Ed.), *Encyclopedia of aging* (pp. 22-23). New York: Springer.

Callahan, D. (1987). *Setting limits.* New York: Simon & Schuster.

Callasanti, T. M. (2002). Work and retirement in the 21st century: Integrating issues of diversity and globalization. *Ageing International,* 27, 3-20.

Daniels, N. (1985). *Just health care.* Cambridge: Cambridge University Press.

Estes, C. (1979). *The aging enterprise.* San Francisco: Jossey-Bass.

_____ (2001). *Social policy and aging: A critical perspective.* Thousand Oaks, CA: Sage.

Falk, G. (2001). *Stigma: How we treat outsiders.* Amherst, NY: Prometheus Books.

Greenberg, J., Schimel, J., and Mertens, A. (2002). Ageism: Denying the face of the future. In T. D. Nelson (Ed.), *Ageism: Stereotyping and prejudice against older persons* (pp. 27-48). Cambridge, MA: The MIT Press.

Greene, V. (1989). Human capitalism and intergenerational justice. *The Gerontologist,* 29, 723-724.

Hendricks, J. (1994). Governmental responsibility: Adequacy or dependency for the USA aged. In D. Gill and S. Ingman (Eds.), *Eldercare, distributive justice, and the welfare state* (pp. 255-285). Albany: State University of New York Press.

_____ (1995). The social construction of ageism. In L. Bond, S. Cutler, and A. Grams (Eds.), *Promoting successful and productive aging* (pp. 51-68). Thousand Oaks, CA: Sage.

Johnson, D. E. and Michaelsen, S. (1997). Border secrets: An introduction. In S. Michaelsen and D. E. Johnson (Eds.), *Border theory: The limits of cultural politics* (pp. 1-39). Minneapolis: University of Minnesota Press.

Kinsella, K. and Velkoff, V. A. (2001). *An aging world: 2001* [U.S. Census Bureau, Series p95/01-1]. Washington, DC: USGPO.

Lamm, R. (2000). *Megatraumas: America at the year 2000.* Boston: Houghton, Mifflin.

Levin, J. and Levin, W. C. (1980). *Ageism: Prejudice and discrimination against the elderly.* Belmont, CA: Wadsworth.

Levy, B. R. (2001). Eradication of ageism requires addressing the enemy within. *The Gerontologist,* 41, 578-579.

Levy, B. R. and Banaji, M. R. (2002). Implicit ageism. In T. D. Nelson (Ed.), *Ageism: Stereotyping and prejudice against older persons* (pp. 49-75). Cambridge, MA: MIT Press.

McCann, R. and Giles, H. (2002). Ageism in the workplace: A communication perspective. In T. D. Nelson (Ed.), *Ageism: Stereotyping and Prejudice against older workers* (pp. 163-199). Cambridge, MA: MIT Press.

Palmore, E. (1999). *Ageism: Negative and positive.* New York: Springer.

_____ (2001). The ageism survey: First findings. *The Gerontologist,* 41, 572-575.

Thompson, E. P. (1964). *The making of the English working class.* New York: Vintage Books.

Vincent, J. A. (1999). *Politics, power and old age.* Buckingham, England: Open University Press.

SONGS

Stephen Sapp

Despite public opinion polls, surveys, focus groups, and other attempts to determine attitudes toward aging and the elderly in the United States, discovering what people really think and feel about growing old, old age, and old people is an ongoing process. The consensus, however, is that this country is not a congenial place for the elderly. The source of these negative attitudes and actions, collectively labeled *ageism,* is difficult to determine, and they clearly stem from many factors. One factor worth investigating is popular music, certainly one of the indicators of—and influences upon—popular thought.

Although ageism in any form and from any source is to be lamented, it is particularly pernicious when manifested in popular music because popular song has served and continues to serve as the "the poetry of the common person." People who never read Keats or Shelley after high school continue to listen to popular music, and attention to the images of aging in such music can give us valuable clues about what our attitudes are and where they come from. It should be noted that the process is a two-way street: Popular songs reflect images of aging held by the songwriters and performers, but they may also help to shape the attitudes held by those who listen to them.

Beyond the cognitive message conveyed in the words of the songs, it is important to be aware that music holds considerable power to evoke emotions and memories, engaging people on a deeper level than words alone. Thus an image or point of view portrayed in a song may have greater impact on a person's psyche than a similar message expressed in narrative form and thus be harder to modify through purely intellectual means of persuasion.

A general discussion of the messages and images of aging found in several representative songs will serve to illustrate the role songs can play in promoting ageism (including more positive images of growing old). Unfortunately, for copyright reasons lyrics of songs cannot be quoted here, but readers can easily find the songs referred to.

"Hello in There" (Prine, 1971), which leads off Bette Midler's 1972 album *Experience the Divine,* offers a particularly discouraging depiction of growing older, beginning with the very title, which suggests it is difficult to "find someone home" when interacting with an older person. A retired couple has failed to keep their relationship alive or to maintain outside contacts, and now that their children have grown and left home, the lack of meaning and hopelessness in their lives is powerfully depicted. Both husband and wife appear to be trapped in the past, with no fulfilling activities in the present and certainly no hope for a worthwhile future. The chorus in particular portrays a decidedly negative image of aging as it compares two natural phenomena (old trees and rivers), which get stronger and wilder as they age, with older human beings, who merely become lonelier as they wait for someone to speak to them. Furthermore, listeners who are familiar with Midler's moving renditions of "Wind Beneath My Wings" and "The Rose" may notice the much less pleasant, nasal voice in which she sings this song. A noteworthy sidelight to this discussion is the fact that John Prine was in his midtwenties when he wrote the song, but the last verse does offer a ray of hope as the songwriter seems to urge listeners *not* to ignore elderly people they encounter, though by the time this important message appears it may well be lost on discouraged listeners.

Another example of songs that depict being old in a negative light is Paul Simon's "Old Friends" (1968), which is presented in Simon and Garfunkel's *Bookends* album together with "Bookends Theme" and provides the focus for that album. Apparently sung by a young man who observes two old men sitting on a park bench in wintertime and tries to imagine his own future, the song is replete with imagery that depicts old age as a time of merely waiting for death. The positive note offered by the fact that the two "old friends" have each other and thus are not completely alone is overwhelmed by their seeming lack of meaningful interaction, as with the relationship depicted in "Hello in There." Here also the negative theme is continued musically as listeners are struck by the somber, even discordant, music and come away from hearing it feeling discouraged and depressed. After a particularly unpleasant musical bridge, "Old Friends" is followed immediately by "Bookends Theme," which in two brief stanzas portrays youth as a time of strength and hope but old age as a period in which the best one can do is hang onto memories of that wonderful past because that is all one has left. People listening to these two songs, especially if they are young, often comment that they can find in them nothing positive about getting old.

A more recent song that illustrates how popular music can foster ageism is Bryan Adams' "18 'til I Die" (cowritten with R. J. Lange in 1996), which appears in the album of the same name. From the expression in the first line of the desire to be young for all his life to the affirmation of the last line that he is going to make his youth last until he dies (fifty-five is the oldest age explicitly mentioned in the song), the singer presents a strong statement that only the things he associates with youth make life worth living, suggesting that the inability to do those things makes life worthless. Although the underlying philosophy reflected in the song may strike some as positive—live for the moment, do not dwell in the past, be willing to try new things constantly so as to "remain forever young"—this message is undermined both by its implication that youth is necessary to such an approach to life and by the implication that a more natural course of aging (including accepting one's aging as inevitable and coming to terms with it) is somehow inappropriate.

Indeed, despite its wonderful successes in making growing old much better for so many people, modern gerontology has contributed to an insidious underlying ageism that says the best way to *age successfully* is to retain the traits associated with youth for as long as possible, an approach that inherently devalues getting old. The song "18 'til I Die" illustrates the problem beautifully.

With just these few examples, the role that popular songs can play in reflecting and fostering ageism becomes clear. Although some songs contain positive notes in their depiction of old age and/or elderly people (e.g., Pete Seeger's "Get Up and Go"; John Lennon and Paul McCartney's "When I'm 64"; Jimmy Buffett's "He Went to Paris"; Stephen Sondheim's "No Time At All"; Kathy Mattea's "Where've You Been?"), even these songs hardly paint a picture of the later years that people in the youth-obsessed culture of the United States of America would look forward to.

See also CULTURAL SOURCES OF AGEISM; PERPETUAL YOUTH

Note: I wish to thank Gail Eisen for alerting me to the importance of popular song as a source of images of aging and for a number of the ideas expressed in this entry.

STAGE THEORY

Erdman B. Palmore

Some gerontologists distinguish between different types of elders by theorizing that elders typically go through different stages in old age. For example, the most popular test in the field of social gerontology (Atchley, 1997) distinguishes between *middle age,* which he says begins around age forty; *later maturity,* which begins in the sixties; and *old age,* which begins in the late seventies. Atchley asserts that these stages are not based on chronological age, but on sets of related characteristics. For example, he says that *old age* is characterized by extreme physical frailty; mental processes slow down; activity is restricted; social networks are decimated; life is unpleasant; and death is near.

Another version asserts the stage theory of the *young old* (those in their sixties), the *middle-old* (those in their seventies), and the *old-old* (those eighty and over). A popularized version of these three stages calls them the *go-go* (young and active), the *slow-go* (slowing down and disengaging), and the *no-go* (feeble and frail).

As appealing as such conceptions may appear on a commonsense level and while they may be useful in pointing out the wide variety among elders, two major problems with these stage theories make them support ageism (Palmore, 1999). First, they are inevitably associated with certain chronological ages. As a result, we end up with a new set of stereotypes associated with certain chronological ages. Even though these stereotypes are purported to apply to smaller ranges of ages, they remain stereotypes nevertheless. As such, they do not fit most individuals in the age range. For example, the majority of persons older than age eighty are not in poor health, do not have organic brain disease, do not have decimated social networks, are not institutionalized, and do not report that life is unpleasant (Rosenwaike, 1985).

Second, these stereotypes emphasize the negative aspects of aging, especially the older stages. They ignore the satisfaction of achieving advanced longevity, and the wisdom, skills, respect, and serenity that often accompany old age.

Thus, on balance, stage theories reinforce the typical negative stereotypes of ageism.

See also DISENGAGEMENT THEORY; STEREOTYPES; THEORIES OF AGING

REFERENCES

Atchley, R. (1997). *Social forces and aging.* Belmont, CA: Wadsworth.
Palmore, E. (1999). *Ageism.* New York: Springer.
Rosenwaike, I. (1985). *The extreme aged in America.* Westport, CT: Greenwood Press.

STEREOTYPES

Erdman B. Palmore

An age stereotype is "a simplified, undifferentiated portrayal of an age group that is often erroneous, unrepresentative of reality, and resistant to modification" (Cook, 2001, p. 5). The word *stereotype* originally referred to the metal plate used in printing. Walter Lippman (1922) is credited with introducing its usage in the sense of a prejudice about a group or type of person.

By definition, any stereotype is erroneous in the sense that it is applied to all members of a category of people, but almost no trait is true of all persons in a category: there are always exceptions to the rule.

I have identified and discussed the evidence for nine major stereotypes that reflect negative prejudice toward elders: illness, impotency, ugliness, mental decline, mental illness, uselessness, isolation, poverty, and depression (Palmore, 1999). In contrast, I have also identified and discussed eight positive stereotypes about elders that many people believe: kindness, wisdom, dependability, affluence, political power, freedom, eternal youth, and happiness. Notice that several of these positive stereotypes are the opposite of corresponding negative stereotypes.

Hummert and colleagues (1994) identify sixty-nine descriptive traits about old people, which they reduce to four negative (severely impaired, shrew/curmudgeon, recluse, despondent) and three positive stereotypes (perfect grandparent, John Wayne conservative, golden-ager).

Extensive evidence from various surveys, such as the Facts on Aging Quiz (Palmore, 1998), the AARP survey (AARP, 1995), and the Harris surveys (Harris, 1981), supports that many Americans believe these stereotypes. In fact, many people hold a mixture of negative and positive stereotypes simultaneously. However, the evidence clearly suggests that none of these stereotypes really applies to most or even to many older persons (Palmore, 1999).

Stereotypes are generally assumed to cause or encourage discrimination against older people. However, the link between stereotypes and discrimination has not been clearly demonstrated.

One problem in measuring stereotypes is the way the questions are phrased. Often the questions ask about "the elderly" or "older persons" as if they were a homogeneous group. Obviously this assumption is false. When respondents are allowed to indicate what proportion of elders have a trait, the amount of stereotyping diminishes. Schonfeld (1982) found that stereotypes about older persons' inflexibility, loneliness, and religiosity diminished markedly when respondents were instructed to indicate which statements were representative of at least 80 percent of the elderly. Also, Kite (1996) found that negative stereotyping of the elderly is reduced when contextual information was provided, especially information about their work-related roles.

- Present fewer exaggerated images and deemphasize the importance of negative characteristics.
- Present facts that counteract false stereotypes such as the assumption that most elderly are senile.
- Balance negative characteristics of elders with positive ones, such as the benefits of aging.

- Show that many stereotypes about elders are actually shared to varying degrees by all ages (such as memory, hearing, and vision problems).
- Show how younger people's prejudice and discrimination tend to contribute to the creation of the stereotype; for example treating the elderly as useless becomes a cause of elders' loss of usefulness.

See also SELF-FULFILLING PROPHECY

- Point out that many stereotypes about elders are outdated because of substantial improvements in elders' situations and abilities.
- Point out that as much variation occurs among elders as among younger people, if not more so. Show that elders are some of the richest and poorest, some of the most athletic and some of the most disabled, some of the most brilliant as well as some of the most disoriented in society.

See also BENEFITS OF AGING; FACTS ON AGING QUIZ; JOURNALISM; TELEVISION; TYPOLOGIES

REFERENCES

AARP (1995). *Images of aging in America.* Washington, DC: American Association of Retired Persons.

Cook, F. (2001). Age stereotypes. In G. Maddox (Ed.), *The encyclopedia of aging.* New York: Springer.

Harris, L. (1981). *Aging in the eighties.* Washington, DC: The National Council on the Aging.

Hummert, M., Garstka, T., Shaner, J., and Strahm, S. (1994). Stereotypes of the elderly held by young, middle-aged, and elderly adults. *Journal of Gerontology: Psychological Sciences, 49,* P240.

Kite, M. (1996). Age, gender, and occupational label. *Psychology of Women Quarterly, 20,* 361.

Lippman, W. (1922). *Public opinion.* New York: Harcourt, Brace, and Co.

Palmore, E. (1998). *The facts on aging quiz.* New York: Springer.

_____ (1999). *Ageism.* New York: Springer.

Schonfeld, D. (1982). Who is stereotyping whom and why? *The Gerontologist, 22,* 267.

SUBCULTURES

Charles F. Longino Jr.

Subcultures are distinctive patterns of cultural traits (including certain values, attitudes, styles, and tastes) associated with particular categories of people facing common problems in a society. They produce ways of life and interpretations of the world that fit the needs of the members (Renzetti and Curran, 1998). In this way, they are broadly functional. Their existence depends on high levels of social interaction. Ethnic and youth subcultures are often given as examples. Corporate culture is a term applying the subculture concept to large businesses when they generate an alignment of values, attitudes, traditions, and general behavioral expectations that become known and often shared by members of the particular corporation.

Rose (1962, 1965a,b) argues that the same principles apply to older persons. Common physiological and economic problems face the elderly, but Rose (1965a) argues that the subculture of the aged arises primarily as a response to status loss. In the United States, old age is culturally defined as so negative that older persons do not want to identify themselves as old (Rosow, 1974). They develop and maintain a subculture, therefore, to insulate themselves from status losses. At the same time, their age-based solidarity may foster a social movement aimed at changing the cultural definition of aging and thereby reducing its negative ascriptive power. The resulting condition, aging-group consciousness, is similar in function to Marx's concept of class consciousness.

Research has provided limited support. A number of studies of age-concentrated housing offered support for Rose's hypothesis that morale and interaction are high in these settings (Hochschild, 1973; Sherman, 1975a,b). An explicit attempt to test this hypothesis (Longino, McClelland, and Peterson, 1980) supported and modified Rose's predictions. This study demonstrated that residents of eight age-concentrated study communities showed (1) qualitatively more positive social integration, (2) distinctive patterns of preference for interaction with and perceptions of the elderly, and (3) an enhanced positive self-conception, relative to demographically comparable age peers in the national population. Evidence for any politically oriented aging-group consciousness, however, was absent. This study concluded that the aged subculture in retirement communities is retreatist in content rather than activist.

A subculture of active retired persons, similar to that envisioned by Rose but without aging-group consciousness, at least not with a negative self-definition, is more likely to define itself as a new subculture formation. Most older people harbor weak or nonexistent age-group identifications (Shanas, 1968). Interest in social support in the 1980s and 1990s seems to have totally eclipsed the older and more political concept of the aged subculture.

This brings us to the dark side of the aged subculture hypothesis. Ryan (1971) notes the use of the concept of *the culture of poverty* as an excuse to blame the victim, to argue that poverty is generated by the subculture of the poor, rather than from outside economic and political forces. In the same way, Levin and Levin (1980) argue that gerontologists see the elderly as a subculture focusing upon the deficits and declines of aging and worrying about their impending frailty and demise. In this way, gerontologists also blame the victim in the sense that they focus their attention away from the positive and more productive aspects of aging: education, volunteering, participation in the labor force, and important caregiving functions that they perform. Instead, the elderly have come to be viewed, primarily as passive, dependent, and self-absorbed and as the objects of care, rather than carers themselves.

Much attention at the turn of the second millennium (Morgan, 1998) has been given to the impending retirement of the baby-boom generation in the United States. From 2008 to 2026 the baby boomers will retire, lowering the median age of the retired population in general, and projecting an image of the concerns of early retirees. A strong possibility exists that the general understanding of aging subculture among gerontologists will be influenced by these population dynamics so that the subculture will be recast in a somewhat more youthful, energetic, and outward-looking image. Their sheer numbers, historical increases in the levels of education, and their weight in the economic and political marketplaces indicate that it will be much more difficult to push the retired population to the sidelines of society. Reading Rose's argument backward, therefore, a corresponding increase should occur in the status and respect accorded to retirees, further diminishing the aged subculture.

See also AGE CONFLICT; AGE NORMS; AGE SEGREGATION; CROSS-CULTURAL AGEISM

REFERENCES

Hochschild, A. R. (1973). *The unexpected community.* Englewood Cliffs, NJ: Prentice-Hall.

Levin, J. and Levin, W. C. (1980). *Ageism: Prejudice and discrimination against the elderly.* Belmont, CA: Wadsworth Publishing Company.

Longino, C. F. Jr., McClelland, K. A., and Peterson, W. A. (1980). The aged subculture hypothesis: Social integration, gerontophilia, and self-conception. *Journal of Gerontology,* 35(5), 758-767.

Morgan, D. (Ed.) (1998). The baby boom at midlife and beyond. *Generations,* 22 (1).

Renzetti, C. M. and Curran, D. J. (1998). *Living soicology.* Needham Heights, MA: Allyn & Bacon.

Rose, A. (1962). The subculture of the aging: A topic for sociological research. *The Gerontolgoist,* 2, 123-127.

_____ (1965a). Group consciousness among the aging. In A. Rose and W. Peterson (Eds.), *Older people and their social world.* Philadelphia: Davis.

_____ (1965b). A subculture for the aging: A framework for research in social gerontology. In A. Rose and W. Peterson (Eds.), *Older people and their social world.* Philadelphia: Davis.

Rosow, I. (1974). *Socialization to old age.* Berkeley: University of California Press.

Ryan, W. (1971). *Blaming the victim.* New York: Vintage.

Shanas, E. (1968). A note on restrictions of life spaced: Attitudes of age cohorts. *Journal of Health and Social Behavior,* 9(1), 86-90.

Sherman, S. (1975a). Mutual assistance and support in retirement housing. *Journal of Gerontology,* 30, 479-483.

_____ (1975b). Patterns of contacts for residents of age-segregated and age-integrated housing. *Journal of Gerontology,* 30, 103-107.

SUCCESSFUL AGING

Meredith Minkler
Martha Holstein

A growing movement in geriatrics and gerontology seeks to replace the earlier *decline and loss* paradigm with a newer emphasis on the potential and likelihood of healthy and *successful* aging. Coined more than fifty years ago but achieving new prominence with the publication of Rowe and Kahn's (1998) landmark book by that title, *successful aging* has become the most popular term used to capture this alternative perspective.

The concept of successful aging has been helpful in focusing renewed attention on health promotion and the prevention of disease and injury as a means of improving the quality, and not merely the quantity, of the later years. The ten-year, $10 million MacArthur Foundation study of successful aging (Rowe and Kahn, 1997, 1998) on which the model rests, further offers impressive evidence for a wide array of health promotion strategies that can help ensure a healthier old age. The model itself is clearly laid out, highlighting three hierarchically ordered characteristics viewed as necessary preconditions for successful aging:

1. avoidance of disease and disability,
2. maintenance of high physical and cognitive functional capacity, and
3. active engagement in life.

Viewed more critically, however, the successful aging model may be seen as contributing to and reinforcing a new form of ageism (Cohen, 1988), in which generalized prejudice against and devaluing of the old is replaced by a more targeted ageism reserved for those who are aging with a disability or in other ways failing to meet the criteria for *aging well* (Cohen, 1988; Minkler, 1990). Indeed, by naming their approach *successful aging* and equating success largely with the achievement of such discreet end points as high-level physical and cognitive functioning, this perspective inadvertently stigmatizes whole groups of people, including those who may be aging with a disability (Minkler and Fadem, 2002). Also largely ignored in the successful aging model are inequities based on race, class, and gender and the importance of losses as well as gains in late life (Baltes and Cartensen, 1996; Scheidt, Humphreys, and Yorgason, 1999).

Ironically, the new successful-aging paradigm has much in common with the century-old Victorian view of a good old age in which robust health symbolized life lived according to the strict dictates of Victorian convention (Cole, 1988). Similar to the earlier view, the new model of successful aging minimizes structural understandings of the *problem* of aging, which would call attention to the lifelong inequalities that help determine health and life chances in late life.

Successful aging has been described as "an inherently normative concept, laden with comparative, either/or, hierarchically ordered dimensions" (Holstein and Minkler, in press). The norms embedded in the notion of successful aging are problematic; first in their tendency to assume the existence of a commonly recognized and accepted end point that makes one person's aging a success and another's *usual* or a failure. Second, even if there were agreement on a desirable and discreet end point (e.g., high physical and cognitive functioning) people clearly differ in the abilities and resources available to them for attaining such a goal. Since how people live—and how they age—is heavily affected by sociostructural factors beyond their control, *success* is more difficult for some to achieve than for others (Holstein, 1998). Older women, people of color, and people with disabilities, in part because of differential life chances, may thus be less likely to meet the criteria for *successful aging* than men, whites, and the able-bodied (Holstein and Minkler, in press). The focus on personal responsibility for health implicit in the successful-aging model further risks ignoring the environmental and policy contexts that can facilitate or severely limit an individual's ability to achieve and sustain high functioning in society (Minkler and Fadem, 2002).

The concept of successful aging has received considerable media attention, where it has been oversimplified and used to reinforce the dominant Western mind-set which frequently measures individual worth in terms of personal accomplishments. Images such as those of astronaut John Glenn orbiting the globe in his late seventies frequently are invoked in such accounts to exemplify what successful aging involves.

The translation of an individualistically couched strategy (e.g., staying fit and vigorous) into a societal vision (e.g., successful aging) risks rendering whole groups of individuals marginal (Blaikie, 1999). As noted previously, such marginalization can encourage damaging comparisons, particularly if one is disabled, or simply old and "not well preserved."

In sum, the concept of successful aging has made an important contribution in focusing renewed attention on health promotion and its potential for a healthier old age. But it is problematic as well in its inadvertent tendency to promote a new form of ageism directed at those who are aging with a disability or otherwise failing to *age successfully.*

See also AGE NORMS; DISABILITY; ROLE EXPECTATIONS; THEORIES OF AGING

REFERENCES

Baltes, M. and Cartensen, L. (1996). The process of successful aging. *Ageing and Society,* 16, 397-422.

Blaikie, A. (1999). *Ageing and popular culture.* Cambridge, UK: Cambridge University Press.

Cohen, E. (1988). The elderly mystique: Constraints on the autonomy of the elderly with disabilities. *The Gerontologist,* 28(Suppl.), 24-31.

Cole, T. (1988). Aging, history and health: Progress and paradox. In J. Johannes, J. Schroots, and J. Birren (Eds.), *Health and aging.* New York: Springer.

Holstein, M. (1998). Women and aging: Troubling implications. In M. Minkler and C.L. Estes (Eds.), *Critical gerontology.* Amityville, NY: Baywood.

Holstein, M. and Minkler, M. (in press). Self, society and the "new gerontology." *The Gerontologist.*

Minkler, M. (1990). Aging and disability: Behind and beyond the stereotypes. *Journal of Aging Studies,* 4, 245-260.

Minkler, M. and Fadem, P. (2002). Successful aging: A disability perspective. *Journal of Disability Policy Studies,* 12, 229-235.

Rowe, J. and Kahn, R. (1997). Successful aging. *The Gerontologist,* 37, 433-440.
_____ (1998). *Successful aging.* New York: Random House.

Scheidt, R.J., Humphreys, D.R., and Yorgason, J.B. (1999). Successful aging: What's not to like? *The Journal of Applied Gerontology,* 18, 277-282.

SUICIDE

Nancy J. Osgood

Compared to other age groups, older adults have the highest suicide rate. Individuals sixty-five and older constitute 13 percent of the U.S. population, but account for approximately 19 percent of suicides (Murphy, 2000). Older adults commit one of every five suicides in America. The suicide rate for older adults is about 50 percent higher than the rate for younger adults. Each year approximately 6,300 older people commit suicide, or eighteen per day. White males eighty-five and older have a suicide rate six times higher than the overall U.S. rate. Firearms are the most common method used. Numerous studies identify two psychiatric disorders that increase the risk of suicide later in life: depression and alcoholism.

Another seldom-discussed factor that may contribute to elderly suicide is ageism. In 1968 Robert Butler coined the term *ageism,* which he defined as "a deep and profound prejudice against the elderly and a systematic stereotyping of people and discrimination against people because they are old" (p. 2). Ageism results in a deep hatred of and aversion toward older people simply because they are old. As a consequence of ageism, older adults in the United States often are isolated and ignored, devalued, disenfranchised, and discriminated against.

Suicide takes place within a particular sociocultural context. The predominant cultural values concerning the meaning and value of life and death, disability and dependency, and aging, influence life-and-death decisions of people living in the culture. American culture is characterized by several major values that favor younger adults over older adults. Ageism is deeply rooted in America's core values.

One such value is an individual-achievement orientation, which places a high value on activity and personal productivity through work, materialism, success, and individual achievement. Older adults who are no longer able to produce due to physical and mental changes or due to social policies that remove them from gainful employment (such as retirement), are at a distinct disadvantage in a society dominated by such a value orientation.

Independence is another predominant value in the United States. Dependency is viewed as a sign of weakness or lack of character. Individuals who cannot earn a living and survive independently in this country are viewed as lazy, incompetent, inferior or worthless, and an economic burden on the rest of society. As individuals age, they experience many physical, mental, social, and economic changes. These changes may make them more dependent—emotionally, physically, and financially—on family members and others in society.

Youth and beauty are also highly valued in the United States. Youth is associated with vitality, activity, and freshness. To be young is to be fully alive, exciting, attractive, healthy, and vigorous. Old age, on the other hand, is associated with decline, disease, disability, and death rather than wisdom, inner peace, and other positive qualities. Older adults living in such a culture are viewed negatively and may come to see themselves as senile and ugly.

Older adults who internalize these negative views of aging and older people may feel they are abnormal, deviant, or marginal members of the culture. They may feel they have a *spoiled identity* (Goffman, 1963). As a result, many disengage from participation in civil, social, and other groups and thus become isolated.

Ageism also contributes to a sense of helplessness and powerlessness among older adults and may increase feelings of low self-esteem and late-life depression. Older adults may view their lives as nonproductive, useless, and meaningless. They may also see their continued existence as a social and economic burden, and a personal burden on family and friends. Low self-esteem, depression, and feelings of uselessness may contribute to suicide in late life.

At the current time in the United States two ageist attitudes are becoming more and more prevalent. First, dependent life is viewed as not worth living; second, there is increased tolerance for suicide and assisted suicide in late life. One ethicist argues for *preemptive suicide,* suggesting that late life is sometimes such a negative experience that people should have the right to end their lives before they are old: "Elective death in advanced age should be recognized as a justifiable alternative to demeaning deterioration and stultifying dependency" (Prado, 1998, p. 5).

Rapidly increasing numbers of older people in our population, coupled with spiraling health care costs, have prompted rhetoric and policy changes aimed at containing health care costs. In recent years an increased call has occurred for health care rationing on the basis of age (Callahan, 1987). Opponents of age-based health care rationing argue that this practice would be an official policy of discrimination against older persons (Kapp, 1989). Today we are hearing increasingly louder cries for the "right to die" and legalization of physician-assisted suicide. It is no coincidence that these positions are gaining momentum at the same time that we are witnessing phenomenal growth in older, more dependent populations. Older adults, especially those age eighty-five and above, place unprecedented demands on limited economic and health care resources in this country. Suicide is viewed as an inexpensive solution to increasingly expensive older adult health care. Prado recognizes that preemptive suicide would have important economic benefits for government-supported health care systems, but does recognize that legislation permitting such suicide depreciates life that is dependent.

In our society we associate old age with morbidity and death, thereby the right to commit suicide may be viewed as a rational choice for older adults. As one well-known thanatologist notes:

"From the view that it is natural for the aged to die, it is not difficult to conclude that they ought to die" (Kastenbaum, 1992, p. 118). He even suggests that if such notions are not challenged vigorously, suicide could become the preferred way of death in America for older adults.

Older adults living in a suicide-permissive culture that devalues them and abhors dependency may come to see their continued existence as unfair to younger people and the society, and as depriving younger people of scarce health care resources. A real possibility exists that older people—who are perceived by family members, physicians, and society as a burden—will be coerced or manipulated into committing suicide or requesting physician-assisted suicide (Battin, 1996; Richman, 1998). It seems easier to eliminate the problem of too many expensive older people to care for, or to encourage the problem to eliminate itself through sanctions encouraging elderly suicide, rather than to face hard moral choices about our spending as individuals and as a society. This view also ignores our appropriate obligations to our older members who have created and improved the society in which we live. Is this the kind of society we want? Harry Moody (1984) expresses his concerns:

> But do we really want a society in which our best answer to the "meaningless" existence of old age is an encouragement for old people to kill themselves? Does this attitude itself not betray contempt for dependency, a feeling that the lives of old people are somehow less than human, and, finally, a secret despair over the last stage of the life cycle? (p. 89)

See also AGE SEGREGATION; BLAMING THE AGED; CULTURAL SOURCES OF AGEISM; ETHICAL ISSUES; SCAPEGOATING; STEREO-TYPES

REFERENCES

Battin, M.P. (1996). *The death debate: Ethical issues in suicide*. Englewood, NJ: Prentice Hall.

Butler, R. (1968). *Why survive? Being old in America*. New York: Harper & Row.

Callahan, D. (1987). *Setting limits*. New York: Simon & Schuster.

Goffman, E. (1963). *Stigma: Notes on the management of spoiled identity*. Englewood, NJ: Prentice Hall.

Kapp, M.B. (1989). Rationing health care: Will it be necessary? Can it be done without age or disability discrimination? *Issues in Law and Medicine,* 5, 337-352.

Kastenbaum, R. (1992). Death, suicide, and the older adult. *Suicide and Life Threatening Behavior,* 22, 1-14.

Moody, H.R. (1984). Can suicide on grounds of old age be ethically justified? In M. Tallmer, E. Prichard, A. Kutscher, R. Debellis, M. Hale, and I. Goldberg (Eds.), *The life-threatened elderly* (pp. 64-92). New York: Columbia University Press.

Murphy, S. (2000). *Deaths: Final data for 1998.* National Vital Statistics Report, 48 (11). Hyattsville, MD: National Center for Health Statistics. DHHS Publication No. (PHS) 2000-1120.

Prado, C.G. (1998). *The last choice: Preemptive suicide in advanced age* (Second edition). Westport, CT: Greenwood Press.

Richman, J. (1998). Euthanasia and physician-assisted suicide in America today: Whither are we going? In J. Kaplan and M. Schwartz (Eds.), *Jewish approaches to suicide, martydom, and euthanasia* (pp. 116-128). Northvale, NJ: Jason Aronson, Inc.

TAX BREAKS

Erdman B. Palmore

Elders enjoy numerous tax breaks (technically called tax expenditures) not available to younger people. This is a form of positive ageism. These tax breaks are justified on the basis of various stereotypes about the aged, such as the assumption that they have higher rates of poverty (not true of the majority); that they are disabled and cannot earn an income (not true of the majority); that they have a fixed income that does not go up with inflation (not true of the majority, because Social Security benefits are indexed to inflation); or that they have "earned" special tax exemptions because of their contribution to society (which may be true of some, but is probably not true of many).

Federal Tax Breaks

Federal tax breaks include the following:

- Exclusion of all or part of Social Security and Railroad Retirement benefits from the federal income tax. This is probably the largest tax break: it cost the government more that $23 billion in 1995 (Hudson, 1995).
- Exclusion of Medicare benefits from taxation. This cost the government more than $13 billion in 1995.
- Raising the threshold for estate taxes to $1 million favors older people more than younger.
- Dependent-care tax credits for employed taxpayers caring for elderly spouses or parents.

- A major tax expenditure (more than \$81 billion) is for pensions and individual retirement accounts (IRAs) that permit contributions to be deducted from present tax obligations by the future elderly population. This is a tax break that helps increase the retirement income of elders.

State and Local Tax Breaks

Elders receive more state and local tax breaks than the general population (Liebig, 2001). However, these breaks have low visibility and so have escaped calls to repeal them. They include the following:

- Special tax treatment is afforded to retirement income and estate and inheritance taxes have been cut, often in an attempt to become retirement havens.
- Most states do not tax Social Security income.
- Almost all states with a personal income tax exclude some pension benefits from taxation.
- Some states have enacted deductions or exemptions for taxpayers caring for older or disabled persons.
- About half of the states favor seniors by providing them with a homestead exemption or circuit breaker program of tax relief from property taxes.
- Some states provide a credit or rebate to elders for part of the sales tax paid.
- The exemption of food and prescription drugs from sales taxes benefit elders more than younger people.

Besides being a form of ageism, these tax breaks tend to favor upper-income elders more than other elders and therefore discriminate against middle- and lower-income elders. Many argue that it would be more effective to help lower-income elders with direct spending on them, rather than using tax credits that are little help to low-income elders.

Many are calling for tax reforms that would eliminate these special tax breaks for elders or extend them to all ages.

See also AGE-SPECIFIC PUBLIC PROGRAMS; BENEFITS OF AGING; GENERATIONAL EQUITY; PUBLIC POLICY

REFERENCES

Hudson, R. (1995). Federal budgeting and expenditures. In G. Maddox (Ed.), *The encyclopedia of aging*. New York: Springer.

Liebig, P. (2001). Tax Policy. In G. Maddox (Ed.), *The encyclopedia of aging*. New York: Springer.

TELEVISION

Erdman B. Palmore

The mass media includes newspapers, magazines, comic books, movies, videos, radio, and television. However, the majority of research on images of the aged in the media has focused on television. This is because TV plays a predominant role in influencing people's attitudes toward aging (Brownell and Mundorf, 2001).

The first conclusion of research on the aged in TV is that they are rarely seen. A review of twenty-eight studies (Vasil and Wass, 1993) concluded that elders were underrepresented in both electronic and print media in terms of their proportion in the U.S. population. Another study (Robinson and Skill, 1995) reported that fewer than 3 percent of the 1,228 adult speaking characters in prime time TV were age sixty-five or older. Of these older characters, less that 9 percent were in lead roles. This shows discrimination both in terms of number and type of roles that elders are allowed to play on TV.

The second conclusion of these studies indicates that elders tend to be marginalized and represented in negative stereotypes. Powell and Williamson's (1985) review of the mass media found stereotypical ageist biases and a trend toward helplessness in the older characters. This is particularly ironic because elders are the group with the greatest exposure time to TV.

The predominant image of older women on TV has been as a nurturer or in the negative role of a nag. However, that changed with the advent of cable TV. Several shows still in syndication featuring older women in positive roles include *The Golden Girls* and *Murder, She Wrote.*

Although the images of aging shown on TV seem to be slowly changing, the usual image is still a negative one that portrays aging as an undesirable experience. This kind of ageism becomes a self-fulfilling prophecy: aging is feared and denied so it becomes fearful and negative.

See also CULTURAL SOURCES OF AGEISM; JOURNALISM; LITERA-
TURE; SELF-FULFILLING PROPHECY; STEREOTYPES

REFERENCES

Brownell, W. and Mundorf, N. (2001). Images of aging in the media. In G. Maddox
(Ed.), *The encyclopedia of aging*. New York: Springer.
Powell, L. and Williamson, J. (1985). The mass media and the aged. In H. Fox (Ed.)
Aging. Guilford, CT: The Duskin Publishing Group.
Robinson, J. and Skill, T. (1995). The invisible generation. *Communication Re-
ports,* 8, 111-119.
Vasil, L. and Wass, H. (1993). Portrayal of the elderly in the media. *Educational
Gerontology,* 19, 71.

TERMS PREFERRED BY OLDER PEOPLE

Erdman B. Palmore

It is a generally accepted principle of social psychology that the
terms we use for people or things tend to affect our perception of
them. Shakespeare was wrong when he said, "A rose by any other
name would smell as sweet." If a rose were called a "stinkweed," for
example, we probably would not think it smelled as sweet (Berelson
and Steiner, 1964).

Thus, one form of ageism is the use of negative terms for older
people, such as old fogey, crone, or hag. In order to avoid such ageism, it would be preferable to use positive or at least neutral terms that
do not offend older people.

However, only a few studies have addressed terms that older people actually prefer. Harris (1975), in a representative survey of older
Americans, found that most expressed strong dislike for terms such
as *old man* or *old woman* or even *aged person.* They preferred the
terms *senior citizen* or *mature American.*

More recently, a survey of 108 Canadians concluded that the majority of those surveyed rated the term *geriatric* as "totally unacceptable" (Frei, 2003). Terms that the study participants reported to be acceptable, but not particularly liked, include *elderly, golden age, older*

adult, older people, and *pensioners.* The preferred terms included *senior, senior citizen,* and *retiree.*

Some gerontologists have suggested that the term *elder* is the most positive of all (Palmore, 2000).

See also LANGUAGE

REFERENCES

Berelson, B. and Steiner, G. (1964). *Human behavior.* New York: Harcourt Brace.

Frei, R. (2003). Individuals older than 65 years dislike the term "geriatric," prefer "senior." *CNS/LTC,* 2(1), 1.

Harris, L. (1975). *The myth and reality of aging in America.* Washington, DC: The National Council of the Aging.

Palmore, E. (2000). Ageism in gerontological language. *The Gerontologist,* 40, 645.

THEORIES OF AGING

Robert Kastenbaum

Do we want to understand or prevent aging? These two motives often are intertwined. Gerontological research is guided by scientific principles such as verifiability and replicability, and its theories evaluated on criteria such as parsimony, coherence, and predictive power. However, it is the quest to prevent or modify aging that attracts both researchers and their funding support. In this sense it might be said that theories of aging are themselves ageist: crafted not from dispassionate objectivity but from antipathy toward the very phenomena it has chosen to study. This situation stands in sharp contrast with studies of infant and child development that seek understanding in order to protect and enhance its phenomena.

The connection between ageism and theories of aging is problematic for other reasons as well. Theories of aging generally focus on changes *within* the individual over time (though environmental factors may also be taken into account). By contrast, ageism usually is regarded as a pattern of perceptions and behaviors directed *toward* the individual by society. Thus ageism and theories of aging tend to bypass each other. Furthermore, none of the major theories of aging were designed to explain ageism, nor has much effort been made to discover possible links.

There is also an implicit contradiction: scientists and activists deplore societal attitudes and practices that discriminate on the basis of age, but at the same time the major research programs are often based on the conviction that aging is a bad thing that should be eradicated or controlled.

Agile gerontologists can distinguish between *people* who are aging and the *process of aging*. People: good. Aging: bad. This neat distinction is perhaps not robust enough to clear gerontology of at least a whiff of its own ageism. Some theorists do emphasize positive facets of aging. The concept of successful aging and the attribution of special wisdom to aged adults are among the attempts to provide an alternative to the prevailingly negative view. These more favorable conceptions, welcome as they might be, nevertheless could be seen as compensatory responses to ageism and, therefore, not entirely free of the subjective element.

Despite the limitations and difficulties that have been noted, it is still useful to explore possible connections between ageism and theories of aging. For perspective, we begin with a brief sampling of biological theories before turning to social gerontology. Biologists are not in a position to give us direct information on ageism, but they can help to keep our social and behavioral science theories from floating away from the physical realities.

Biological Theories of Aging

Somatic mutation theory (Curtis, 1965) was part of the first crop of biological explanations to sprout from modern gerontological research. Aging begins at the cellular level. Each generation of somatic cells within our body produces the next generation—but not perfectly. Errors pile up. Basic functions are disrupted. As individual cells become less efficient, so do tissues and organ systems. It becomes increasingly difficult to coordinate complex activities, cope with stress, and adapt to changing conditions. We slow down: in fact, slowing might be considered the primary sign of aging (Vercruysen, 1993). We also become more fallible. One can imagine millions of cells experiencing *senior moments*.

Other theories arrived at a similar conclusion through somewhat different paths. For example, Walford (1965) proposed that we age because our immune system turns against us. Cell populations lose their uniformity and become more diverse, no longer recognized as friends by our immune defenses. An evolutionary perspective also found its voice:

> We probably age because we run out of evolutionary program. In this we resemble a space probe that has been designed to pass Mars, but that has no further built-in instructions once it has done so, and no components specifically produced to last longer than that.
>
> It will travel on, but the failure rate in its guidance and control mechanisms will steadily increase—and this failure of homeostasis, of self-righting, is exactly what we see in the aging organism. (Comfort, 1964, p. 93)

This biological perspective implies that we humans, as with other species, have been designed to function just long enough to procreate after our kind and protect our young. After reaching our physical prime, then, we do not have anything much to do or anything much to do it with. The landmark research of Leonard Hayflick (1971, 1994) reinforced this view, although he believes that the biological sciences will eventually discover a way to moderate the aging process. Hayflick overturned the prevailing belief that the individual cell is immortal (that is, if conditions are congenial). It turns out that cells flourish through a certain number of divisions (depending on the species), and then demonstrate clear signs of structural and functional decline. One can say either that our constituent cells have programs with a relatively brief shelf life (Comfort) or that we are actually programmed to age and die (Hayflick).

Proponents of these seminal theories could find nothing pleasant to say about aging from the standpoint of either the individual cell or the individual person. Some biologists maintain that aging is a tonic for the species because it winnows out the weak. This dubious application of the "survival of the fittest" principle, however, poses the question: Wouldn't it be more useful if people who have developed skills and understanding through many years of experience continue to serve society unhobbled by aging?

Several inferences can be drawn from biological findings and theories:

1. Physical decline over time is a characteristic of our life form, but neglect, abuse, or animosity toward aging persons has no basis, no justification in biology.
2. The underlying biological process of aging is gradual and occurs at different individual rates. A societal attitude that labels a person as old at a particular chronological age is at odds with a wealth of research and cogent theory.
3. Biological theories of aging have not yet dealt adequately with the cognitive, interpersonal, and cultural achievements of a long life. The fact that some people continue to function at a very high level at an advanced age suggests an ability to compensate or transcend physical impairment—a kind of heroism that deserves respect rather than ageist scorn.

Social Gerontology Theories of Aging

The first two theories to attract wide attention quickly became locked in such an adversarial contest that one can hardly be considered without the other. The Kansas City Study of Adult Life produced *disengagement theory* (Cumming and Henry, 1961; Henry, 1965). Disengagement was seen as a "normal" process of mutual withdrawal between an aging person and society. The aging individual becomes increasingly aware of the diminished time remaining in life and is ready to become free from obligations. A heightened interiority occurs as people reflect on the meaning of their lives, followed by a reengagement in which individual and society connect again, but in a more selective way. By implication, disengagement was a positive development because it was thought to occur under favorable circumstances and serve as part of the natural life course. Furthermore, society also benefited from this process because it opened opportunities for younger people.

Opponents viewed this theory in a less favorable light. Disengagement looked too much like justification for removing older adults to the sidelines, although this implication was strongly denied by founding theorists Elaine M. Cumming and William E. Henry. Enter *activity theory*. People are better off if they remain involved in social transactions and other forms of activity as they grow older. This position was not developed into a formal theory comparable with the numerous principles and subprinciples articulated by disengagement theory. Instead, it consisted largely of (1) protest against the suspected ageism of disengagement theory, and (2) the prevailing cultural value that people fare best when they keep themselves busy. Thomas G. McGowan (1996) notes that activity theory argued that disengagement is not part of a natural biological process because most elders still function well until their terminal decline. Rather, withdrawal from significant roles is compelled by an ageist society. (These competing theories were fresh and feisty at a time when most employed Americans were still required to retire at a fixed age, usually sixty-five. It therefore seemed inappropriate to speak of a natural process of "mutual withdrawal.")

The disengagement/activity controversy generated abundant research. It was found repeatedly that elderly people with active life styles reported greater life satisfaction or morale. However, this connection held true only for especially meaningful activities. Being just "busy, busy, busy" did not have much value in itself. Morale was also higher for people classified as "active" rather than "disengaged." These findings did not resolve the controversy, however. Good health might be the most significant factor, making it possible to be more active and derive more enjoyment from life. Furthermore, activity theory does not escape its own possible ideological taint. The United States has often been characterized as a *doing* rather than a *reflecting* society (as compared, for example, with India, where meditation is a traditional value and elders are cherished for their spiritual development) (Maduro, 1981). Disengagement theory aroused opposition because it seemed to play into ageist exclusion from societal power. Activity theory was vulnerable to the charge of trying to keep aging people busy, even if in trivial ways, because of the establishment's distrust and discomfort with the inner life. If cultivating the inner life is a natural part of the life course, then activity theory seemed intent on denying that experience to its elders.

Modernization theory offered a historical perspective on ageism. Anthropologist Leo Simmons (1945) suggested that elders have a more powerful and protected role in societies with a low level of industrial development. Emphasis shifts from tradition to innovation and productivity, gradually marginalizing elders who represent a used-up rather than sacred past. Elders also become more abundant as longevity increases, so are apt to become less special and revered. More recent scholarship sets forth a more complex picture of modernization and its effect on the aged. The main thesis of modernization remains of keen interest, though: the desire to live a long and full life has come into conflict with the perception of aging as a "social problem." There was probably always some ambivalence in society's attitude toward the aged (Kastenbaum, 1974; Kastenbaum and Ross, 1975) but full-fledged ageism may indeed be a by-product of modernization.

Exchange theory provides still another perspective that regards individual experiences within the framework of large-scale sociocultural dynamics. All interactions involve an exchange of benefits or values. Relationships thrive when the transactions result in equitable benefits: people feel they have received good value for what they have given. Families, organizations, and even nations also function more effectively when all the members believe they are being fairly treated. In practice, though, many people do feel victimized in the pattern of societal exchanges. Some gerontologists have applied exchange (or equity) theory to the exchange interactions that are experienced by many people as they grow older (Antonucci, 1990; Cook, 1992). There is a tendency for people to lose some of their power to obtain what they want or need from their interactions with family, friends, and even store clerks. At the same time, those who interact with elders may anticipate that *they* will derive little benefit from the interactions. Accordingly, both the elder and the transactional partner may enter a situation with attitudes that have a negative influence on the outcome.

Does exchange theory and research explain ageism? Societal barriers to services and opportunities do increase with age. Younger people often do talk down to elders. It could be argued, though, that this pattern of inequality is dictated by reality—the diminished function of elders—rather than ageism. Less can be expected of old people, so one must make adjustments. This argument can be tested in both the scientific and the ethical realms. Is it fact or ageist stereotype that elders cannot participate in equitable relationships and transactions? Are exchange and equity to be evaluated in terms of the immediate situation or from the larger perspective of all that an elderly person has contributed to society over the years?

Several other theories focus more intensely on the individual aging person, though not to the exclusion of sociocultural influences. As we age we will be—ourselves! This, somewhat simplified, is the central thesis of *continuity theory* (Atchler, 1997). Our personalities are shaped by early experience and then revised a bit and fine-tuned in adolescence and early adulthood. We bring our distinctive view of the world and ourselves with us wherever we go, including the far reaches of adult life. Research has in fact demonstrated that basic personality endures through the adult years. The relationship styles and coping techniques we have practiced throughout our lives will still be evident. Ageism looks rather peculiar in the light of continuity theory. People are still fundamentally their old (that is, young) selves through the years—so what sense does it make to treat them differently and worse?

Developmental theories at first were concerned only with the early years of life. Eventually the perspective enlarged to encompass the full life course. The question of how a person develops from infancy through advanced age was almost invariably accompanied by the question: how *should* we move through the entire compass of our lives? *Stage theories* were the first type to become popular, notably Eric Erikson's (1950, 1959) conceptualizations. He viewed human lives as marked by stages, each of which confronts the individual with a developmental challenge. The final stage involves the challenge of achieving "a sense of integrity" instead of "a sense of despair." Erikson's theory did much to encourage people to think beyond childhood and youth. It also found value in old age and emphasized that both the individual and society share responsibility to create the conditions for a good life.

Nevertheless, "stages," whether Erikson's or that of other theorists, have not fared well under research conditions or critical inquiry. The idea of stages across the life course has literary and philosophical appeal but has made little progress in the direction of established fact. In addition, despite its generous outlook on young and old alike, there may still be a hint of ageism in its assignment of specific tasks for specific times of life. To see life as a series of tasks or dragons to slay also bears the mark of social values and habits rather than objective findings.

Psychoanalytic theory brought some excitement to gerontology with its psychosexual development perspective. (Erikson's theory pushed off from its Freudian model to become psycho*social* rather than psycho*sexual*.) Freud himself had little to say about aging, and most of that little was pessimistic. Some later psychoanalysts did take up the challenge. Helene Deutsch (1945) believed that women entered crisis and lost social value when they passed the age of child-bearing. Fertility and ageism were therefore closely related. The prevailing psychoanalytic view was that the biological aging process undermined the inhibitions and other defensive strategies that people had relied upon. Forbidden sexual and aggressive impulses threatened to escape control and cause mischief in various directions. Conflicts that had been more or less swept under the rug surfaced again. Aging adults needed help to keep the whole circus of infantile and neurotic impulses under control, given their weakened ego strength.

This was certainly a negative take on aging, although it had more the character of a clinical diagnosis than a societal stereotype. It was also a poorly informed position because (1) few psychoanalysts had actually devoted themselves to treatment of elderly adults, (2) their attention was focused almost entirely on people in serious distress, and (3) the nascent field of gerontology had produced few facts in support of their theoretical and therapeutic nihilism.

Some psychoanalytically oriented therapists eventually did undertake therapy with elderly people and discovered their considerable potential for insight and symptom relief. Stanley Cath's (1972) concept of *depletion anxiety* identified a problem that seemed to occur most frequently in the later adult years as individuals attempt to cope both with their remaining life and the prospect of death, while having fewer resources to call upon. With concepts such as depletion anxiety, psychoanalytic theory had the beginnings of an age-relevant but nonageist approach.

Another branch of developmental theory focuses on the relationship between the individual and situation. *Old behavior,* for example, is seen as a phenomenon cocreated by person and situation (including expectations). For example, *slow behavior* was a function of the match between the individual's pace and the pacing set by the environment, and a multitude of other old behaviors could be generated by depriving people of the opportunity to have their words and actions have effect (Kastenbaum, 1974). It is not age so much as certain types of behavior that mark a person as old and expose that person to ageism. Modify the relationship between individual and environment and much of the negative kind of old behavior vanishes—or use altered environments to give young people personal experience with being caught in an old situation and thereby revise their attitudes.

Habituation is another facet of developmental-field theory (Kastenbaum, 1993). Mental and emotional development become evident in infancy when the child habituates, that is, shows that it recognizes it has seen or heard something before. Aging begins when *hyperhabituation* creeps in: the tendency to treat new people, situations, and events as though already so familiar that nothing can be learned from them. The tendency of some elderly people to treat the new like the old is regarded as one of the main cues that touch off or confirm ageism. Actually, whether people become hyperhabituated with advancing age depends upon the kind of person they are—and the kind of person the world has made them.

Concluding Word

All the theories identified here and much of the research confirms the common observation that aging is often accompanied by stress, loss, and challenge. Nothing in either the biological or social-psychological theories, however, supports ageism as either a necessity or an adaptive response on the part of society. We still have limited control over the biological processes that comprise aging but we have unrealized potential for replacing ageism with a more accurate, effective, and compassionate response.

See also CULTURAL SOURCES OF AGEISM; DISENGAGEMENT THEORY; GERONTOLOGY; MODERNIZATION THEORY; PERPETUAL YOUTH; SELF-FULFILLING PROPHECY; SOCIAL PSYCHOLOGY; STAGE THEORY; SUCCESSFUL AGING

REFERENCES

Antonucci, T. (1990). Social supports and social relationships. In R. H. Binstock and E. Shanas (Eds.), *Handbook of aging and the social sciences* (Second edition) (pp. 94-128). New York: Van Nostrand Reinhold.

Atchler, R. (1997). *Social forces and aging.* Belmont, CA: Wadsworth.

Cath, S. (1972). Psychoanalytic viewpoints on aging—An historical survey. In D. P. Kent, S. Sherwood, and R. Kastenbaum (Eds.), *Research, action, and planning for the elderly* (pp. 279-314). New York: Behavioral Publications.

Comfort, A. (1964). *Processes of aging.* New York: Signet.

Cook, K. S. (1992). Exchange theory. In E. F. Borgatta and M. L. Borgatta (Eds.), *Encyclopedia of sociology,* Volume 2 (pp. 606-610). New York: Macmillan.

Cumming, E. M. and Henry, W. E. (1961). *Growing old.* New York: Basic Books.

Curtis, H. J. (1965). The somatic mutation theory of aging. In R. Kastenbaum (Ed.), *Contributions to the psychobiology of aging* (pp. 69-80). New York: Springer.

Deutsch, H. (1945). *The psychology of women,* Volume 2. *Motherhood.* New York: Grune and Stratton.

Erikson, E. (1950). *Childhood and society.* New York: Norton.

_____ (1959). *Identity and life cycle.* New York: International Universities Press.

Hayflick, L. (1971). The longevity of cultured human cells. *Journal of the American Geriatrics Society, 22,* 1-12.

_____ (1994). *How and why we age.* New York: Ballantine Books.

Henry, W. E. (1965). Engagement and disengagement: Toward a theory of adult development. In R. Kastenbaum (Ed.), *Contributions to the psychobiology of aging* (pp. 19-36). New York: Springer.

Kastenbaum, R. (1974). Should we have mixed feelings about our ambivalence toward the aged? *Journal of Geriatric Psychiatry, 7,* 94-107.

_____ (1993). Habituation: A key to lifespan development and aging? In R. Kastenbaum (Ed.), *Encyclopedia of adult development* (pp. 195-200). Phoenix: Oryx Press.

Kastenbaum, R. and Ross, B. (1975). Historical perspectives on care of the aged. In J. G. Howells (Ed.), *Modern perspectives in the psychiatry of old age* (pp. 421-448). New York: Brunner/Mazel.

Maduro, R. (1981). The old man as creative artist in India. In R. Kastenbaum (Ed.), *Old age on the new scene* (pp. 71-101). New York: Springer.

McGowan, T. G. (1996). Ageism and discrimination. In J. E. Birren (Ed.), *Encyclopedia of gerontology,* Volume 1 (pp. 71-80). San Diego: Academic Press.

Simmons, L. W. (1945). *The role of the aged in primitive societies.* New Haven: Yale University Press.

Vercruysen, M. (1993). Slowing of behavior with age. In R. Kastenbaum (Ed.), *Encyclopedia of adult development* (pp. 457-467). Phoenix: Onyx Press.

Walford, R. L. (1965). Immunology and aging. In R. Kastenbaum (Ed.), *Contributions to the psychobiology of aging* (pp. 81-86). New York: Springer.

TRANSPORTATION

William A. Satariano
David R. Ragland

Transportation is defined as a means or system of personal or mass conveyance, designed to enable individuals to reach destinations beyond walking distance. This includes access, use, and/or operation of different forms of transportation, such as the private automobile, public transit (e.g., city bus and subway), and commercial travel (e.g., airline).

Automobile driving in older populations has received particular attention. In the United States the automobile represents the most common form of transportation for older people (Marottoli et al., 2000). Despite the overall significance of automobile travel, the percentage of older people who drive declines with age (Foley et al., 2002; Lyman et al., 2001). Seniors experience the highest crash rate per miles driven as well as the highest crash-injury and crash-fatality rates, i.e., probability of injury or death holding constant the force of the crash (Evans, 2000; Dellinger, Langlois, and Li, 2002). Overall, automobile crashes represent the second leading cause of accidental death among seniors age sixty-five and older. Automobile crashes and injuries are associated with the number and type of chronic health conditions, cognitive dysfunction, visual impairments, and reduce physical performance (Waller, 1991; Ball et al., 1993).

The aging driver situation has led to an important public policy issue. With the aging of the population, an increase has occurred in the percentage of older individuals operating automobiles and a growing concern about a corresponding increase in traffic crashes and injuries. A need exists, therefore, to develop the best strategy to balance the rights of individuals and the benefits they derive from driving with concerns about public safety. Although public policy in this area should be based on scientific research, consideration of this issue has been colored by ageism.

Ageism may affect access to and/or use of various means or systems of transportation through the formal or informal adoption of stereotypes, prejudice, or misinformation about the association between chronological age and functional capacities. This ageism is based on the premise that a uniform relationship exists between increasing chronological age and the number, type, and severity of functional limitations. This, in turn, implies that once people reach a particular age, they are functionally limited in the performance of basic tasks such as operating an automobile or negotiating a bus, rail, or subway system. This position serves to justify proposals for special licensing to limit the timing or location of driving for older people of a particular age.

Although proponents of this position may accept that chronological age is only a marker, they argue that it is the best available marker, given that no other functional screens have been developed, with the notable exception of standard tests of visual acuity. It is worth noting that recent evidence indicates that visual acuity is not an effective screening test. Better measures or markers include useful field of view tests, some cognitive assessments, and certain medical conditions such as stroke (McGwin et al., 2000; Wood, 2002).

Ageism is also reflected in the absence of technological and environmental designs that accommodate age-related functional limitations. Although considerable variability occurs between chronological age and functional capacity, as noted previously, chronological age is, in fact, associated with an increased incidence and prevalence of functional limitations. In this case, ageism is reflected in the failure to develop innovative technological and environmental designs that accommodate these functional limitations and extend the time in which older people can drive automobiles or make use of other forms of transportation. The underlying assumption is that older people with functional limitations are not worth the commitment of time and resources to develop such systems. This position also may explain in part the reasons why priority is not given to the development and dissemination of more sophisticated and more comprehensive licensing screens based on functional capacity.

Future Research

Future research in this area should address the following concerns:

- It would be useful to determine whether perceived ageism (e.g., perception that family members do not consider it safe for people to drive or use other means of transportation once they have reached a particular age) is associated with a person's decision to stop driving or change his or her use of other forms of transportation. In addition, it would be useful to investigate the extent to which other factors (e.g., race/ethnicity, gender, socioeconomic status, and geographic region) affect the association between ageism and transportation.
- Research is needed to determine the more parsimonious sets of measures to assess multiple, integrated functional capacities

(e.g., useful field of vision and hand-eye coordination) to safely operate different forms of transportation. This information would be useful to determine more effective screening strategies to judge competence to operate an automobile, regardless of chronological age.

- A related area of research would be to assess which technological and environmental designs affect transportation use among people of different ages and levels of functional competence. This research may lead to the development of new transportation vehicles and systems that would enable people to be mobile for as long as possible.
- Research in community planning could be designed to assess the feasibility of developing multiple, integrated systems of transportation in communities. This would include studies of the effective *transitioning* from one form of transportation to another. When a person can no longer operate an automobile under particular situations, other forms of transportation should be in place to ensure continued mobility. To the extent that ageism is based on stereotypes and misinformation, research of this kind would lead to strategies that ensure older people can maintain their mobility safely for as long as possible.

See also DRIVER'S LICENSE TESTING; FACTS ON AGING QUIZ; FUNCTIONAL AGE; STEREOTYPES

REFERENCES

Ball, K.C., Owsley, et al. (1993). Visual attention problems as a predictor of vehicle crashes in older drivers. *Investigative Ophthalmological and Visual Science*, 34, 3110-3123.

Dellinger, A.M., Langlois, J.A., and Li (2002). Fatal crashes among older drivers: Decomposition of rates into contributing factors. *American Journal of Epidemiol*, 155, 234-241.

Evans, L. (2000). Risks older drivers face themselves and threats they pose to other road users. *International Journal of Epidemiology*, 29, 315-322.

Foley, D.J., Heimovitz, A. et al. (2002). Driving life expectancy of persons aged 70 years and older in the United States. *American Journal of Public Health*, 92, 1284-1289.

Lyman, J.M., McGwin, B. et al. (2001). Factors related to driving difficulty and habits in older drivers. *Accident Analysis and Prevention*, 33, 413-421.

Marottoli, R.A., de Leon, C.F.M., et al. (2000). Consequences of driving cessation: Decreased out-of-home activity levels. *Journal of Gerontology: Social Sciences,* 55, S334-S340.

McGwin, G., Chapman, V., et al. (2000). Visual risk factors for driving difficulty among older drivers. *Accident Analysis and Prevention,* 32, 735-744.

Waller, P.F. (1991). The older driver. *Human Factors,* 33, 499-505.

Wood, J.M. (2002). Age and visual impairment decrease driving performance as measured on a closed-road circuit. *Human Factors,* 44, 482-494.

TYPES OF AGEISTS

Erdman B. Palmore

Ageism entails two different dimensions: prejudice and discrimination (Palmore, 1999). When these two dimensions are cross-classified, they result in four types of persons related to ageism. Each of these types requires a different strategy to reduce ageism.

1. *Unprejudiced nondiscriminators.* These have been called the *all-weather liberals* who thoroughly accept the American creed in both belief and action (Merton, 1949). They believe discrimination or prejudice against elders is wrong. Such people should be the leaders of effective campaigns to reduce ageism. However, their effectiveness may be diminished by the *fallacy of unanimity.* This illusion of consensus in the community is produced by the tendency of liberals to talk only to one another. When they assume unanimity against ageism, they may become complacent and inactive.

2. *Unprejudiced discriminators.* These are the *fair-weather liberals* who, despite their own lack of prejudice, support discrimination against elders because it is easier or more profitable to discriminate than to take a stand against discrimination. These people may go along with a policy of discrimination against elders in employment in order to secure their own promotion or other personal advantage. These people may suffer from some feelings of guilt because of the discrepancy between their beliefs and actions. Therefore they are strategic persons for the all-weather liberals to work on.

3. *Prejudiced nondiscriminators.* These are the *fair-weather ageists* who reluctantly conform to laws or other pressures against age discrimination. These individuals can be kept from discrimination, not by appeal to democratic values, but by making discrimination costly or unpleasant. They may be persuaded by education and propaganda to reduce their prejudice against elders and thus move toward becoming unprejudiced nondiscriminators.

4. *Prejudiced discriminators.* These are the *all-weather ageists* who are consistent in belief and practice. The strategy for dealing with this type depends on the issue and the situation. If their discrimination can be made costly through legislation or boycotts, they may move into Type 3. If they can be educated or persuaded to give up their prejudices, they may be moved into Type 2 or even Type 1.

"Different strokes for different folks" is a saying that applies to these different types, who require different strategies.

See also TYPOLOGIES

REFERENCES

Merton, R. (1949). Discrimination and the American Creed. In R. MacIver (Ed.), *Discrimination and national welfare.* New York: Harper & Row.
Palmore, E. (1999). *Ageism.* New York: Springer.

TYPOLOGIES

Erdman B. Palmore

The three major types of ageism may be categorized as cultural, individual, and institutional (Palmore, 1999). Cultural ageism is listed first because it is the basic cause of individual and institutional ageism. Crosscutting these three types is the positive/negative dimension. Most people are aware only of negative ageism: prejudice or discrimination *against* older people. Few are aware of positive ageism: prejudice or discrimination *in favor* of older people. However, government programs that are examples of positive ageism, such as tax breaks for the aged, Supplemental Security Insurance (SSI), Medicare, and senior centers, are becoming more controversial because of the mounting budget deficit.

Cultural agism is found in our language, literature, humor, songs, and mass media. Our language encourages ageism through equating chronological age with various negative or positive characteristics. For example, *aging* or *getting old* usually involves negative situations such as becoming frail, inactive, senile, or disabled. Similarly, *staying young* usually involves such positives as remaining strong, active, alert, and capable.

On the other hand, *old* sometimes has positive connotations such as mature, venerable, or experienced, as in the expression, "an old master" or "an old hand." Similarly, *young* sometimes has negative connotations such as immature or inexperienced.

Literature presents a mixture of negative images (e.g., *King Lear*) and positive images (e.g., Santa Claus). The majority of humor and songs about aging are negative and much of humor about aging is ambivalent, but positive humor is rare.

The images of elders presented on television are clusters of stereotypes, sometimes positive (as in *The Golden Girls*), but more often negative (as in commercials for health remedies) or simplistic stereotypes.

Individual ageism can be divided into prejudiced attitudes and discriminatory behavior. Negative attitudes include the stereotypes that most aged are sick, impotent, ugly, senile, mentally ill, useless, isolated poor, and depressed. Several studies using the Facts on Aging Quiz (FAQ) have shown that the majority of people believe several of these stereotypes. These stereotypes are common among all ages, races, regions, and both sexes. The only variable making a substantial difference in their frequency is education: educated persons are less prejudiced against the aged.

Some widely shared positive stereotypes include beliefs that most elders are kind, wise, dependable, affluent, politically powerful, free, and serene. Evidence supports some of these positive stereotypes but as with all stereotypes, they are not true of all elders.

Individual discrimination against the aged includes refusal to hire or promote, elder abuse, or mistreatment by long-term care personnel and other health professionals. Positive individual discrimination in favor of elders includes voting in favor of older candidates (our political leaders tend to be older individuals), retirement communities that discriminate against younger people, and family power exploited by older persons.

Institutional ageism can be negative or positive discrimination: negative discrimination is found in employment and compulsory retirement policies, government programs that exclude the aged, and long-term care institutions that neglect or otherwise mistreat older patients.

Positive discrimination by institutions includes senior centers, special employment opportunities for elders only (such as the Senior Community Service Employment), special tax breaks, discounts, income-maintenance programs, and Medicare. These huge programs involve hundreds of billions of dollars annually.

Whether one views such positive discrimination as desirable depends on one's political orientation and value judgments.

See also AGE-SPECIFIC PUBLIC PROGRAMS; CULTURAL SOURCES OF AGEISM; DISCOUNTS; FACTS ON AGING QUIZ; HUMOR; LANGUAGE; LITERATURE; PUBLIC POLICY; SENIOR CENTERS; STEREOTYPES; TAX BREAKS; TELEVISION; TYPES OF AGEISTS

REFERENCE

Palmore, E. (1999). *Ageism*. New York: Springer.

UNCONSCIOUS AGEISM

Becca R. Levy

Ageism operates on two levels: conscious (aware, controlled, or explicit) and unconscious (unaware, automatic, or implicit). Both levels apply to the targets as well as the targeters. That is, individuals can perpetuate ageism or be victimized by it, whether or not they are aware of the process.

Although exploration of the unconscious has a venerable history, extending back to the nineteenth century, it is only recently that computer methods have been developed to examine unconscious prejudice in a systematic way. Previously, studies of ageism relied on self-report measures and interviews. The assumption has been that individuals are aware of their age biases. However, a growing body of research suggests that prejudice can also operate below awareness. Most of the research on unconscious prejudice has focused on sexism and racism, but ageism has received increasing attention.

Several studies demonstrate a dissociation between unconscious and conscious stereotypes in the realm of race (e.g., Devine, 1989); gender (e.g., Banaji and Hardin, 1996); and age (e.g., Hummert et al., 2002). Consistent with this dichotomy, the two levels of stereotypes appear to draw on different parts of the brain (e.g., Hart et al., 2000). Furthermore, in individuals with moderate Alzheimer's disease, unconscious processes continue to operate whereas the conscious processes no longer seem to function (Levy and Benaji, 2002).

One type of unconscious ageism research has concentrated on the targeters. Perdue and Gurtman (1990) were the first to show that ageism has what they call an "automatic cognitive component" (p. 199).

They found that after college students were subliminally primed with the word *old*, they made decisions about negative traits more quickly and positive traits more slowly than after being subliminally primed with the word *young*. The authors suggest the following:

> Age-related biases in person perception may have become so routinized that they may influence social judgments at a level below that at which we consciously ascribe traits to others. Such "automatic" ageism may be hard to eradicate if it has been incorporated in our implicit personality theories or social schemata and is evoked without awareness on our part. (p. 201)

Another type of unconscious ageism research has concentrated on the targets. Specifically, this line of research focuses on the consequence of activating either positive or negative age stereotypes in older adults without their awareness. A premise of these investigations is that stereotypes of aging are internalized from the time of childhood and into adulthood—before these stereotypes, which are predominantly negative, become relevant to the individual as an older person. Therefore, elders do not have the psychological defenses against stereotypes about their group (i.e., self-stereotypes) that are available to members of groups that have been stigmatized from birth. Because of their resultant vulnerability, it is assumed that elders harbor aging self-stereotypes that can be unconsciously activated to influence cognitive and physical spheres.

In the first of a series of studies based on these assumptions, we considered whether a priming intervention (that subliminally presented either positive or negative age stereotype words on a computer screen) could affect memory performance (Levy, 1996). We found that older adults exposed to positive age stereotypes demonstrated better memory performance than older adults exposed to negative age stereotypes. The effect of the words on the performance was one indication that the participants' images of old age had been primed. Another indication was their reaction times: it took longer to recognize the positive words than the negative words. Apparently, a resistance to the positive stereotypes of aging occurred because there are fewer of them to internalize and they are therefore less accessible for activation. The same experiment included conscious interventions that were found to have no effect on memory performance.

In subsequent studies using the same unconscious priming method, we found that exposure to positive age stereotypes had a beneficial effect on a range of outcomes, including will to live and cardiovascular response to stress (Levy et al., 2000; Levy, Ashman, and Dror, 2000). When the studies included younger as well as older participants, the predicted unconscious ageism effects only emerged for the latter. We concluded that it is necessary for these unconscious primes to be self-relevant in order to have a cognitive or physical effect.

However, a subsequent study found that college students who were consciously exposed to negative stereotypes of aging had a slower walking speed compared to those who received neutral primes (Bargh, Chen, and Burrows, 1996). We found that older adults who were subliminally exposed to positive age stereotypes had a faster walking speed than older adults who were subliminally exposed to negative age stereotypes (Hausdorff, Levy, and Wei, 1999). Further light on these two sets of findings is shed by a recent study that concluded self-relevance explains why their targets responded to primes that were administered below awareness but did not respond to recognized primes; whereas nontargets only responded to recognized primes (Shih et al., 2002).

A survey approach to unconscious ageism has been conducted with the Implicit Association Test (IAT). This measure assumes that individuals will make associations faster for judgments that are congruent with unconscious associations and slower for judgments that are incongruent with unconscious associations (Greenwald, McGhee, and Schwartz, 1998). Several types of age IATs have been developed: including a nonverbal one with photographs of younger and older adults; and a verbal one using names that were popular with older cohorts but are rarely used anymore (e.g., Gertrude) as well as names that have recently become popular and are mostly used by younger adults (e.g., Britney). Both age IATs produced similar findings, giving credence to the assumption that the IAT validly measures unconscious ageism.

IAT research has yielded a number of striking findings. In a study of more than 60,000 participants it was found that unconscious prejudice against the elderly is consistently negative from ages eight to seventy-one and that older adults express a greater unconscious identification with the young than with the old (Nosek, Banaji, and

Greenwald, 2001). This suggests that unconscious ageism overrides one of the most consistent findings in psychology: in-group preference (Levy and Banaji, 2002). In addition, IAT research demonstrates that unconscious age bias is stronger than racial and gender biases (Nosek and Banaji, 2004).

Unconscious ageism is able to identify social psychological processes that would otherwise go unrecognized by both researchers and participants. Without this recognition, both targets and targeters are deprived of a basis for countering the negative effects of unconscious ageism. As the field develops, hopefully it will contribute to a time when there is less to study.

See also MEASURING AGEISM IN CHILDREN

REFERENCES

Banaji, M . R. and Hardin, C. D. (1996). Automatic stereotyping. *Psychological Science,* 7, 136-141.

Bargh, J. A., Chen, M., and Burrows, L. (1996). Automaticity of social behavior: Direct effects of trait construct and stereotype activation on action. *Journal of Personality and Social Psychology,* 71, 230-244.

Devine, P. (1989). Stereotypes and prejudice: Their automatic and controlled components. *Journal of Personality and Social Psychology,* 56, 5-18.

Greenwald, A. G., McGhee, D. E., and Schwartz, J. L. K. (1998). Measuring individual differences in implicit cognition: The implicit association test. *Journal of Personality and Social Psychology,* 74, 1464-1480.

Hart, A. J., Whalen, P. J., Shin, L. M., McInerney, S. C., Fischer, H., and Rauch, S. L. (2000). Differential responses in the human amygdala to racial outgroup vs ingroup face stimuli. *Neuroreport: An International Journal for the Rapid Communication of Research in Neuroscience,* 11, 2351-2355.

Hausdorff, J., Levy, B., and Wei, J. (1999). The power of ageism on physical function of older persons: Reversibility of age-related gait changes. *Journal of the American Geriatric Society,* 47, 1346-1349.

Hummert, M. L., Garstka, T. A., O'Brien, L., Greenwald, A. G., and Mellot, D. S. (2002). Using the implicit association test to measure age differences in social cognitions. *Psychology and Aging,* 17, 482-495.

Levy, B. (1996). Improving memory in old age by implicit self-stereotyping. *Journal of Personality and Social Psychology,* 71, 1092-1107.

Levy, B., Ashman, O., and Dror, I. (2000). To be or not to be: The effect of stereotypes of aging on the will to live. *Omega: Journal of Death and Dying,* 40, 409-420.

Levy, B. and Banaji, M. (2002). Implicit ageism. In T. Nelson (Ed.) *Ageism: Stereotypes and prejudice against older persons.* Cambridge: MIT Press.

Levy, B., Hausdorff, J., Hencke, R., and Wei, J. (2000). Reducing cardiovascular stress with positive self-stereotypes of aging. *Journal of Gerontology: Psychological Sciences,* 55, 1-9.

Nosek, B. A., Banaji, M. R., and Greenwald, A. G. (2001). Harvesting implicit group attitudes and beliefs from a demonstration website. *Group Dynamics,* 6, 101-115.

Nosek, B. A. and Banaji, M. R. (2004). (At least) two factors moderate the relationship between implicit and explicit attitudes. In R. K. Ohme and M. Jarymowicz (Eds.), *Natura Automatyzmow.* Warszawa: WIP PAN and SWPS.

Perdue, C. W. and Gurtman, M. B. (1990). Evidence for the automaticity of ageism. *Journal of Experimental Social Psychology,* 26, 199-216.

Shih, M., Ambady, N., Richeson, J. A., Fujita, K., and Gray, H. M. (2002). Stereotype performance boosts: The impact of self-relevance and the manner of stereotype activation. *Journal of Personality and Social Psychology,* 83, 638-647.

VOICE QUALITY

Erdman B. Palmore

Some changes in voice qualities are age-related. The larynx becomes a less-effective sound generator with advancing age. Reduction in the elasticity and strength of the laryngeal musculature reduces vocal intensity and produces several other effects, such as vocal jitter and shimmy that contribute to the stereotype of the aging voice (Palmore, 1999). Experiments show that most people can usually distinguish between the voices of older and younger persons.

Ageism comes in when the sound of an older person's voice triggers negative attitudes. For example, when undergraduate college students listened to tapes of younger and older male speakers reading identical material, they rated the older speakers as less competent, less flexible, more old-fashioned, and from lower social classes (Stewart and Ryan, 1982).

In a somewhat similar study, McCall (1993) found that when college students responded to slides of either an older or a younger adult reading a prerecorded passage (which was identical for both ages), the students underestimated the number of words spoken by the older person, had less interest in the older person, and answered fewer content questions correctly for the older person. Thus, even though the voice quality was the same, the students' prejudice against older persons was reflected in their assumptions that older persons read more slowly, that they are less interesting, and are not worth paying attention to.

REFERENCES

McCall, T. (1993). Listener perceptions of older versus younger adult speech. *Educational Gerontology,* 19, 503.

Palmore, E. (1999). *Ageism: Negative and Positive.* New York: Springer.

Stewart, M. and Ryan, E. (1982). Attitudes toward younger and older adult speakers. *Journal of Language and Social Psychology,* 1, 91.

Index

Order a copy of this book with this form or online at:
http://www.haworthpress.com/store/product.asp?sku=5303

ENCYCLOPEDIA OF AGEISM

_____in hardbound at $59.95 (ISBN: 0-7890-1889-6)

_____in softbound at $39.95 (ISBN: 0-7890-1890-X)

Or order online and use special offer code HEC25 in the shopping cart.

COST OF BOOKS_____

☐ **BILL ME LATER:** (Bill-me option is good on US/Canada/Mexico orders only; not good to jobbers, wholesalers, or subscription agencies.)

☐ Check here if billing address is different from shipping address and attach purchase order and billing address information.

POSTAGE & HANDLING_____
(US: $4.00 for first book & $1.50 for each additional book)
(Outside US: $5.00 for first book & $2.00 for each additional book)

Signature_____

SUBTOTAL_____

☐ **PAYMENT ENCLOSED: $_____**

IN CANADA: ADD 7% GST_____

☐ **PLEASE CHARGE TO MY CREDIT CARD.**

STATE TAX_____
(NJ, NY, OH, MN, CA, IL, IN, PA, & SD residents, add appropriate local sales tax)

☐ Visa ☐ MasterCard ☐ AmEx ☐ Discover
☐ Diner's Club ☐ Eurocard ☐ JCB

Account # _____

FINAL TOTAL_____
(If paying in Canadian funds, convert using the current exchange rate, UNESCO coupons welcome)

Exp. Date_____

Signature_____

Prices in US dollars and subject to change without notice.

NAME_____
INSTITUTION_____
ADDRESS_____
CITY_____
STATE/ZIP_____
COUNTRY_____ COUNTY (NY residents only)_____
TEL_____ FAX_____
E-MAIL_____

May we use your e-mail address for confirmations and other types of information? ☐ Yes ☐ No We appreciate receiving your e-mail address and fax number. Haworth would like to e-mail or fax special discount offers to you, as a preferred customer. **We will never share, rent, or exchange your e-mail address or fax number.** We regard such actions as an invasion of your privacy.

Order From Your Local Bookstore or Directly From
The Haworth Press, Inc.
10 Alice Street, Binghamton, New York 13904-1580 • USA
TELEPHONE: 1-800-HAWORTH (1-800-429-6784) / Outside US/Canada: (607) 722-5857
FAX: 1-800-895-0582 / Outside US/Canada: (607) 771-0012
E-mail to: orders@haworthpress.com

For orders outside US and Canada, you may wish to order through your local sales representative, distributor, or bookseller.
For information, see http://haworthpress.com/distributors

(Discounts are available for individual orders in US and Canada only, not booksellers/distributors.)

PLEASE PHOTOCOPY THIS FORM FOR YOUR PERSONAL USE.
http://www.HaworthPress.com   BOF04